The Clinical
Nurse Specialist
in Theory
and Practice

The Clinical Nurse Specialist in Theory and Practice

Edited by

Ann B. Hamric, R.N., M.S.

Assistant Director of Nursing for Education
Medical College of Virginia Hospitals
Richmond, Virginia

Judy Spross, R.N., M.S.

Clinical Specialist, Oncology Nursing
Dartmouth-Hitchcock Medical Center
Hanover, New Hampshire

Grune & Stratton
A Subsidiary of Harcourt Brace Jovanovich, Publishers
New York   London
Paris   San Diego   San Francisco   São Paulo
Sydney   Tokyo   Toronto

Library of Congress Cataloging in Publication Data

Main entry under title

The clinical nurse specialist in theory and practice.

    Includes bibliographic references and index.
    1. Nurse practitioners.   I. Hamric, Ann B.
II. Spross, Judy. [DNLM   1. Nurse clinicians. WY 128
C639]
RT82.8.C573   1983   610.736   82–12134
ISBN 0–8089–1519–3

Contents

Acknowledgments

This volume owes its existence to the Clinical Nurse Specialist Section at Dartmouth-Hitchcock Medical Center, Hanover, New Hampshire, sponsor of the regional CNS conference where many of these ideas were generated. The editors are grateful to this group for their hard work and unwavering faith in the worth of this endeavor.

We thank Cheryl Wilson, Laura Stancs, and Dee Smith for their assistance and patience in typing and retyping chapters. Special thanks are owed Jeanette Kissinger, R.N., Ed.D., who carefully reviewed numerous manuscripts, and Doris Bloch, R.N., Dr.P.H., for her valuable critique of Chapter 12. We express heartfelt appreciation to Carol Wolfe for her interest and considerable support in the preparation of this book. Finally, we thank our contributors for their willingness to grapple with these important but difficult issues.

Foreword

This volume is a comprehensive analysis of the clinical nurse specialist (CNS) role as it is being assimilated into the nursing mainstream in the 1980s. Current nursing theory and clinical practice issues are uniquely blended. The content is timely in relation to professional priorities, consumer demands, and economic constraints. The role is critically examined from the viewpoint of CNSs, administrators, and educators.

CNSs will readily identify with the hard-hitting analysis of this multifaceted role made by those who are experiencing it firsthand. Practicing CNSs relate obstacles and strategies for implementing theory-based practice, teaching, consultation, and research; they share the satisfactions and frustrations of juggling a joint appointment; and they tackle the thorny issue of CNS performance evaluation. CNSs describe the price of freedom within a traditionally structured environment.

Nursing administrators emphasize preparing the environment for the CNS, preserving the CNS's autonomy, and justifying the CNS's existence in the harsh reality of budget negotiations. Professional bonding is promoted through shared goal setting and mutual support among the various hierarchical levels within nursing. A conceptual framework for the supervision of motivated, self-directed nursing professionals is eloquently stated.

Nursing educators examine the CNS role from the standpoint of systems theory and role theory. They stress preparation for the reality shock inherent in implementing a nontraditional role. Essential content for graduate education in nursing is defined, and increased consistency across programs is advocated.

Hamric and Spross not only provide a thought-provoking picture of the present CNS role, they also challenge us to consider the potential of the CNS. The editors anticipate professional nursing practice privileges becoming the norm, specialization aligning with a nursing model rather than a medical model, and role convergence of the CNS and nurse practitioner unifying advanced nursing practice.

This book has something to offer everyone connected with the CNS role. It should be required reading for administrators and educators of CNSs. It will be a valuable resource for graduate students preparing for the CNS role and interviewing for their first position. It will be an essential reference and indispensable source of support for the beginning CNS. It will stimulate lively discussion among practicing CNSs who are experiencing the perpetual challenges of their multidimensional role. It is intriguing to speculate on the influence that *The Clinical Nurse Specialist in Theory and Practice* will have on the continuing evolution of the CNS role.

Ann Paulen, R.N., M.S.N., F.A.A.N.
Clinical Specialist in Oncology Nursing
Center for Health Sciences
University of Wisconsin
Madison, Wisconsin

Preface

It is both timely and important to re-examine the clinical nurse specialist (CNS) role in terms of theory and practice. Previous CNS literature identified a general framework within which the role was developed and established the CNS's versatility and flexibility in responding to patient needs. This latter, pivotal aspect of the CNS has proved to be both a bane and a blessing. Early writers gave little specific information concerning the realities of role implementation. As a result individual specialists were left to define and develop their own position within institutions. These efforts have produced widely differing practice modes, role confusion as well as role diversity, and varying degrees of success in achieving the original goal of improved nursing practice.

It is both significant and disturbing to note that the CNS role is not identified either as a problem or as a solution to nursing's concerns in the preliminary findings of the National Commission on Nursing. The nursing professional in general and the perceived shortage of nurses were subjects of much testimony. One might consider implied acknowledgment of the CNS role in the commission's statement discussing the status and image of nursing. "Lack of recognition and understanding of the nurses' role in health care delivery—by the public, other health care professionals and nurses themselves—was considered by many who presented testimony to be a key contributor to current nursing-related problems."* This statement may suggest that role confusion and lack of a recognized impact of the CNS on the health care system continue to exist throughout the country. For the status and image of nursing to

---

*National Commission on Nursing's Summary of Public Hearings, The Hospital Research and Education Trust, Chicago, Illinois, 1981, p. 9.

improve, nursing's most advanced practitioners must decrease this confusion and demonstrate their effect on health care.

This book is an effort to speak directly and definitely to CNS roles, functions, contributions to nursing practice, and crucial issues facing CNSs in the current health care environment. Theoretical role prescriptions are examined with regard to practice experience, so that more realistic expectations and more effective role expression can be implemented.

This volume includes the beliefs and experiences of successful CNSs and administrators or educators who have worked closely with CNSs. A major assertion throughout the work is the conviction that the CNS role is not only viable but necessary to nursing's continued professional growth.

The contributors to this volume examine current trends and future directions in CNS practice. The first section, "Theoretical Implications," explores the conceptual and theoretical bases of CNS practice and role development. The second section, "Aspects of CNS Practice," deals with specific functions, such as direct care, independent practice, research, and consultation, that have been challenging to integrate into practice. The third section examines the CNS from an administrative perspective and focuses on the issues of placement of the CNS within an organizational structure, administrative support, and effective administrative utilization of the CNS. The evaluation section proposes a model for developing evaluation strategies for the CNS and discusses two evaluation methods that have been operationalized: staff evaluation and peer review. The final section explores future directions in advanced practice, education, and administration as they relate to CNS role development. A model for future practice based on these trends is presented.

The book will be of interest to practicing specialists, administrators employing or considering the employment of CNSs, and faculty and students in graduate specialty programs. This volume is a resource for understanding the versatile and complex CNS role. In addition, *The Clinical Nurse Specialist in Theory and Practice* is a guide enabling CNSs to strengthen their practice and increase their effectiveness.

Ann B. Hamric, R.N., M.S.
Judy Spross, R.N., M.S.

Contributors

Anne-Marie Barron, R.N., M.S.
Former Clinical Specialist
Psychiatric Liaison Nursing
Dartmouth-Hitchcock Medical Center
Hanover, New Hampshire

Sarah Jo Brown, R.N., M.S.
Former Associate Director for Clinical Affairs
Dartmouth-Hitchcock Medical Center
Hanover, New Hampshire

Lucy Feild, R.N., M.S.
Clinical Nurse Specialist
Medical Nursing Division
Brigham and Women's Hospital;
Assistant Professor
Graduate Medical Surgical Nursing Department
School of Nursing, Boston University
Boston, Massachusetts

Lauren A. Felder, R.N., M.N.
Director of Patient Services
Director of Nursing
The Shepherd Spinal Center for Treatment of Spinal Injuries
Atlanta, Georgia

Shirley Girouard, R.N., M.S.N., C.S.
Clinical Specialist
Medical-Surgical Nursing
Dartmouth-Hitchcock Medical Center
Hanover, New Hampshire

Mary L. Gresham, R.N., M.S.N.
Practitioner/Teacher
Gerontological Nursing;
Assistant Professor
College of Nursing
Rush University
Chicago, Illinois

Ann B. Hamric, R.N., M.S.
Assistant Director of Nursing for Education
Medical College of Virginia Hospitals
Richmond, Virginia

Eileen Callahan Hodgman, R.N., M.S.N., F.A.A.N.
Consultant, Special Projects
Former Director of Nursing Research
Beth-Israel Hospital
Boston, Massachusetts

Harriet Kitzman, R.N., M.S.
Doctoral Candidate
University of Rochester
Rochester, New York

Susan Leibold, R.N., M.S.
Clinical Specialist
Pediatric Nursing
Medical College of Virginia Hospitals
Richmond, Virginia

Cecilia Martinez, R.N., M.N.
Clinical Nurse Specialist
University of California
Department of Psychiatry
The Curtis W. Gifford Mental Health Clinic
San Diego, California

Marilyn P. Prouty, R.N., M.S.
Administrator for Nursing
Dartmouth-Hitchcock Medical Center
Hanover, New Hampshire

Sister Callista Roy, R.N., Ph.D., F.A.A.N.
Associate Professor of Nursing
Mount St. Mary's College
Los Angeles, California;
Adjunct Associate Professor of Nursing
University of Portland
Portland, Oregon

Sally A. Sample, R.N., M.N.
Associate Director for Nursing
University of Michigan Hospitals;
Assistant Dean for Clinical Affairs
University of Michigan School of Nursing
Ann Arbor, Michigan

Judy Spross, R.N., M.S.
Clinical Specialist, Oncology Nursing
Dartmouth-Hitchcock Medical Center
Hanover, New Hampshire

Duane Walker, R.N., M.S., F.A.A.N.
Associate Administrator, Hospital and Clinics
Director of Nursing Service
Stanford University Medical Center
Palo Alto, California

I. THEORETICAL IMPLICATIONS FOR THE CLINICAL NURSE SPECIALIST ROLE

1. A Conceptual Framework for CNS Practice

Sister Callista Roy
Cecilia Martinez

During the 1960s and 1970s, nursing developed rapidly as a scientific and practice discipline. Building on more than a century of evolving concepts for nursing practice, nurse scholars and practitioners are clarifying the major concepts of the field. Through theory development, research, and practice nurses observe, classify, and relate the factors involved in helping persons to positively affect their health status. This notion of nursing science is further discussed by Roy (in press). New roles have emerged to provide particular services based on this evolving scientific knowledge. The emergence of the role of the clinical nurse specialist (CNS) has been a significant development in this process.

This chapter proposes a conceptual framework for clinical specialist practice as a way of looking at the roles, functions, and other issues discussed in this book.

SYSTEMS FRAMEWORK FOR CLINICAL SPECIALIST PRACTICE

A conceptual framework identifies and relates major concepts to help visualize what cannot be observed. A number of conceptual frameworks for nursing practice have been described in recent years. For example, one text (Riehl and Roy 1980) presents 11 such frameworks. As various frameworks have been analyzed and critiqued, a commonality of major concepts for nursing has emerged. Newman (in press) identifies these major concepts as (1) person, (2) health, (3) environment, and (4) nursing. Each conceptual framework for nursing practice identifies and relates these major concepts in such a way that one can depict the elements of nursing practice ideally, then apply this conceptualization to real clinical practice situations.

Conceptual frameworks generally have an identifiable theoretical and philosophical base. The nursing practice frameworks currently in use are most frequently rooted in systems, developmental, or interaction theories (DeBack, 1981). A common thread of humanistic values permeates these recent writings.

The framework for the CNS proposed in this chapter is based on systems theory and on humanistic values. A system is a set of units so related or connected as to form a unity or whole. It is characterized by inputs, outputs, and control and feedback processes. Systems theory helps us to see how a person or group functions as a whole within a changing environment. Furthermore, systems theory moves beyond single causal relationships to provide a way of dealing with the multiple variables affecting any situation the CNS may encounter. Using an explicitly humanistic value base reinforces nursing's heritage of providing caring persons within the health care setting. Belief in each person's creative power, in the importance of one's dynamic purpose rather than simple cause and effect relations, in a holistic approach to human behavior, in the importance of each person's point of view, and in the significance of interpersonal relationships are all notions explored in humanistic philosophy and psychology that have particular relevance in building this conceptual framework.

Figure 1-1 presents a diagram of a systems framework for clinical specialist practice. The input side of the figure lists some of the more significant internal and external inputs that influence the individual CNS in her or his practice. Such internal influences as education and experience are significant in the functioning of any professional person. For the CNS, master's level education and expert clinical skills are prescribed. Each nurse will also bring to the role her or his own particular education and experience. The wide variations of kinds of education and experience that nurse specialists have had are reflected in their functioning as systems.

A number of personality factors internally affect the functioning of the CNS. In Chapter 10, Brown discusses the strong motivation toward high achievement observed in many nurse specialists. The American Nurses' Association's operational definition of the nurse specialist's role (1976), which is discussed in detail in Chapter 3, implies a number of other personality factors relevant in the role. The definition describes a person who exercises judgment, demonstrates leadership ability, and is assertive and creative enough to act as an advocate and influence change, at the same

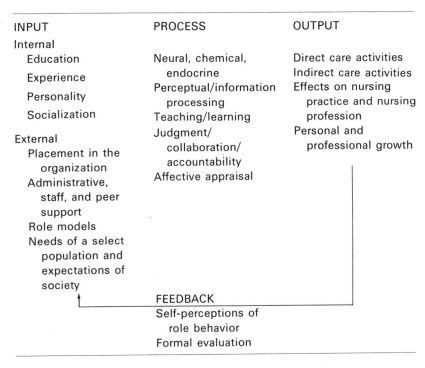

INPUT	PROCESS	OUTPUT
Internal		
Education	Neural, chemical,	Direct care activities
Experience	endocrine	Indirect care activities
Personality	Perceptual/information	Effects on nursing
Socialization	processing	practice and nursing
	Teaching/learning	profession
External	Judgment/	Personal and
Placement in the	collaboration/	professional growth
organization	accountability	
Administrative,	Affective appraisal	
staff, and peer		
support		
Role models		
Needs of a select		
population and		
expectations of		
society	FEEDBACK	
	Self-perceptions of	
	role behavior	
	Formal evaluation	

Figure 1-1. A systems framework for clinical specialist practice.

time that she or he can engage in effective interpersonal relations within the health care delivery system.

The last internal input listed in our systems framework is socialization. The experience that the CNS has as she or he is initiated into the role influences how the individual performs the role. Hamric discusses, in Chapter 3, anticipatory socialization as a way of enhancing positive role socialization.

Our framework indicates a number of significant external factors that are input for the functioning of the specialist. The placement of the CNS within the nursing service administration is a crucial variable for the person in the role (hence the emphasis on this factor in Part III of this volume). Other external factors that have great consequence for the clinical nurse specialist are administrative, staff, and peer support. One aspect of peer support, which also affects the socialization process, is the presence or absence of role models for the CNS to emulate.

The final external input listed in Figure 1-1 is the needs of a select population and the expectations of society. The American Nurses'

Association highlighted this factor in their operational definition of the CNS. The Association's statement emphasizes the fact that the needs of a select patient population and the expectation of the larger society both act to define the role of the nurse specialist (1976 p. 5).

The output of the system consists of the role behaviors of the nurse specialist. The next section of this text includes a number of chapters dealing with the roles and functions of the clinical nurse specialist. These role behaviors include, first, direct and indirect patient care activities. Table 3-1 identifies the subroles related to direct and indirect care functions. Direct care functions involve being an expert practitioner, role model, and patient advocate. Indirect care functions include functioning as a change agent, consultant/resource person, clinical teacher, supervisor, researcher, liaison, and innovator. These functions are discussed in detail in later chapters, and some examples from the practice of one CNS are provided later in this discussion.

Two additional types of output of CNS practice, produced by both the direct and indirect care activities of the specialist, are particular effects on nursing practice in general and on the nursing profession as a whole. The improvement of nursing practice was an explicit goal of the development of the role of the expert clinical practitioner (Bullough & Bullough, 1977, p. 9). The achievement of this goal, in turn, can obviously affect the image, authority, and autonomy of the nursing profession. Finally, another predictable output of CNS practice is the frequently observed personal and professional growth of the individual nurse specialist.

Given the input of this system and the diverse role behaviors that are its output, how can we conceptualize the processes within the system? The processes listed in Figure 1-1 are derived from Roy and McLeod's work on the "regulator" and "cognator" processes of the person as an adaptive system (Roy & McLeod, 1981). Roy proposes a nursing science perspective on how persons respond to the changing environment. The regulator coping mechanism responds automatically through neural, chemical, and endocrine processes, while the cognator uses complex processes of perception, information processing, learning, judgment, and emotion. The regulator and cognator can be viewed as interacting subsystems of the person that process the input received to produce the behavioral output that is observed. For the purpose of describing the internal processes most relevant for clinical specialist practice, the general "regulator" category of neural, chemical, and endocrine processes is listed first. Secondly, an adapted listing of "cognator" processes is included: perceptual/information processing, teaching/learning, judgment/collaboration/accountability, and affective appraisal.

The nurse specialist is a person with innate and acquired abilities to deal with the changing world. On the most primitive level, there are the automatic and reflexive neural, chemical, and endocrine processes that ready the person for coping by means of approach, attack, or flight. Anyone can identify with the sensation of speeded up or slowed down physiological processes in a situation of extreme fright. The type of situation that causes such stress is not unknown to the CNS in practice. Aside from extreme situations, neural, chemical, and endocrine processes are, of course, a constant part of the internal processing of all the input with which the CNS deals on an ongoing basis.

In addition to these more elementary responses, the CNS has highly developed cognator processes. Through education and experience, the nurse specialist has a well-developed ability to perceive and process both overt and covert information from the environment. Skills of teaching and learning also are expanded through constant use. The next category of cognitive processes, judgment/collaboration/accountability, is the one that perhaps most definitively distinguishes the practice of the CNS. The nurse specialist possesses mature clinical and professional judgment processes, high-level ability to collaborate with colleagues in the health care field, and a well-developed sense of accountability for patient care that does not vary with external lines of authority. Finally, the particular expertise of the clinical specialist provides her or him with an ability to make affective appraisals, with both sensitivity and objectivity.

As the system we have described operates in practice, the output of the system produces two major types of feedback that return as input to the system. The nurse specialist observes and reflects on the role behaviors involved in her or his practice. These self-perceptions of role behavior form a significant part of the feedback loop for the total system of CNS practice. In addition, formal evaluation, as discussed in Part IV of this text, is a second channel of feedback regarding the behaviors of those practicing in the role of the CNS.

ILLUSTRATION OF THE SYSTEMS FRAMEWORK

Let us now illustrate the framework we have been describing with a real-life example from the practice of one particular CNS. In doing so, we will try to use both the humanistic and the systems theoretical approach to CNS practice.

The nurse specialist used in this example, whom we will call Carol, holds a master's degree in psychiatric nursing.

At the time Carol was interviewed and observed in practice, she had 10 years of experience, having first held the position of CNS at a Veterans'

Administration hospital for 2 years and then taken up her current position at a university mental health clinic, where she had been for 8 years.

From her graduate education, this specialist identifies the factors most influential in her current role as the supervision she received from her instructors in graduate clinical courses, the readings provided for her course work, and the research that she did on the role of the nurse specialist while she was preparing for her comprehensive examinations. Another educational experience that she found meaningful was a course in group dynamics where students had formed a therapeutic group and alternated playing the roles of therapist and participant. These initial educational experiences remain with her as internal input for her CNS practice.

Since her master's education, Carol has had a wealth of experiences that contribute to her expertise in functioning in the role of psychiatric CNS. Because she has worked in teaching institutions, she has had the advantage of having 10 years of individual supervision for her case load. Carol works with interdisciplinary teams for patient intake and disposition as well as for case conferences. In addition, her own psychotherapeutic skills are further sharpened as she supervises trainees from a number of disciplines by working with them to analyze videotaped therapy sessions or presentations of their cases. She subscribes to relevant journals, and she also reads textbooks and papers recommended by her supervisor or by the medical faculty and guest speakers that provide didactic teaching for the psychiatric residents.

This background of education and experience is enhanced by certain of her personality characteristics. Carol is the kind of person who can engage quickly in a relationship, yet she also remains objective, so that she is aware of others' feelings and her own. When questioned about how her personality makes her effective in dealing with others, Carol says that her own clear philosophy and purpose in life seem to come across to others as they deal with critical issues. She is highly committed to her patient population and to quality patient care. She is a gifted person and an analytical thinker who takes initiative aggressively and is highly motivated. She is responsible and can work without being told what to do or being given constant reassurance.

In discussing her socialization into the role of nurse specialist, Carol notes that in her first position at the veterans' hospital she was able to create the position out of her understanding of the role and the possibilities she saw in the situation. Her role emerged as she saw particular needs, assessed them, proposed responses to the needs, and found her plans accepted. Her supervisor had set up a program for consultations by the psychiatric CNS with the nurses on the medical–surgical services. Being initiated into this function was one part of her socialization to the role. In addition, her socialization was aided by collaboration with four other mental health nurse specialists in parallel positions.

In regard to her placement within the administrative organization, this nurse specialist began in a position that made her directly responsible to a nursing supervisor who reported to the assistant chief of nursing. Her current position is a staff-level position reporting, for her direct care activities, to a coordinator who is responsible to the medical director of the clinic. In addition, for her administrative duties in a crisis clinic she reports to a coordinator directly responsible to the administrator of the clinic. Both coordinators are licensed clinical social workers.

As Carol spoke of administrative, staff, and peer support, she reflected some contrasting levels of support. Her first nursing supervisor, at the Veterans' Administration hospital, had graduated not long before from the same program Carol graduated from; this created a rapport between them. This supervisor provided administrative backing as well as peer support. The other four nurse specialists at the hospital also provided support for one another. This CNS felt the support and respect of the nursing staff and personnel in other disciplines here, particular from the faculty and residents in psychiatry.

In her more recent position at the university mental health clinic, the administrators immediately above her are most supportive and respond to her high degree of competence. The higher-level administrators have respect for her skills but have interfered with certain aspects of her work. For example, the clinic administrator, who had a different philosophy about crisis intervention, introduced different forms for patient intake at the crisis clinic, discarding those that Carol had developed. Carol finds the peer support at this clinic less strong than at the Veterans' hospital. Generally the staff consult one another in areas of a given expertise and provide support when working as an intake team, but their interaction is limited. In this geographic area, there is a society of specialists in psychiatric mental health nursing. Some members of this group get together informally occasionally, outside of meeting times, to share concerns.

The role models for this CNS have been the nurse specialists with whom she has worked and the experts in psychotherapy from other disciplines on the staff or on the faculty.

We noted that significant factors affecting CNS practice are the needs of a select population and the expectations of society. As stated above, Carol's functioning within her role emerged as she saw particular needs in her area of expertise and responsibility. For example, at the veterans' facility Carol set up an outpatient group for alcoholics and their spouses. In regard to expectations from society, Bullough and Bullough (1977) point out that the advent of the nurse specialist in community mental health centers and psychiatric wards created few serious problems. Psychiatrists and the public at large had already dealt with the entry of social workers and clinical psychologists into this domain. Carol reports that her skills are most appropriate to the needs of the current outpatient population that she serves and that her services are readily accepted as within the expectations of the patients applying to the clinic.

Carol demonstrated the highly developed cognator processes described earlier. She identified her perceptual/information processing skills as perhaps her greatest strength. In evaluating the condition of patients, for example, she takes in a great deal of information and quickly sifts the relevant variables, seeing them as a dynamic whole with themes that give meaning to the situation. This keen ability to assess and diagnose makes her a recognized expert in determining appropriate disposition for patients. In the teaching/learning situation, she finds herself forced to find workable solutions; she pursues data relentlessly until she finds how they can be put together and communicated to trainees and patients. Within these two cognator processes, she conceptualizes, synthesizes, and communicates.

Just as in the process of perceiving and sorting information, so in the process of judgment this nurse specialist can quickly consider a wide range of knowledge and treatment modalities and come to a judgment about the best possibility. Because of well-developed collaborative skills, she also is open to new data, to refocusing her analyses and judgments, and possibly letting go of initial judgments. Carol's judgment and collaboration skills are also shown in her ability to set priorities for her involvement in individual patient care and her administrative responsibilities. We have already mentioned this nurse specialist's high-level of commitment to quality patient care. She knows that she is consistent and reliable in handling her case load and in the running of the crisis clinic, including getting the necessary paperwork done.

As for affective self-appraisal, Carol reports that both positive and negative feelings are aroused in her direct care activities with patients and in her indirect care activities with colleagues. Her recognition of these feelings and their effect upon the goals of the interaction makes it possible for her to handle them well. In the case of strong negative or positive countertransference to a patient, she has had the patient reassigned to another therapist when this was warranted. Her ability to recognize and deal with these feelings provides the objectivity important for staff members of a teaching institution.

To give a few examples of the output side of our framework, we can describe some of the role behaviors of this nurse specialist. In her initial CNS position in the veterans' facility, Carol spent 80 percent of her time in the direct care activities of the expert practitioner. Individual and group therapy were her major focus. In the university clinic, she worked for 7 years with her role defined as 100 percent clinician. This involved 22 hours each week in individual and group therapy particularly the young women's identity groups and marital and other cojoint or two-person therapy. Currently, she has decreased her expert practitioner activities to 16 hours each week of individual and group therapy, and about one-third of her position now involves administration of the crisis clinic. This change in patient contact hours resulted largely from financial exigencies at the agency. In addition to these somewhat more limited direct care activities at the clinic, Carol is also involved in private practice. She conducts group sessions for a class of graduate students in psychiatric nursing, works with individuals and couples, and is forming a group concerned with women's identity for those who have not dealt effectively with the problem of obesity.

In both of her full-time positions, this nurse specialist has contributed greatly in the role model and patient advocate subroles of her direct care functions. Her peers, superiors, and trainees from many disciplines recognize her expert modeling of the therapist role and of the role of a professional person. Her patient advocate activities have ranged from making efforts to adjust sliding scale charges for the patient to discussing a patient's medication with an overseas embassy when called about the person being detained for carrying drugs. Clear communication with other · community agencies on behalf of her patients is an important priority. In her roles as an administrator of the crisis clinic, she has organized a system to check on continuity of follow-through for all patients who originally contact the clinic. She personally reviews the case load to ascertain that dispositions indicated by the staff and trainees are in the best interests of the patient.

In direct care activities, Carol has acted as an agent for change in several instances. At the veteran's hospital, she designed and implemented an assessment tool based on a conceptual framework for nursing. At the university clinic, she redesigned the crisis program when given this responsibility. The roles of consultant, resource person, clinical teacher, and supervisor have been ongoing in her role functioning. She provides lectures and workshops on given topics, such as suicide prevention, helps to teach trainees how to write up cases, and supervises trainees in both individual and group therapy. Her well-recognized clinical expertise is called upon by both peers and trainees. The trainees with whom she has worked include professionals from many disciplines—nursing, social work, and medicine. The trainees from the field of medicine have included medical students, family practice residents, and residents in psychiatry.

As a researcher, this CNS designed and conducted a project to determine better methods for case dispositions. This survey study at the

Veterans' hospital related individual and group patient intake to the treatment recommended and to patient follow-through. Currently she is involved in a study to systematically evaluate the use of the crisis clinic. In regard to liaison activities, Carol has served as her clinic's representative to the nearby university inpatient service.

When asked about her role as an innovator, Carol quickly asserted that she has leadership abilities that are recognized as effective. She initiates the best approach she knows, whether she feels sure it will be accepted or not, as in the case of the forms she designed for the crisis clinic.

From what has been said about the practice of this CNS, one can readily infer that nursing practice in her area of mental health care, as well as the status of the nursing profession, have been enhanced by her activities. The graduate nursing students who work with Carol have observed themselves to be increasingly more self-aware, to have better interpersonal skills and greater knowledge and skill in group therapy process than prior to their work with Carol. This nurse specialist's own practice and that of those she affects contributes to better nursing care. In turn, her role performance affects how others look at nurses. She feels that by acting as a peer or supervisor for those in other disciplines she is helping to change the image of nursing.

The personal and professional growth of this individual CNS is also reflected in her functioning. In her 10 years in this role she has developed a sense of professional identity and security, along with enhancing her skills. As noted, her opportunities for supervision of her own case load and acting as a supervisor for others continuously contribute to her ongoing professional development. In addition, her deep professional involvement motivates her to attend the various lectures and other learning opportunities available at the university. To function well as a CNS is to continue to grow as a person and as a professional.

As for the "feedback" into the system from her role behaviors, when asked about her self-perceptions in the role of CNS Carol responded that she feels self-assured and can validate herself. She has the confidence to "forge ahead and can give it because I've got it." She finds that her patients and colleagues believe in her because she believes in herself.

With regard to formal evaluation as feedback, she stated that these processes have not been particularly influential in her own performance. In the first facility, her supervisor evaluated her every 3 months, and she read and signed the evaluation. Currently she has an annual review by her clinical coordinator. In addition, this second agency has a system of peer review done each month. This review involves selecting a file from her case load and filling out a checklist on the "bare bones" of care, such as whether or not the intake record is complete, medications recorded, a diagnosis listed, and progress reports entered. She sees her review of other's records as a perfunctory duty and assumes that their review of her is handled similarly. Nonetheless she acknowledges the necessity of such reviews in a teaching situation.

A CNS APPROACH TO INDIVIDUALS AND GROUPS

Systems Frameworks for Individuals and Groups

The CNS is involved in direct and indirect care activities that focus on both individuals and groups. We may expand on the systems framework that has been presented by providing parallel systems frameworks showing how the nurse specialist can visualize the individuals and groups with whom she works.

In earlier writings, Roy (1976, Roy & Roberts, 1981) has described the person as an adaptive system. This framework is modified in Figure 1-2 to describe, in a more general way, the input, processes, output, and feedback of individuals viewed as a system. When the CNS views the individual patient as a system, relevant internal input for this system will include growth and development, family background, culture, coping mechanisms, and health status. At the same time, the nurse specialist will consider the

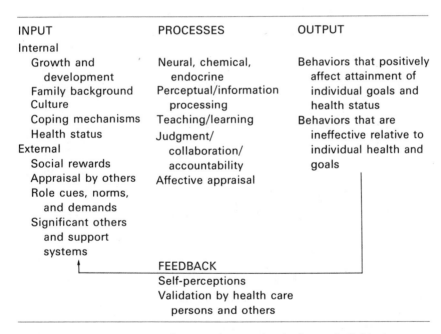

Figure 1-2. A systems framework to use in viewing an individual.

external factors affecting the individual, such as social rewards; appraisals by others; role cues, norms, and demands; and availability of significant others and support systems.

The center portion of Figure 1-2 remains the same as that of the systems framework for clinical specialist practice. The CNS recognizes in other persons the basic processes for handling input that were described for the nurse specialist, that is, neural, chemical, endocrine; perceptual/ information processing; teaching/learning; judgment/collaboration/ accountability; and affective appraisal.

What output of the individual as a system is relevant in the view of the CNS? In a role that involves promoting health status and attainment of individual goals, it would seem that the nurse specialist would view as output behaviors related to these two outcomes. Thus Figure 1-2 indicates that from the point of view of the CNS the internal and external input for the person are processed by the regulator and cognator mechanisms to yield behaviors that either result in attainment of individual goals and improved health status or that are ineffective in relation to goals and health. For example, the CNS might observe the life-style changes of a post-coronary patient. Certain changes can decrease the risk of further cardiac disease at the same time that the person is able to accomplish personal and career goals.

Feedback mechanisms within this framework can be stated most simply as the individual's self-perceptions and validation by health care persons and others regarding achievement of goals and improved health.

To develop a systems framework for the CNS to use in viewing a group, we may draw upon some unpublished work by Roy (1979) in which she described the family, organization, and community as a system. Figure 1-3 represents a composite and modification of Roy's earlier models of these three types of groups. Internal input that is significant for groups include the individual needs of each person in the group; the group's available energy, material resources, and information; the goals and objectives of the group, both explicit and implicit; and the general level of group co-hesiveness. As the clinical specialist views any group, she or he recognizes external inputs such as the political, economic, and legal climate sur-rounding the group; any current changes in the environment; and the kinds of outside support and threats that are operating to affect the group. The CNS assesses input to any group she deals with. For example, in conducting a health teaching group for postcoronary patients, she or he is aware of both the individual needs of each group member and the cohesiveness of the group as these affect the functioning of the group and support for individual group members.

Based on some general notions of group dynamics, the following group processes are identified as important to the nurse specialist's view of

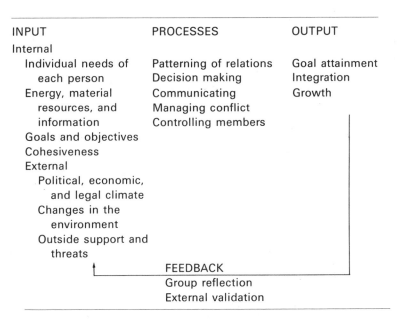

INPUT	PROCESSES	OUTPUT
Internal		
Individual needs of each person	Patterning of relations	Goal attainment
	Decision making	Integration
Energy, material resources, and information	Communicating	Growth
	Managing conflict	
	Controlling members	
Goals and objectives		
Cohesiveness		
External		
Political, economic, and legal climate		
Changes in the environment		
Outside support and threats		
	FEEDBACK	
	Group reflection	
	External validation	

Figure 1-3. A systems framework to use in viewing a group.

the group: patterning of relations, decision-making, communicating, managing conflict, and controlling members of the group. For example, in dealing with the postcoronary patient group, the CNS will note who relates to whom, and how group members communicate verbally and non-verbally.

The types of output that can be expected as a group processes its varying internal and external input have been summarized as varying levels of goal attainment, integration, and growth. This output is fed back into the system by group reflection and external validation.

In the nurse specialist's approach to individuals and groups, the basic frameworks presented in Figures 1-2 and 1-3 may be useful. Although the diagrams are a simplification of many complex concepts, each portion of either framework may be extended, validated, or modified by the CNS in her or his practice.

Examples of Clinical Practice

Here is an example of a case in which the nurse specialist used the systems framework for individuals as a way of approaching assessment and treatment of one patient.

J. W., a 25-year-old woman comes to the mental health clinic complaining of listlessness, irritability, insomnia, depression, crying, poor concentration, and loss of appetite. The nurse specialist agrees to see J. W. In approaching this case within the framework presented in Figure 1-2, the CNS assesses the behaviors noted as output, the internal and external factors that are affecting these behaviors, and the processes that the person is using in dealing with the input.

The nurse specialist notes that J. W. is distracted, has poor eye contact, and is worried about not meeting her own standards for her work. Only last month the patient was top salesperson in her division at work. In the past two weeks she has spent long hours at work, but her sales record has been dwindling. Getting to know J. W. better, the CNS identifies her as a developmentally generative adult. She comes from a family in which both parents were highly motivated, successful professionals. J. W.'s parents were away from home much of the time. Because of this, J. W. spent long hours after school alone in an empty house. She has no memory of how she felt at those times. However, she does recall that in order not to be aware of her feelings, she ate a lot and watched television.

Throughout most of her life she has tended to isolate negative and painful feelings. At this time she is unable to put this defense to use, since she is overwhelmed with all kinds of feelings that are foreign to her. J. W. recently lost her cohabiting boyfriend when he became interested in another woman. Since this happened, her usual coping mechanisms have become ineffective. She does not understand why she cannot pull herself together and do her work.

With further exploration it was discovered that spending longer hours at work was a way of avoiding the "empty house" and many hours alone now that her boyfriend had gone. Staying at work also affected J. W.'s other support systems. Her friends complained that she was never at home and often gave up trying to reach her. In addition, J. W.'s closest brother and his family had recently moved out of state.

Behaviors that the nurse specialist observed showed the effect of neural, chemical, and endocrine changes as J. W. attempted to cope with loss. In some ways, J. W. has well-developed cognator processes, but there is a deficit in affective appraisal. The self-perception that J. W. is feeding back to herself is inadequacy, since her identity is tied to her work, in which she feels she is failing.

Viewing this person within the systems framework, the nurse specialist is able to plan with J. W. for dealing more effectively with the changes in her life. The CNS will provide alternative self-perceptions for J. W. at the same time that she helps her to feel and express the losses she has been through. Through her contact with the nurse specialist, J. W. will be able to experience the importance of significant others and support systems in her later life and then will be able to develop ways to enhance these relationships. The hoped-for outcome for nursing intervention is that J. W.'s symptoms of depression will decrease, while her general health status increases. Likewise she will feel more comfortable in handling the demands of work and balancing these with meeting her own emotional needs.

Moving from the individual level to that of the group, we may cite an example of a CNS responding to a local disaster. This example shows how the CNS viewed the local community in terms of the systems framework presented in Figure 1-3.

Carol, whose practice was cited earlier in this chapter, was on the staff of the university mental health clinic when a plane crashed within a few miles of the clinic. Numerous health care workers responded to the immediate emergency and its aftermath.

The plane crash occurred during the daytime over a residential area of small homes in an older section of the city. At least 140 persons were killed on board the plane and in the neighborhood. Wreckage was spread over a one-mile-wide area, and 10 homes were destroyed and others damaged. The staff of the mental health clinic felt the impact of the disaster so close to their offices personally. They immediately began to organize a way of being of service to the local community. They recognized that this response was one way of working through their own feelings of a threat to their integrity, yet they also felt that the impact on them personally could be useful in identifying with the needs of the community.

Carol and other clinic staff set up meetings in the community. Within a week after the disaster, she met in a local school with about 10 survivors from the area. Her aim was to assess where the members of the group were in the process of dealing emotionally with the incident and to move them along in this process as a means of primary prevention of more serious mental health problems at a later time.

In assessing behavioral output, Carol noted that the group was expressing frustration and anger. At times they had not been able to get to their homes or remaining belongings because the police had roped off the area. Later they had had to show identification in order to be able to move about. Large crowds of the public coming to view the area angered them. They were most indignant about the looting that had taken place and were fearful about what would happen when police protection was taken away. Their anger also focused on the airline company, their various insurance companies, and the politicians they thought were responsible for ignoring the air traffic problems in the area over a 15-year period.

The external input to the group included the dramatic incident of the crash as well as the whole complex of political, economic, and law enforcement factors that preceded and followed the incident. The additional threats of the onlookers and looters added to the input the group had to cope with. Internally, each person in the group bore the burden of his or her own experience at the time of the crash. Basic resources of food and shelter had been cut off for some. The situation provided new perspectives on the goals and objectives of the group and its cohesiveness. Throughout the group session the CNS observed the processes of relations and decision making in the group.

An initial approach was to deal with the practical concerns and share with the group information about the outside help that was available for them and others in the community. Emergency shelter, relocation, and rebuilding were discussed. In the next part of the session, the group shared their experiences. All of them recounted where they had been, what happened to them, and how they felt at the time of the crash. The nurse specialist noted that no one reported crying, yet within the session many became tearful. It was evident that some persons needed support and wanted to be able to talk with others about their experience. They were concerned about members of their family or neighbors who would not talk about the crash. There was a sense of common shock, loss, and trauma. They wanted to help others in the area and were particularly concerned for the elderly who were withdrawn and too fearful to leave their homes. The group received validation from the CNS that their anger, sadness, and guilt were expected and appropriate feelings.

Carol noted a cohesiveness and bonding within the group. The group leaders were soon absorbed as insiders who had experiences to recount as well.

Surprisingly, the group moved beyond the integration to seeking new goals. The issue of the future of the crash site became important for them. They began working with the decision of whether to build a memorial on the site or to rebuild homes. This decision provided a common goal, and helping others was a common coping mechanism.

The group received the feedback of their own reflection and external validation. Carol reported that for her the experience had been one of personal growth and greater concern for the local community. In the year following the airplane crash, the mental health clinic provided individual follow-up therapy for the people of the area who needed this additional help.

These two clinical examples show how the CNS may use the two systems frameworks we have presented in her approach to individuals and groups. It can be noted that in applying the group framework to her work setting—for example, the nursing staff of a given unit—the CNS may be dealing with group processes that are listed in Figure 1-3 but were not prominent in the example of the community group. That is, attention to processes of communicating, managing conflict, and controlling members may be relevant.

THE SYSTEMS FRAMEWORK AND RESEARCH

In addition to guiding nursing practice, a conceptual framework can be used to generate nursing research. The three systems frameworks presented in this chapter for clinical specialist practice and for the nurse specialist to use in viewing individuals and groups suggest many possibilities for research. Examples of the kinds of questions that might be asked include:

What input within each system relates to what outputs? For example, does anticipatory socialization for the nurse specialist role affect direct care activities, indirect care activities, effect on nursing practice and the profession, or personal and professional growth?

With regard to inputs to the individual system, we might investigate the question of what coping mechanisms correlate with improvements in the health status of patients, and under what circumstances. For example, one study (Roy, 1977) suggested that increased levels of decision making by patients lead to increased levels of adaptation only for middle-aged groups and those not seriously ill. Furthermore, the study showed a hint of a relationship between psychosocial adaptation and levels of wellness for patients in a nonacute, long-stay hospital.

We might also ask what kind of experience leads to more effective cognator–regulator activity for the individual (either CNS or patient) or to more effective processes for the group. Research projects related to teaching and learning would provide some information to use in answering this question. Similarly, research efforts aimed at identifying how to teach affective skills as well as cognitive skills are relevant here.

In looking at specific concepts from the systems framework for groups, we might pose such questions as these: Will meeting the individual needs of persons in the group enhance goal attainment, integration, or growth for the group? What types of outside supports are helpful for group integration and growth? Do increased group skills of managing conflict lead to greater goal attainment for the group?

Specific hypotheses can be generated on the basis of these questions and numerous others implied in the three frameworks. Empirical indicators for the variables can be determined and measurement procedures developed. Research projects may be initiated to test the hypotheses. In this way, new knowledge may be developed to guide the practice of the clinical specialist.

SUMMARY

In this chapter, we have proposed a conceptual framework for clinical specialist practice. Systems theory and humanistic values form the basis of the framework. Two related frameworks were introduced for the clinical nurse specialist in viewing individuals and groups. Examples were given to illustrate the concepts of the frameworks. Some research questions, derived from the framework, were posed. The frameworks are offered as broad outlines to help the reader conceptualize in an integrated way the complexity of interacting factors within CNS practice.

REFERENCES

American Nurses' Association, Congress of Nursing Practice, Description of practice: clinical nurse specialist. *The scope of nursing practice*, Kansas City, Mo.: American Nurses' Assn., 1976.

Bullough, B. & Bullough, V. (Eds.) *Expanding horizons for nurses*. New York: Springer Publishing Co., 1977.

DeBack, V. The relationship between senior nursing students' ability to formulate nursing diagnoses and the curriculum model, *Advances in Nurs Science*. 1981, *3*, 51–66.

Newman, M.A. The continuing revolution: a history of nursing science. In N.L. Chaska (Ed.) *The nursing profession: a time to speak*. New York: McGraw-Hill Book Co., in press.

Riehl, J.P. & Roy, S.C. *Conceptual models for nursing practice*. New York: Appleton-Century-Crofts, 2nd ed., 1980.

Roy, S.C. *Introduction to nursing: an adaptation model*. Englewood Cliffs, N.J., Prentice-Hall, Inc., 1976.

Roy, S.C. *Decision-making by the physically ill and adaptation during illness*. Dissertation, University Microfilms, Ann Arbor, 1977.

Roy, S.C. Preliminary thoughts on the use of the roy adaptation model in community/environment socialization, First Annual Graduate Conference, *Planned change in nursing practice*. Unpublished paper. The University of Portland, School of Nursing, 1979.

Roy, S.C. *Introduction to nursing: an adaptation model*. Englewood Cliffs, N.J.: Prentice-Hall, Inc., 2nd ed., in press.

Roy, S.C. & McLeod, D., Theory of the person as an adaptive system. In S.C. Roy & S.L. Roberts, *Theory construction in nursing: an adaptation model*. Englewood Cliffs: Prentice-Hall, Inc., 1981.

Roy, S.C. & Roberts, S.L. *Theory construction in nursing: an adaptation model*. Englewood Cliffs: Prentice-Hall, Inc., 1981.

2. Theory-Based Practice: Functions, Obstacles, and Solutions

Shirley Girouard

Nursing practice, if it is to complete its evolution from a task-oriented vocation to a goal-directed profession, must be based on theory. Clinical nurse specialists (CNSs), as leaders in the profession, have an obligation to promote theory-based practice for the sake of both the nursing profession and for themselves. Such practice will contribute to clarity and identity for the profession as a whole and for the CNS in particular.

One may ask why it is important for the CNS to practice from a theoretical base. The answer to this question is, in part, the same as that for any professional nurse. Theory-based practice can contribute to role definition and to the knowledge base of nursing. Theory also provides direction for day-to-day practice. Although all nurses can practice from a theoretical base, it is the CNS, with her or his advanced education and expert knowledge and skill, who must guide other nurses in their use of theory. Nursing theories and theories from other disciplines can also be used to develop methods for implementing and evaluating the CNS role. CNSs may find that practice based on theory helps them to see their activities and goals in broader perspective, so that the day-to-day frustrations of the role do not cause them to lose sight of their overall objectives.

If the CNS does not utilize theory, how would practice be directed? If we look at professional nursing practice, we can see that many nurses operate according to habit, tradition, and directives. The CNS may also be seduced into functioning in this manner. The multiplicity of activities and pressures on the CNS can result in responsive behaviors that are task-oriented, rather than being the expression of a coherent and goal-directed approach to nursing. Theory can provide consistency and coherence.

If we are to develop theory-based practice, we must give attention to both nursing theories and theories from other disciplines. Nursing theories are those that can be applied to the delivery of patient care. An example of this type of theory is Roy's adaptation theory, in which the nurse uses biopsychosocial mechanisms to evoke positive responses in clients in order to effect internal or external change (1980). Other theories of use to nurses are those relating to role, organization, and supervision. For example, nurses can use change theories in a variety of situations to implement a role or effect change.

This chapter will discuss the importance of theory-based practice for the CNS and describe one theory that the author found especially useful in analyzing and putting into practice the clinical specialist role. Obstacles encountered when one attempts to practice from a theoretical base will be described, and the major factors influencing the clinical specialist's use of theory in her or his practice will be defined.

It is important to note that the CNS can use nursing theory (as well as theories from other disciplines) in a variety of ways. For example, the CNS could use Roy's adaptation theory as the basis for direct patient care activities. If she or he wished to guide other nurses to use the adaptation theory, the CNS would then use change theory to implement such an effort. Research activities could focus on testing some aspect of the adaptation theory or testing one's ability to function as a change agent.

If one is to practice from a theoretical base, it is necessary to have a commitment to this goal. Without such a commitment, clinical specialists may find that their practice is based more on habit, tradition, and the directives of others than theory. Choosing a theoretical base that is consistent with one's own values and those of the people in one's environment will make theory-based practice easier to accomplish. Obviously one must come to value theory first. I would like to share with the reader the process which resulted in my own commitment to theory and its usefulness to the nursing profession.

A TESTIMONIAL TO THEORY

After 4 years of practice in nursing, I was "burned out." I was discouraged about nursing and my ability to practice in the way I thought I should. While pursuing a baccalaureate degree, I had been exposed to sociological theory. This was my first significant contact with theory, and I viewed it then as an intellectually stimulating process. Social theory helped me to conceptualize, classify, and describe human behavior. I also began to realize that social theory provided explanations for phenomena that I had observed. For example, Durkheim's theory of suicide enhanced my understanding of this phenomenon and helped me to better understand the role of the nurse in caring for persons who attempted suicide. An introduction to medical sociology and the application of theory to health care increased my commitment to the value of theory. I saw how theory could be used in health care to plan interventions (programs) that would have predictable outcomes. This recognition encouraged me to consider nursing theories and those of other disciplines as means by which I could begin to think about nursing and its impact on health care. Hoping to explore nursing theory in a more meaningful way and to learn ways of influencing nursing practice, I enrolled in a graduate program to prepare for the role of the CNS.

I had my next significant encounter with theory in my graduate nursing program. Initially, it seemed like an encounter of the third kind. The world of nursing was more complex than ever. As I was learning new knowledge and skills, reflecting on my past experiences, and intensively reading the nursing literature, my perception was that nursing was in a state of chaos. Webster defines chaos as "any confused collection or state of things." To me, nursing was a confused collection of knowledge, tradition, habits, titles, roles, and organizational structures.

Contributing to my sense of chaos in nursing was the new role for which I was preparing. As described in the literature, the CNS role included the following components: direct care provider, role model, collaborator, change agent, consultant, teacher, and researcher. The literature stated that the CNS, as expert clinician, is to foster improved nursing practice. As Holt states, "The concept of the CNS evolved from a need to improve the quality of nursing care. It was envisioned that a master's prepared nurse with expertise in clinical practice would influence quality care, not only of the patients she gave direct care to, but all patients within her realm of influence" (1975, p. 83). These goals were compatible with my motivations for becoming a CNS, but I was struggling with the question of how one could ever put such a broad definition into practice.

Continued exposure to nursing authors such as Chapman (1976), Roper (1976), Abdellah (1971), Reilly (1975), and McFarlane (1977), who emphasized the need for theory-based nursing practice, resulted in my recognition that theory could provide a framework for understanding and practicing the CNS role, in particular. Interestingly, the literature relating to nursing theory presented the first obstacle I encountered in my efforts to practice from a theoretical base. It contributed to my confusion: terms were defined differently by different authors, there were microtheories and macrotheories, and numerous different theories of man as the basis for practice. There were also theories from other disciplines to examine (provided one subscribed to the school that said nurses could use theories from other disciplines). If I was to identify a useful theory, I had to make sense of this theoretical chaos.

The work of Dickoff, James, and Wiedenbach (1968) provided a framework I could use to begin to organize my thinking about nursing theory. They defined four categories of nursing theory:

1. Factor-isolating: Basic, descriptive theory that names real-world phenomena.
2. Factor-relating: Descriptive theory that suggests connections among factors (concepts).
3. Situation-relating: Predictive or explanatory theory that attempts to predict relationships.
4. Situation-producing: Prescriptive theory that identifies what activities will produce certain results.

As a CNS student, I was most interested in the fourth level, situation-producing theory. How could I enhance the quality of nursing care provided by staff nurses? It was clear, from my own experience and from reports in the literature, that nursing practice was often less than ideal. As a CNS, I had to find a way to make quality nursing care happen.

The Linker Theory of planned change (which I will discuss shortly), a situation-producing theory, provided me with a theoretical framework for implementing the role of CNS. I tested the theory for my thesis research, convincing myself that theory could reduce chaos and provide direction for my practice in the CNS role. Admittedly, during the reality shock phase of my first CNS role, I lost sight of my theoretical base. The early phase of my role saw me struggling to survive, not promote change. As I adjusted to the role, however, my theoretical perspective returned and I developed a more holistic view of my practice. This confirmed for me the importance of theory for my CNS practice.

THE LINKER THEORY

The Linker Theory of planned change developed by Havelock (1976) is a sociological rather than a nursing theory. Because I view the CNS's function as change-agent as the most significant aspect of the role, it was appropriate for me to use a theory of change as the basis for my practice. This illustrates how the CNS can utilize a theory from a non-nursing discipline to provide a cohesive framework for practice.

Havelock's Linker Theory describes a relationship between the change agent and the user of the change and offers a method for effecting change. It unites classical change theories—problem solving, research/development/ diffusion, and diffusion through social interaction. The Linker Theory requires the change agent to function in a variety of ways, thus allowing the CNS using it to implement all components of the CNS role.

The Linker Theory, as I applied it to the CNS role, focuses on the user/client—in this case the staff nurse—as problem solver, with the change agent—here the CNS—given a more significant role than in other theories of change. The CNS is identified by the nursing staff as an outsider because she or he is not a staff nurse. The CNS using this theory would be the link between resources and the nursing staff. Figure 2-1 shows the relationship between the user and change agent and identifies the key concepts. Most nurses are familiar with these concepts (e.g., felt need, problem diagnosis, and implementation), which are comparable to the nursing process. Havelock derives a number of propositions from the relationships among the concepts, describing the conditions that are necessary if change is to be effected.

When applied to the interaction between the CNS as change agent and the nurse as the user of change, Havelock's propositions take the following form:

1. The nurse (client) experiences a felt need and diagnoses a problem.
2. The change agent (CNS) stimulates the nurse's (client's) problem-solving ability.
3. The nurse seeks alternatives and considers resources.
4. The nurse appreciates the resource knowledge and understands how this knowledge is generated and validated.
5. The nurse retrieves data relating to the problem.
6. The nurse considers the alternatives presented by the CNS.
7. Reciprocal feedback is necessary.
8. The nurse implements the planned change.

Havelock's propositions concerning the change agent, when applied to the CNS as resource, give the following set of requirements:

9. The change agent (CNS) assists with the diagnosis of the problem by further exploration and the use of more remote resources.
10. The CNS's knowledge is applied to the situation.
11. The CNS offers solutions and presents alternatives.
12. The CNS must have links to a variety of resource systems.

IMPLEMENTING THE LINKER THEORY: OBSTACLES AND SOLUTIONS

A discussion of my experience in attempting to apply the Linker Theory to my CNS practice follows and is summarized in Table 2-1. I encountered various obstacles to meeting the conditions required by the

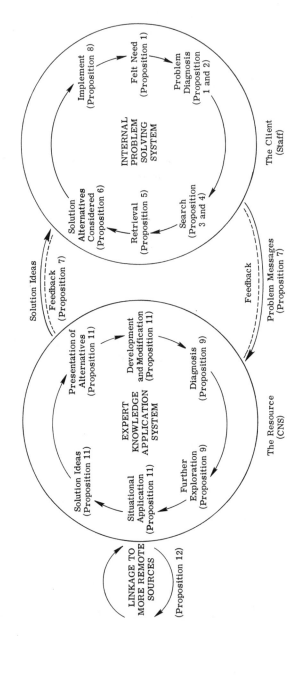

Figure 2-1. Linkage model. (Adapted from Havelock, R., & Havelock, M. Training for change agents. Ann Arbor, Mich.: University of Michigan, Institute for Social Research, 1978, p. 23.)

propositions and devised solutions to use in overcoming the obstacles. In the process, I became aware of a set of factors that affect CNS practice that I believe will also be encountered by other practitioners, whether they are using the Linker Theory or any other theoretical approach.

Propositions Relating to the Staff Nurse as User

Proposition 1. The first proposition states that the change process begins when the user (nurse) experiences a need affecting health care and diagnoses the problem. In my CNS role, I found that many of the nurses I worked with, even if they were generally aware of problems in health care delivery within their institution, were unable to articulate specific needs. Both the new graduate in "reality shock" and the experienced nurse overwhelmed by the needs of patients (and of new nurses) were unable to identify their needs. This was a significant obstacle to utilizing the Linker Theory to promote change. Thus I began to assist the nurses to identify and articulate their needs. For example, the new graduates wanted "how to" information, so I found myself teaching classes on management of tubes and drains, tube feedings, and so forth. More experienced nurses also needed how-to information about new procedures and equipment. This represented a beginning, but not the ultimate goal of my practice as a change agent.

The CNS will often find that she or he identifies needs that the staff do not see, and this can be another large obstacle. According to the Linker model, the staff must feel the need if change is to be effective. If the staff do not feel the need to change, they will not sustain the change. I identified a need to improve the quality of preoperative patient teaching provided by nurses but the staff were not perceiving this need. By my demonstrating (role modeling) the benefits of preoperative teaching and discussing the literature supporting it, the staff came to perceive the same need. This was a slow process but more long-lasting than other approaches, as demonstrated by the fact that the preoperative teaching tools are in use two years after their introduction to the staff.

Proposition 2. In this proposition, Havelock points out that in order to be most useful and helpful, the change agent must be able to stimulate the user's own problem-solving ability. Often the nurses the CNS works with may not wish to be stimulated. The situation of "burnout" can present a formidable obstacle to theory-based CNS practice. The specialist's excitement about new approaches may not be well received, so she or he must find ways to stimulate the nursing staff. In an effort to do this in relation to problem solving, I would wait until the staff expressed frustration about

Table 2-1

Relationship of Theory, Obstacles and Solutions

Focus	Proposition	Obstacle(s)	Solution(s)
Nurse (user)	1. Nurse experiences a felt need and diagnoses a problem.	Staff nurses are unable to articulate a specific need; CNS identifies a need staff do not see.	CNS assists staff to identify needs through dialogue and role modeling.
CNS	2. Change agent (CNS) stimulates nurse's problem-solving ability.	Nurses are "burned out" and do not wish to be stimulated.	CNS utilizes nurses' frustrations by channelling them into problem solving to relieve frustration.
Nurse	3. Nurse seeks alternatives and considers resources.	Nurses lack knowledge and experience in identifying and using resources.	CNS uses self as role model to demonstrate specialist's availability as a resource; CNS identifies and uses other resources in her or his practice.
Nurse	4. Nurse appreciates the resource knowledge and understands how this knowledge is generated and validated.	Nurses lack knowledge of theory and research and its application.	CNS explains theory and research and how it can be used in day-to-day problem solving.
Nurse	5. Nurse retrieves data relating to the problem.	The assessment skills of nurses are weak.	Through education, role modeling, and supervision, CNS improves knowledge and skill of staff.
Nurse	6. Nurse considers the alternative solutions presen~d.	Nurses are threatened when CNS offers alternatives.	Maintain contact, role model as consultee, and discuss feelings.

Nurse and CNS	7. Reciprocal feedback is necessary.	No system for giving feedback exists.	Establish expectation for feedback; develop system of supervision; encourage staff to evaluate CNS formally and informally.
Nurse	8. Planned change is implemented.	Poor communication (written and verbal) between nurses.	Have nursing leaders on unit follow up on changes introduced; reinforce value of clear communication.
CNS (resource)	9. CNS assists with diagnosis of problem by further exploration and use of more remote resources.	Resistance of other health care providers.	Maintain dialogue and demonstrate benefits of collaborative interactions.
CNS	10. CNS's knowledge is applied to the situation.	Insecurity of CNS; knowledge deficit.	Utilize support of other nurses (CNSs, etc.); admit ignorance to others and use other resources.
CNS	11. CNS offers solutions and presents alternatives.	Little time to do necessary research; staff not interested in lengthy discussions.	Prioritize problems and focus on those of most significance (to staff and/or patient); summarize information and present in usable format.
CNS	12. CNS has links to a variety of resource systems.	Use of other resources make CNS feel inadequate.	CNS receives support of others and makes continued efforts to gain self-confidence.

something that had happened on the unit. For example, I overheard a group of nurses complaining about how demanding a patient, Mr. S., had been the previous night and that morning. I discovered that Mr. S was scheduled for gastroscopy later in the day. When I asked the nurses if perhaps he was worried about the procedure and what it might show, they agreed. From this conversation the nurses realized that we were not preparing our patients well psychologically for gastroscopy procedures because we were not helping them to cope with their anxiety. Further exploration and discussion of the issue resulted in plans to develop a slide tape program to prepare patients for gastroscopy. The nurses were guided to develop and use their own problem-solving skills to meet this felt need.

Proposition 3. If the nurse is to seek alternatives and resources for solving a problem, the nurse must know that alternatives exist. Many of the nurses I worked with were unfamiliar with research and theory and were not experienced in using many such resources to solve problems. They had no experience with using a resource such as the CNS, which, according to Linker Theory, was essential. I spent much time initially, helping the nurses to learn who I was and what a CNS was. Having established some identity, I next had to demonstrate my knowledge and skills as a resource person. This can be very difficult when as a new CNS you are unsure of your role!

Proposition 4. This proposition states that if the nurse is to use the CNS most effectively, the nurse must appreciate the special knowledge that the CNS has and understand how this knowledge is generated and validated. Once again, it was necessary to do some groundwork, because few of the nurses were knowledgeable about nursing theory and research. Fewer still were able to appreciate how to use theory and research in their practice. Thus it was necessary to introduce theoretical and research concepts into everyday situations. Rather than present "grand theory" or isolated research findings, it was useful to bring such knowledge to bear on real problems the nurses were encountering. For example, when confronted with the question of how best to prepare laryngectomy patients for discharge, I could introduce theory and research relating to patient teaching, body image, and self-care. Not only is this more acceptable to the staff than doses of pure theory; it forces the CNS to increase her or his ability to apply theory and research to practice.

Proposition 5. This proposition requires the nurse to collect data relating to the problem. An extreme example of one nurse's weakness in data collection involved a patient who had undergone a Whipple procedure. The nurse was having a difficult time managing the patient's physiological and psychological response to the surgery. When we sat down to discuss the patient, I learned that the nurse did not know what the procedure was or that the patient had cancer. Again, I found myself working to establish the conditions (knowledge and skills) so that the change process described in the theory could take place. Obviously, developing data collection skills was a focus of my early efforts. In-service programs and one-to-one supervision of documentation were two methods utilized to improve the nurses' practice in data collection.

Proposition 6. This proposition calls for the nurse to consider alternative solutions to the problem offered by the CNS. If the issue of threat is a significant one, this proposition may not be met. I found that my proudly held image of the CNS as an expert created feelings of inadequacy and resentment in many of the staff. Compounding this was the resentment experienced by some of the head nurses, physicians, and other care providers who viewed me as infringing upon their spheres of influence. For example, I was once accused by a physician of issuing an order to the nursing staff not to give a certain dose of a drug to a patient. Interestingly, I had been out of the hospital when the incident occurred. Still, the rumor was that I was responsible for this situation. When perceived as threatening, one cannot expect to have others easily consider one's ideas. By establishing a good working relationship with the nurses and explaining and discussing my actions, I slowly overcame this obstacle.

Proposition 7. This essential proposition states that reciprocal feedback is necessary for effective utilization of the CNS; that is, both the CNS and the nurse need to benefit from the interaction. I see this as the key to the CNS's ability to be accepted and thus begin to function as a change agent. Perhaps if I had looked carefully at my theory, I would have recognized earlier that this factor was crucial. Feedback (particularly positive feedback) can contribute to the formation of significant professional relationships and trust. A beginning CNS could meet regularly with individual staff nurses to provide them with feedback about their practice. This could also be done while making patient rounds and participating in patient care conferences. I also asked the leadership staff to evaluate my performance so that they could give feedback to me. This experience, discussed in detail later in this volume (Chapter 13), provided a climate in which feedback was expected and utilized.

Proposition 8. Obviously the staff nurse must implement the planned change accurately if change is to take place. In order for proposition 8 to be met in a complex environment, communication is essential. I found poor written and verbal communication among the staff nurses to be a major obstacle to my change-agent role. An example was a decubitus care regime that another nurse and I had developed for one of our patients. We documented the plan of care carefully and communicated it to the oncoming nurse. Sometime within the next 16 hours the plan was changed. This went on for a few days until we discovered the source and were able to discuss the problem. Certainly, that staff nurse was discouraged. I expect that all of us see the problems associated with poor written and verbal communication. Once again, I had to improve communication if I was to be a successful change agent. One way this was accomplished was by my communicating to the unit leadership and asking them to follow through on suggestions. It was also necessary for the leadership group to accept the notion that a well-developed proposal for change needed to be given an adequate trial before being discarded. Repeated emphasis on these ideas in discussions and practicing accordingly can gradually reduce the problems of communication and resistance to change.

Propositions Relating to the CNS as Resource

Proposition 9. This proposition states that the CNS assists with the diagnosis of a problem through further exploration of the problem and the use of more remote resources. "More remote resources" refers to resources not immediately available to the staff nurse in her or his work environment. Health care literature, other care providers, other CNSs, and administrative support are all examples of such resources. Administrative support for both the CNS and the staff is important if change is to take place. Fortunately this resource was readily available to me and did not present an obstacle. One significant obstacle, already mentioned, was the resistance of some other health professionals. It is difficult to use them as resources when they are not supportive of the role. For me, time and patience was the solution to overcoming such resistance. Perseverance was also required.

Proposition 10. This proposition states that the CNS applies her or his knowledge to the situation to enhance change. I, like most new nurse specialists, came to my role eager to use my specialized knowledge and skills. As is evident, I encountered many obstacles in attempting to do this. Application of one's knowledge and skill is difficult when one is feeling very unsure of oneself in a new role. I also found that my knowledge and skills did not exactly fit the situation in all cases. For example, one of my units had plastic surgery patients, including burned patients. I had not taken care of a burned patient in 12 years. Thus, *I* had to gain some knowledge if I was to be able to assist the nurses to problem solve in this area. New nurse specialists must learn early that they will never have all the knowledge they need for any given situation. They must be willing to admit their ignorance and seek outside help. Although difficult to do when one is supposed to be an "expert," this behavior both models desirable resource seeking and decreases the staff's resistance to the CNS.

Proposition 11. According to this proposition, the CNS who wishes to effect change must be able to offer solutions and present alternatives. Some of the problems in doing this include deficits in knowledge and skill required by the situation, the demands of the institution, and other professional and personal obligations. Lack of time is probably the major obstacle I encountered here. It was time-consuming for me to collect data, research problems, and formulate solutions to present to the staff. Even more discouraging was the fact that sometimes after I had spent 10 hours preparing some alternatives the staff were too busy to discuss them. Although time will always be an obstacle, one does learn to set priorities, thus making things more controllable. Once the staff recognizes that the CNS can be helpful, they often make time to discuss the issues with the specialist.

Proposition 12. This proposition states that the CNS must have access to a variety of resource systems. CNSs need to assist the nursing staff to develop reciprocal and collaborative relationships with resources other than themselves if the change agent role is to be fulfilled. In attempting to do this, I encountered an unexpected obstacle within myself—jealousy. When I encouraged nurses to use other resources (especially other CNSs), I found that I was jealous when they did so. Also, when I suggested resources other than myself, I could almost hear the staff saying, "You're supposed to be our CNS;" they seemed to feel that in sending them to another CNS I was not fulfilling the expectations they had of me in the CNS role. This obstacle can be overcome as one develops confidence in oneself. Also, the value of the support of other nurse specialists in the setting cannot be underestimated.

In summary, the Linker Theory of planned change was useful to me as I learned to perform the role of CNS. Awareness of the propositions, or ideal conditions for my work, allowed me to identify the obstacles to my ability to function as a change agent. Once the obstacles were identified, I was able to develop strategies to overcome them, and the desired changes began to happen. The pattern of propositions, obstacles, and solutions discussed in this section is outlined in Table 2-1.

FACTORS INFLUENCING THE USE OF THEORY

As mentioned earlier, many of the factors that influence the ability of the CNS to function from a theoretical base are shared with other professional nurses. Some examples of these factors are one's knowledge base, one's skill and experience in applying theory to practice, the multiplicity of demands in the practice setting, and the lack of clarity in the definition of nursing. As a nursing leader, the CNS must not only deal with the above-mentioned factors her- or himself but also find ways to assist others to practice from a theoretical base. Compounding the clinical specialist's dilemma are the problems of role preparation, administrative and organizational issues, the management of more complex activities and increased demands, the need for evaluation of one's performance, and the experimental nature of the role. Although the influencing factors the CNS has in common with all nurses attempting to use theory as a base for practice are significant, I would like to focus on the particular factors influencing the CNS just mentioned. Hopefully the clinical specialist will have dealt with some of the commonly experienced problems prior to assuming the CNS role.

Most graduate programs preparing nurse specialists believe that they prepare their students to function from a theoretical base. As most nurse specialists know, this is not always true. Theoretical knowledge and, more important, guidance in using theory in practice would be meaningful additions to the curriculum. Once the CNS is in a practice setting, continuing education and contact with colleagues can assist in role development. Discussion of theoretical models and the experiences of the CNS in using theory can provide opportunities to explore a variety of theoretical approaches to practice and role implementation.

Administrative and organizational factors also affect the CNS's ability to use theory in practice. Poor definition of role and responsibilities make it difficult for the CNS to evaluate the appropriateness of her or his theoretical perspective in a given setting. Administrative support is also important. A nursing department that rewards task-oriented performance more than creative thinking presents a significant obstacle to the CNS wishing to utilize a theoretical base for nursing practice. As Shaefer (1973) points out, a lack of administrative support was found to be significantly related to CNS job dissatisfaction. Certainly if one's department is not interested in or supportive of practice oriented toward theory, the CNS attempting such practice will have significant problems overcoming this obstacle. I would suggest that clinical specialists choose work settings where their values can be supported. Those with great energy could, of course, seek to utilize change theory and alter the value system of an entire department.

The multiplicity of activities that most CNSs find themselves engaged in represent a significant factor affecting their performance. Establishing priorities and managing one's time carefully are critical skills. Time to think and analyze is important if one wishes to utilize theory in practice. Woodrow and Bell (1971) discuss this by pointing out that managing time and setting priorities are difficult when one's responsibilities are broad and vaguely defined. As they mention, limiting the CNS's scope of responsibility can help. Aradine and Denyes (1972) noted that the nurse specialists they studied had difficulty setting priorities. Priority setting could be made easier if one were able to look at the numerous demands in relation to a theoretical framework. For example, a CNS using the Linker Theory might focus initially on establishing relationships with those she or he intends to influence. Then the more significant issues could be tackled first.

If the CNS is to practice from a theoretical base, evaluation and feedback are crucial. By using a theory basis, CNS evaluation and performance can be evaluated against the theory. Without such feedback, the CNS will not know if the chosen theory is appropriate. Such testing of theory can enhance the CNS's research and critical thinking abilities.

The newness of the CNS role presents an interesting set of obstacles that are important factors affecting theory-based practice. Because so little research has been done to justify or document the effect of the nurse specialist on patient care, theories about it remain unsupported. If we can substantiate the theoretical justification of the CNS role through research, we will then able to better define the role by demonstrating role components that affect patient care. A case can then be made for removal of obstacles inhibiting role performance.

Role descriptions of the CNS always include the component of the role model. In theory, this makes sense. But, as Woodrow and Bell point out (1971), nurses may not want one. These authors go on to say that there are few ways for nurses who emulate the CNS to be rewarded. A clinical ladder represents one way to accomplish this. The clinical specialist can also make significant contributions to rewarding behaviors by using such informal feedback mechanisms as giving positive feedback, publishing with staff nurses, and contributing to their individual growth and development.

Although the obstacles limiting the ability of the CNS to use theory in practice are indeed real, they can, as illustrated above, be overcome. An awareness of the obstacles and development of strategies to overcome them is the first step. One way to overcome obstacles is to articulate a theory and then apply it to a clinical problem. For example: if the CNS and the leadership staff on a given unit recognize the need to improve documentation on the unit, they could utilize the Linker Theory in an attempt to make a change in current practice. Initially they would guide the staff to experience the need for improved documentation and to diagnose the reasons why the problem is occurring. The CNS would then assist the staff in using their problem-solving skills to assess and plan to overcome the problem. Alternatives would be considered and other resources utilized. When the planned change is implemented, feedback would be utilized to modify the solutions attempted and sustain the desired change.

CONCLUSION

Dickoff et al. (1968, p. 415) state: "Theoretically speaking, anyone capable of speech is capable of theorizing." If one agrees with this statement, theory-based practice is possible. Theory-based practice is critical to professional nursing practice. Identification of a theory upon which to base one's practice is the initial step toward such a goal. As obstacles are anticipated or arise, the nursing process can be used to overcome them. The CNS would assess the situation, make a diagnosis of the problem, plan strategies to overcome the problem, implement them, and then evaluate progress.

Perseverance is required. But if one believes that theory can contribute to knowledge, define nursing roles, and provide the CNS with direction, theory must be utilized by persons in the role. As Dickoff et al. state, "theory is born in practice, refined in research, and returns to practice" (1968, p. 415). The CNS is in an ideal position to provide critical links between theory and practice. The CNS can also demonstrate the value of practice to the development and testing of nursing theory. As John Gardner states in an essay on excellence: "The society [profession] which scorns excellence in plumbing [practice] as a humble activity and tolerates shoddiness in philosophy [theory] because it is an exalted activity will have neither good plumbing [practice] nor good philosophy [theory]. Neither its pipes [practice] nor its theories will hold water." (1961), p. 86)

REFERENCES

Abdellah, F. Foreward, in Murphy J. F. (Ed.), *Theoretical issues in professional nursing.* New York: Appleton-Century-Crofts, 1971.

Aradine, C., & Denyes, H. Activities and pressures of clinical nurse specialists. *Nurs Res.*, 1972, *21*, 411–418.

Chapman, C. The use of sociological theories and models in nursing. *J Adv Nurs*, 1976, *1*. 111–127.

Dickoff, J., James, P., & Wiedenbach, E. Theory in a practice discipline: P. 1. *Nurs Res.* 1968, *17*, 415–435.

Dickoff, J., James, P., & Wiedenbach, E. Theory in a practice discipline: Pt. 2. *Nurs Res*, 1968, *17*, 545–554.

Gardner, J. *Excellence.* New York: Harper & Brothers, 1961.

Havelock, R. *Planning for innovation.* Ann Arbor, Mich.: Institute for Social Research, 1976.

Holt, F. Clinical Nurse Specialist—Super Nurse?? *Symposium on the clinical nurse specialist.* Sigma Theta Tau Monograph Series, 1975, *75*, 83–89.

McFarlane, J. Developing a theory of nursing. *J Adv Nurs*, 1977, *2*, 261–270.

Reilly, D. Why a conceptual framework? *Nurs Outlook*, 1975, *23*, 566–569.

Roper, N. A model for nursing and nursology. *J Adv Nurs*, 1976, *1*, 219–227.

Roy, S. C. The Roy adaptation model. In J. Riehl & S. C. Roy (Eds.), *Conceptual models for nursing practice*. New York: Appleton-Century-Crofts, 1980.

Shaefer, J. A. The satisfied clinician: Administrative support makes the difference. *J. Nurs Adm*, 1973, 3, 17–20.

Woodrow, M., & Bell, J. Clinical specialization: Conflict between reality and theory. *J Nurs Adm*, 1971, *1*, 23–27.

3. Role Development and Functions

Ann B. Hamric

The idea of specialists in nursing is not new to the profession (American Nurses' Association, 1980). Private duty nurses could be considered early specialists. Persons with extensive experience in one clinical area have traditionally considered themselves specialized. The idea of a specialist in clinical nursing prepared at the master's level, however, represented a significant variation from these traditional practitioners. Developed for the purpose of improving the quality of nursing care provided to patients, the clinical nurse specialist (CNS) role is a relatively recent development, having appeared in the mid-1960s. Another trend in specialization has occurred in primary care with the development of nurse practitioners. Although some nurse practitioners are master's prepared, many are not. (This and other differences between these two specialty "types" will be explored in Chapter 17.) For the first half of the 20th century, specialization in graduate education in nursing consisted of functional rather than clinical preparation. Nurses who wished to become specialized took courses in administration, teaching, or supervision rather than an aspect of clinical practice (Smoyak, 1976). As recently as 1970 Edith Lewis wrote, "No one is yet quite sure of exactly who the clinical specialist is: how she should be prepared; what are her functions and responsibilities; or where and how she fits into institutional or agency structure" (p. vii). Many of the early writings on the role in the 1960s were speculative, general statements about definitions and qualifications. Writers concerned themselves with broad conceptual definitions rather than with concrete role prescriptions. They sought to justify the need for a master's-prepared nurse remaining at the patient's bedside. Nomenclature varied from article to article: *nurse clinician, clinical associate, liaison nurse,* and *clinical supervisor* were all used to describe a master's-prepared specialist working to improve nursing care (Lewis, 1970, p. vii).

This chapter will describe the overall role of the CNS as presented in the literature, along with some complications that may occur in applying these general descriptions. The process of role development will then be examined in detail, in terms of a model which suggests that the CNS encounters a variation of "reality shock" in attempting to implement this complex role.

OVERVIEW OF THE CNS ROLE

It is safe to say that the CNS role is still developing, although it has achieved some legitimacy and some fairly stable role prescriptions in the last 10 years. Underlying all the diverse and divergent descriptions there runs a common thread: a belief that the CNS is an expert clinical practitioner in a specialized area of nursing, with expanded authority and autonomy, who directs her or his efforts toward the improvement of patient care and nursing practice. Specialists may function in any setting, although most are employed in tertiary health care centers. As Geraldine and Gilbert Padilla have stated, "The clinical nurse specialist is an agent of change in nursing practice and . . . through her advanced education and practice, she represents a new role model for nursing that stresses clinical expertise as the basis for leadership and innovation in patient care" (1979, p. 2). The American Nurses' Association (ANA) formalized an operational definition of the CNS that articulates this belief. Although rather broad and open to some differing interpretations, the definition is a positive step in delineating and differentiating the CNS role from other expanded roles. The ANA states:

The clinical nurse specialist (CNS) is a practitioner holding a master's degree with a concentration in specific areas of clinical nursing. The role of the CNS is defined by the needs of a select client population, the expectation of the larger society, and the clinical expertise of the nurse. By exercising judgment and demonstrating leadership ability, the CNS functions within a field of practice that focuses on the needs of the client system and encompasses interaction with others in the nursing and health care systems serving the client. . . . The function of the CNS is unique with respect to the particular use of clinical judgment and skills regarding client care, service as an advocate when the client is unable to cope with a particular situation, and influence for change as necessary in the nursing care and in the health care delivery system. The CNS is obligated to operate within and affect nursing care delivery systems and the total health care delivery system. While roles may change by circumstances for a certain period of time, this practitioner ceases to be recognized as a CNS when the patient–client–family ceases to be the basis of practice (1976, p. 5).*

This last statement is probably the most significant one in the operational definition because it clearly differentiates the CNS from master's-prepared nurses in educational or strictly administrative positions.

There are two major aspects of the ANA's definition. First, the CNS is described as an expert practitioner in a specific area of clinical nursing, a direct caregiver to patients. Second, the CNS is a change agent within the health care system. This latter aspect involves a variety of indirect activities undertaken to improve the overall quality of patient care. Using these categories of direct and indirect functions, the role of the CNS can be further understood as a constellation of subroles, as shown in Table 3-1. There are numerous theoretical descriptions of the CNS, each giving a differing emphasis to these behaviors (Baker & Kramer, 1970; Fagin, 1967; Georgopoulos & Christman, 1970; Kramer, 1974; Reiter, 1966; Riehl & McVay, 1970). In the direct care role, the CNS functions as an expert practitioner by virtue of her or his advanced education and expanded practice base. The CNS is capable of giving highly expert nursing care to patients with complex health problems. She or he functions as a professional role model for staff nurses, demonstrating desirable practice behaviors for others to emulate. Third, the CNS is a patient advocate. The patient is the focus of the clinical specialist's activities, and her or his primary commitment is to helping the patient rather than the institution, physicians, or staff members.

Indirect care functions include that of change agent. It is expected that CNSs, through their influence and authority, will improve nursing care practices in their specialty areas. Another is consultant or resource person. Briefly, consultation is a process in which an individual with recognized expertise is invited by another to assist in resolving a problem. This important subrole will be discussed in depth in Chapter 7. The CNS is also described as a clinical teacher of nursing personnel as well as nursing students on the clinical unit. A third function is that of supervisor, with the CNS responsible for clinical and, in some cases, administrative supervision. Some authors go to great lengths to make it clear that the CNS should not have to be a supervisor. But even if this term is not used, the CNS is still seen as a leader, a motivator, and a monitor of the quality of care given by

---

*Reprinted with permission from American Nurses Association. Congress for Nursing Practice, The Scope of Nursing Practice—Description of Practice—Clinical Nurse Specialist. May, 1976.

Table 3-1
Subroles of the CNS

Direct Care Functions	Indirect Care Functions
Expert practitioner	Change agent
Role model	Consultant/resource person
Patient advocate	Clinical teacher
	Supervisor
	Researcher
	Liaison
	Innovator

staff nurses. All of these are traditionally considered supervisory functions. Another indirect activity is that of researcher. The CNS is expected to initiate relevant clinical studies, as well as translate research findings into routine clinical practice. Again, this aspect will be considered at length in subsequent chapters. The liaison function involves the CNS being a link of communication between nursing staff and nursing administration, between patients and staff, between nursing and other disciplines, even between inpatient and outpatient services. The CNS is often seen as a bridge of continuity within a fundamentally discontinuous health care system. The last indirect care function identified is that of innovator. CNSs bring bold new ideas to bedside nursing. They are not afraid to try new approaches to "shake up" the system for the sake of improved patient care.

At this point, the reader may be thinking that this all sounds lovely, but where are the problems? There are many, only a few of which will be highlighted here. The first occurs when the CNS is not the clinical expert she or he is promoted as being. In the late 1960s and early 1970s, pressure on the nursing profession led some nursing leaders to encourage students to move directly from baccalaureate to master's programs. The resulting graduates were often too weak in technical aspects of bedside care to function as clinical experts. While technical skills are not necessarily the most important nursing skills, they are often the ones staff nurses use to judge another's competence. Generally, master's programs emphasize theoretical content and its relationship to practice, and attempt to amplify and strengthen a student's practice base. A student with weak or negative practice experience may graduate without the skills needed to practice at an advanced clinical level. As a result, nursing staff are understandably dismayed and even hostile if they have a CNS who knows less about bedside care than they do.

Even if the CNS is an expert practitioner, she or he can experience problems in other areas. Early writers assumed that the expert-practitioner functions of the CNS would inevitably result in the enhancement of total patient care through the process of role modeling. This assumption can be easily challenged by anyone who has spent some time in the role. Although role modeling has some validity, it is not the only factor in achieving the transition between giving good care oneself and influencing other nurses to give good care. Certain conditions must be present for role modeling to be effective. Situational, attitudinal, and behavioral factors in the nursing service organization can all influence CNS effectiveness. For example, an autocratic supervisor who disagrees with the CNS may cancel out the latter's role modeling effectiveness. Further, there seems to be an implicit assumption that role modeling will be effective for all levels of staff, even though professional and motivational levels differ markedly between different levels of staff and between individuals at the same level. When CNSs attempt to model professionally oriented behavior, they may find that many of their staff members are technically oriented or lack motivation to change their behavior.

There are other factors that make the theoretical descriptions of the CNS difficult to attain in practice. The CNS may experience conflict in attempting to prove her or his worth to nursing staff, physicians, and nursing administrators and still function as a patient advocate. The individual's interpersonal skills and ability to promote new knowledge and elicit compliance by staff are among the variables influencing the CNS's effectiveness as a change agent. Many of the indirect care subroles such as change agent, consultant, and clinical teacher, cannot be effectively implemented if the CNS does not have a strong power base. Although power can be formally or informally derived, the CNS must have legitimate authority before her or his suggestions will become established practice. Too often CNSs are placed in advisory positions with minimal administrative support. In such a situation, the individual CNS is likely to be frustrated, and the role may be labeled as ineffective. Even with administrative support, the CNS must confidently demonstrate patient-care skills and independent judgment and actively develop sources of power in order to maximize her or his effectiveness.

One of the reasons role definition is so difficult for this nurse is the innovative component of the role. Flexibility is inherent in and essential to CNS function. The CNS can change priorities and attendant activities on the basis of needs identified and develop different strategies that will meet those needs. As a result, within a given institution, CNSs may be functioning very differently from one another. This fact frustrates those seeking to identify discrete activities that can be expected of all CNSs.

One final point is worth mentioning in this discussion of some difficulties in applying theory to practice. Although a nurse, the CNS is described as a nontraditional nurse who does not fit the usual conceptions of staff nurse, head nurse, or supervisor. This feature makes the CNS's intraprofessional relationships delicate, since she or he may be viewed with suspicion or even hostility by those in traditional nursing roles. Often this means that individual personality variables become very important in determining role effectiveness. It is a common phenomenon with new roles that people consider one's personality as much as one's activities. Although this phenomenon no longer occurs with the traditional positions of head nurse and supervisor, the newness and flexibility of the CNS role causes personality and other individual variables to be inordinately important to success. Consequently, considerable responsibility is placed on the individual CNS to "sell" the role, especially in an institution that has not previously employed such a nurse.

ROLE DEVELOPMENT

Because of the complexity and newness of the CNS role, a process of role development must occur before the new CNS is able to function with maximum effectiveness. On the basis of interviews with 4 clinical specialists, Baker identified 4 phases of role development: orientation, frustration, implementation, and reassessment (1979). These bear a very interesting similarity to Kramer's phases of reality shock (1974). In addition, Oda described 3 phases of specialized role development that parallel 3 of Baker's stages: role identification, role transition, and role confirmation (1977). Oda described the phases well, but she did not discuss them in terms of their affective or emotional components, often the most difficult components with which the CNS must deal. Further, Oda felt that all phases could be completed in six weeks, an unreasonably short period. For those reasons, the author feels that Baker's phases offer a more realistic framework for consideration. (For a comparison of the phases defined by Baker, Kramer, and Oda, see Table 3-2.) Many of the anecdotal reports in the literature of individuals attempting to implement the clinical specialist role lend support to Baker's framework (Aradine and Denyes, 1972; Barrett, 1972; Scully, 1967; Woodrow & Bell, 1971). The idea that clinical specialists experience a form of reality shock is an emerging notion and has not been submitted to rigorous analysis. It has, however, been the author's recurring experience as a practicing CNS, a teacher of specialist students, and a consultant to beginning CNSs that this form of reality shock occurs regularly. Those who have survived reality shock as staff nurses are discouraged to experience this distressing phenomenon again as CNSs, often in a more complex form. It is worthwhile, therefore, to examine the CNS brand of reality shock as described by Baker and experienced by many

Table 3-2
Phases of Role Development

Veronica Baker	Marlene Kramer	Dorothy Oda
Orientation	Honeymoon	Role identification
Frustration	Shock or rejection	
Implementation	Recovery	Role transition
Reassessment	Resolution	Role confirmation

beginning CNSs. Some strategies that can be employed to enhance positive resolution will be presented.

Phase 1 is described by Baker as the orientation phase, by Kramer as the honeymoon, and by Oda as the role identification phase. Baker felt that this phase lasted three to four months for the clinical specialist. New specialists are fresh from graduate programs or new to the institution. Their clinical skills have been sharpened and enhanced, and their professional orientation has been strengthened. In addition, they may have been away from the rigors of the work environment long enough that they remember mostly positive experiences and are ready to return to the "real" world of practice. They are eager to begin the CNS role with freedom to finally perform patient care in the best possible manner. They may feel a pioneer spirit, that they are "breaking new ground" in patient care. As Baker described this phase, the new specialist is enthusiastic, zealous, optimistic, and anxious. Baker's interviewees "began with the idea that they wanted to prove to the nursing staff that they could give nursing care just like any of them . . . . They hoped to bring about change by being role models" (1979, p. 58). One of the major tasks of this phase is to clarify the role, first to oneself and then to others in the setting (Oda, 1977, p. 375). One reason the phase lasts so long for the CNS is that clarifying a nontraditional role takes a number of months. This process may be shortened in an institution where CNSs have been effectively employed for some time.

Phase 2 is called the frustration phase by Baker; shock or rejection by Kramer. Oda did not describe this phase, but it is extremely common and very important. Baker found that this period of frustration lasted six weeks to three months in the clinical specialists she interviewed. "As time passed and no apparent change was perceived by any of the clinical specialists, they then went through a period of depression and frustration" (Baker, 1979, p. 58). To the individual CNS, everything seems to be wrong. Comments are heard such as, "I don't even know where to start, this place is such a mess." The specialist is suddenly overwhelmed by the size of the problems that must be faced, the resistance encountered, and the necessity to effect immediate change in all areas of practice. Kramer found that phase 2 in the new baccalaureate graduate was brought on by the realization that school-bred values conflicted with work-world values (1974, p. 4). To some extent that same conflict occurs in the new specialist. Professional values have been heightened by the graduate school experience. It is difficult justifying one's professional self in a task-oriented system, especially with such perceived ambiguity of tasks and functions as are associated with the CNS role. For example, it is very difficult to urge consideration of such nebulous and diverse professional functions as acting as a change agent or liaison upon a task-oriented person concerned about the number of different activities that she or he has to accomplish in a specific period of time. The CNS begins to feel pressure to prove her or his worth to the staff and to others, on their terms.

There seem to be other components to the CNS variant of the shock phase, too. The first is the jarring realization that a number of cherished assumptions and self-expectations are unrealistic. New specialists are often saddled with unrealistically high performance expectations. They begin to realize that one person cannot perform all the role functions described in the literature, much less simultaneously. One week the CNS may be a good direct caregiver but a poor consultant to the staff; the next week she or he may be a superb liaison but patients complain that they never see the CNS. Second, it takes considerable time to integrate these role functions into one's repertoire. Many of the role functions described in the literature for the CNS are unfamiliar to most nurses. Staff nurses have not been expected to be liaisons or researchers or consultants; it takes time to learn these activities, much less to feel comfortable with them as part of one's everyday business. Third, there are very real impediments to the utilization of the CNS's skills by nursing personnel. These obstacles have been well described by Woodrow and Bell in their article on the conflict between reality and theory (1971). Contrary to being welcomed with open arms by an admiring staff, many CNSs find doors shut in their faces. One of the impediments that Woodrow and Bell identified was time pressure on nurses. The staff they worked with did not want added duties such as patient teaching. They felt overwhelmed with the duties they already had and thought the CNS should take problems off their hands rather than advising them and leaving the implementation with the staff. If the CNS tries to avoid this by taking on all of the problem patients or problem situations, she or he runs the risk of what can be called the "dumping syndrome," in which the staff dump their problems on the CNS and no real change occurs in the staff's behavior. Another impediment Woodrow and Bell identified was the lack of mutual responsibilities among nursing administrators, nursing educators, and the CNS. The CNS may find her- or himself left alone to develop and sell the role to the rank-and-file nurse. Impediments to role modeling were also identified by Woodrow and Bell, as was the degree of threat inherent in the role. When one nurse is given the title of specialist, this may threaten and alienate staff nurses who feel that they do an excellent job of giving specialized care. Another problem identified by Woodrow and Bell was the experimental nature of the role. The fact that the CNS is relatively new in the health care system may cause administrators and other nurses to say, "We will watch this person for 6 months. If this individual doesn't make it, we will eliminate the position." This attitude results in a lack of commitment to help the CNS successfully deal with problems (1971, p. 23–28).

The strategies for overcoming these impediments are complex, and it may take more than a year for the individual to see the results of her or his efforts. In addition, effecting lasting change within a large system takes a long time and requires sustained effort. This slowness in getting results can be extremely frustrating for the new specialist.

Other factors may complicate the CNS's sense of frustration. Lack of administrative power or authority can be a problem. The CNS often has a nebulous position within the formal hierarchy of the institution. Lack of peer support, if the CNS is the only one in the institution, can also increase the sense of frustration. Lack of meaningful contact with peers can occur even when there are other CNSs in the institution because of geographic and specialty separation. The lack of role models to imitate and of validation of one's behavior are real problems in this phase. Another difficult problem in this phase is beginning doubts about one's clinical expertise. When staff nurses bring overwhelming problems to the new CNS and the CNS finds it impossible to solve them easily, the specialist may begin to doubt her- or himself. Baker described the emotions of this phase; first comes "a period of frustration in which the clinical specialist considers her value to the position. This is a period of rude awakening. The frustration is followed by depression brought on by the slowness of her progress, the resistance that is met, and the feelings of inadequacy in the role" (p. 161). Kramer has described other reactions in the new graduate of regression, rejection of school values or oneself, protective isolationism, hostile or hypercritical attitude towards work, moral outrage, and excessive fatigue (pp. 5–7). Any of these may be experienced by the clinical specialist as the individual struggles to align her or his conception of the role with the reality constraints being experienced.

Phase 3 is characterized by Baker as implementation, by Kramer as recovery, and by Oda as role transition. It is important to note that according to Baker's time frame, the CNS has been functioning in the position for 6 months before she or he enters phase 3. Baker found that phase 3 lasted from 4 to 6 months, with the result that the first year of employment was taken up with these first three phases. Baker described the phase of implementation as a period of organization and reorganization, of rethinking and clarifying one's position to the staff and the health team. Oda discussed this phase similarly and emphasized that the specialist is interacting with others and beginning to modify her or his approach in response to the feedback received from other health care professionals and from staff nurses (p. 375). Baker's subjects developed specific projects during this phase—visible tasks with tangible results for which they could be rewarded (pp. 58–59). Kramer described a beginning sense of humor as the first sign that the new graduate was entering the recovery phase. She found that there was a lessening of tension, along with the beginning of an ability to objectively assess and predict situations (pp. 7–8). The CNS is developing feelings of being accepted, and enthusiasm is returning. The sense of returning perspective on one's situation is an important aspect of the implementation phase. The CNS is continuing to clarify her or his role but is beginning to get a sense of the specific role configuration that suits the particular setting and her- or himself. Phase 3 is a critical phase because it can lead to either positive or negative resolution.

Phase 4 is called reassessment by Baker, resolution by Kramer, or role confirmation by Oda. Baker found that this was reached in her subjects after 12–18 months. All 4 of her subjects had been employed only 12–18 months, and they all felt that they were currently in the reassessment phase. Baker did not have any idea of how long this phase lasted because her subjects had not been in their roles long enough. Both Baker and Oda described phase 4 in positive terms. Negative resolution can and does occur, however, and can have deleterious effects on patient care. Kramer's work with new graduates resulted in four possible categories of resolution, three of which may be seen in CNSs. Kramer described three negative categories and one positive category of resolution (Table 3-3). She organized these on the basis of the bureaucratic and professional role conceptions of the individual. Each category will be discussed in terms of CNS resolution. Descriptions of the three negative resolutions come from Kramer's work because she is the only writer who has identified these categories.

The first negative category Kramer identified were the "rutters." She found that these people had withdrawn from everything and were just doing a job. They had given up and tended to be indifferent, minimally conforming to the behavioral and performance requirements of the job. This category of negative resolution is rarely seen in CNSs because most "rutters" do not have sufficient drive to go on to graduate school.

The second negative resolution was that of the "organization woman." This individual accepted and integrated bureaucratic values but had minimal or no integration of professional values. This nurse was influenced

Table 3-3
Categories of Resolution

	Low Professional Role Conception	High Professional Role Conception
High Bureaucratic Role Conception	Organization women	Bicultural troublemakers
Low Bureaucratic Role Conception	Rutters	Lateral arabesquers

Reproduced with permission from Kramer, M. *Reality Shock: Why Nurses Leave Nursing.* St. Louis: C. V. Mosby, 1974.

by work-centered role models and adopted a stance of adaptive conformity, of valuing the bureaucratic system and maintaining order and the status quo. Kramer found that these individuals were happy and contented but were not change agents in the health care setting. In terms of the CNS, this resolution can occur as individuals begin to search for more traditional role expression. Some people may develop a resolution pattern that centers around supervisory or administrative activities, especially those that place emphasis on maintaining the system. The CNS may still keep the same title but takes on more and more administrative functions and becomes increasingly removed from clinical contact. She or he begins to advocate the institution rather than the patients. Interestingly, the CNS may decry this process in others but not move to change the pattern developing in her- or himself.

The next category that Kramer identified as a negative resolution was that of the "lateral arabesquer." She found that lateral arabesquers were hurt, confused, and morally outraged by what they were encountering in the institution. They placed a high value on formal education. Many wished to return to school; some withdrew or were asked to withdraw from the system because their behaviors were unacceptable to the administration. These individuals experienced high role deprivation, and they tended to be job hoppers to safer, more idealistic environments. In terms of the CNS, a variety of resolutions are variations of the lateral arabesque. In one, the CNS leaves the hospital setting to become a faculty member of a school of nursing or returns to school for more graduate study. In another resolution, the CNS may stay in the setting but become a staff developer not directly responsible for patient care or remove her- or himself from the clinical realities of the setting by decreasing the level of personal involvement. Other CNSs may become independent of the setting by becoming involved in independent practice or working with a group of physicians. (It must be noted that these changes in career pattern may also occur in CNSs who are effective in the role. Obviously, the author is not referring to those individuals.) While not necessarily negative for the individual, the ultimate result of each of these resolutions can be negative for the role and for the system, in the sense that the individual CNS does not have a significant impact on patient care or on staff rendering that care. In some cases, nurses, administration, and other health care professionals may generalize from the individual's lack of effectiveness to conclude that the CNS role does not have a favorable impact on patient care. The net result of these negative resolutions is that the system continues unchanged.

The positive resolution category that Kramer describes for recent baccalaureate graduates is that of "bicultural troublemakers." Kramer found that bicultural troublemakers exhibited behaviors consistent with the expectations of both professional and bureaucratic groups. They were highly functional and, even though they experienced high role deprivation, they also had high job satisfaction. They were risk takers. They evidenced growth-producing conflict resolutions; they were creative and welcomed challenge. She found that fewer new graduates were in this category, possibly because it took a period of time to go through the phases of reality shock to reach resolution. In addition, she found that more bicultural troublemakers than any other category returned to school to become CNSs. The reader will recall that Baker and Oda described phase 4 in positive terms, analogous to Kramer's description. Baker found greater insight and further refinement of the role occurring in the CNSs she interviewed. All of her subjects were presently in the resolution phase. (Baker had originally hoped to interview 5 subjects. One of them left her position during the phase 2 experience, so that by the time of Baker's interview 4 specialists remained.) Oda feels that the role confirmation phase involves reinforcement of the role definition established earlier. "The degree to which the staff accept her and administrators recognize her, indicates the extent to which the role is confirmed" (p. 375). During this phase, significantly less time is spent clarifying the role, and others in the work setting may assist in implementing the role. Baker describes the affective aspect of this period as one of "morale rearmament—renewed enthusiasm and optimism" (p. 61). In my own experience, phase 4 was the most productive one, when my activities began to show some really positive impact on patient care. Staff nurses and other health care personnel understood and supported my functions and came appropriately to refer patients, discuss nursing care problems, or suggest conferences. Much of the energy expended in role clarification was actually taken over by the nursing staff, who would explain to patients and new staff what the CNS's role was and how the specialist could be utilized. This freed a great deal of time and allowed me to function as a CNS rather than constantly having to explain to others in the setting what I was supposed to be doing.

After phase 4, what? The literature gives no guidelines because most writers have had less than two years of experience with the CNS role. One of Baker's subjects felt that the phases were cyclical. Interestingly, she had had the least experience at the time of the interview. On the basis of 3 years in the role, I tend to disagree with this position. Although aspects of each phase do recur as changes occur within the system, the specialist's own clear role definition and established place within the setting lend stability to role expression. I found that implementation and role reassessment continued but that the anxiety of the orientation phase and the turmoil experienced during the frustration phase were not repeated with the same intensity. There may be exceptions, however. I have worked with CNSs who experienced a radical change in nursing administration philosophy, from one of support to one of threatening nonsupport. This did lead to a cyclic repetition of the phases and, unfortunately, culminated in the resignation of a number of CNSs from the institution. Another exception could be CNSs who move from one setting to another. Unfortunately, there is no data on whether they go through the phases of role development again in the new setting. It is likely that they do to some extent. The process of role development would probably be shortened, however, because of the clear role conceptions and experience that they bring to the new position.

Given this fairly lengthy process of role socialization, what can be done to enhance positive resolution? A number of suggestions spring directly from aspects of the CNS's reality shock. One of the most important ways to enhance positive resolution is through "anticipatory socialization," to use Kramer's terminology. This preparation for the realities of the role should occur in graduate education and be continued in the administrative supervision that the new specialist receives in her or his first position. There are many components of socializing students to the CNS role. Although it is important to prepare students to be expert clinicians, this is not sufficient. They must also be exposed to theoretical and practical aspects of the CNS role. This would involve giving realistic assumptions to students so that they understand, for example, that the process of change is very slow and that role modeling, although important, is probably not a sufficient strategy to effect lasting change. Other assumptions from the literature need to be challenged and debated within graduate programs so that students have a good grasp of what they can expect as practicing specialists. One such assumption is that all nurses will be receptive to advice from a colleague with advanced knowledge. Another is that staff nurses will view the CNS as their peer, as well as their advocate (on the contrary, they often distrust the specialist in both respects). Strategies for beginning one's work as a new

CNS should be identified and discussed. Another aspect of anticipatory socialization is to teach students to evaluate the process of their activities, rather than the product. One characteristic of a school environment is that one performs certain activities, achieves a product, and is evaluated, usually in a semester's time. The student tends to take that same expectation into the work setting. One CNS was heard to remark, "I've been here three months, and I want my grade now." The new CNS looks for results of his or her activities, such as a consistent change in staff behavior or improvement in patient outcomes. Such measurable changes rarely occur in the first year of role development. Indeed, the author believes that the new CNS and the employer should not evaluate the effectiveness of the specalist's strategies, or performance in terms of products achieved, until the CNS has held the job for one year. The CNS needs to understand, however, that she or he can still evaluate the process of her or his activity (for example, the improved attitude of one staff member). Patient advocacy activities are often tangible sources of satisfaction. The CNS may need help to develop concrete, short-term goals and to prioritize those goals to achieve a realistic performance level.

Another aspect of anticipatory socialization involves learning to creatively exist within the system. Theoretical material can be very helpful in preparing students to analyze problem situations that they will encounter in practice. Specifically, readings on leadership, problem solving, motivation, power, change, organizations, and conflict resolution can all be useful when applied to specific problem situations. It is the author's experience that students need help seeing the relevance of theory to specific practice problems. This gap between reality and theory, if not bridged while in graduate school, will be difficult for the student to bridge once she or he becomes a practicing specialist. A clinical example may serve to illustrate these points. One graduate student devised a clinical experience in which she served as a respiratory CNS helping to develop an outpatient program. She was known to the institution and the physician in charge of the program, who gave her verbal assurances that they were delighted to have her participate in setting up this program and hoped she would stay to run it after graduation. Eventually, however, she became extremely frustrated by the failure of the physician to act on her suggestions, even though they were supported by the literature and by others in the setting and even though the doctor agreed with her in meetings. What she failed to see was the underlying conflict over the issue of power. The physician, who had formal authority, was threatened by her assertiveness and informal power with other staff members. After reading about formal and informal power, she was able to develop strategies to decrease his feeling of threat and to enhance her power base. She was also able to understand that some of her ideas were not likely to be implemented as long as she had only advisory status.

There is one additional aspect to anticipatory socialization for the CNS role. It is important to be honest about the fact that there are factors that will impede role development and to address these factors. Students need to understand the inevitability of encountering resistance and to learn some strategies to use in overcoming resistance. The perceived ambiguity of role tasks and functions must be minimized. This process should begin in the school environment by having students formulate realistic performance expectations for themselves, through exercises such as developing a written job description, or formulating short-term and long-term goals for a certain position. These activities should include prioritizing. Such exercises enhance the student's own clarity regarding the role she or he is to assume. In addition, a realistic job description or objectives for a position can be an important aid in the job interview. These expectations should continue to be refined later with experience and through dialogue with peers and superiors in the work setting. Knowledge of CNS role development should help both the new CNS and the employer to develop evaluation strategies that emphasize process achievements and the attainment of short-term goals.

Besides anticipatory socialization, provisions for ensuring clinical competence and a healthy sense of the limits to one's knowledge base are very important before entering the CNS role. The author believes that students should have sufficient positive clinical experience so that they have mastered staff nursing in their specialty before entering a graduate school. Then their master's degree student experiences can focus on deepening their clinical knowledge, practicing various CNS roles, and increasing use of independent judgment and autonomy. Students who leave graduate programs feeling that they are established clinical experts may have a hard time confronting the limits of their own knowledge once they are expected by staff or others to "have all the answers." The resultant questioning of one's expertise is one of the more difficult components of the frustration phase.

Another factor that enhances positive resolution is administrative support—specifically, concrete expressions by nursing administrators of willingness to support the role. In a survey of CNSs, Shaefer (1973) found that this evidence of tangible support in the face of resistance was the single most important factor in a CNS's job satisfaction. Any institution that contemplates hiring a CNS should examine their expectations. Are they realistic and achievable by one individual? Do structural and systemic factors allow for success, or do certain changes need to occur within the system before the specialist will be able to be effective? Can administration clarify the CNS's position within the organization? And, an important question, has the specialist been given the authority to carry out the responsibilities that she or he has been given? These questions should be addressed before the role is introduced, rather than after problems appear. The issue of administrative support, a crucial ingredient in the success or failure of the CNS, is examined at length in Chapter 10.

Another factor enhancing positive resolution is the provision for peer support and role models. Beginning CNSs need consensual validation and feedback a minimum of every three months during the first year. Specifically, they need help with setting limits, with understanding how to cope with problem situations, and with maintaining a sense of perspective—of seeing the forest and not just the trees. They need support in dealing with the painful affective responses such as feelings of inadequacy and depression experienced during the frustration phase. If the new CNS does not have peers to utilize for such feedback, then she or he needs a trusted advisor, someone in nursing administration, a former teacher, or even a friend knowledgeable about the problem the CNS is encountering who can provide objective analysis of problem situations. The author tells her students that they get one collect phone call every three months for the first year after they graduate. Thankfully, not all of them use this resource. But the ones that do really need it. This ability to feel that there is someone to whom to turn for objective advice is crucial to successful completion of each phase of role development.

Finally, if a CNS is moving toward a negative resolution pattern such as "organization woman" or "lateral arabesquer," she or he should be helped to look closely at her or his own needs and career goals. Allowing a specialist to continue to function ineffectively as a CNS is a disservice to both the individual and the title.

There are many issues in the future development and strengthening of the CNS role. As a profession, nursing is beginning to develop consistency in parameters of CNS role preparation and role expression. Research is needed on the phases of role development and factors that enhance positive resolution. Strategies for managing each phase creatively should be explored. Most major writings on the CNS date from the mid-1960s to the early 1970s, and there has been little amplification or specification of problems encountered since that time. As previously noted, very little has been written by anyone who has been in the role longer than 2 years. Undoubtedly there are individuals who have practiced for 5 to 10 years who have a wealth of experience to share. It is hoped that they will begin writing their experiences with role development.

"Specialization is the inevitable result of new knowledge within fields and demands from the public for new service" (Smoyak, 1976, p. 678). The ANA has stated that "specialization in nursing is now clearly established" and that it represents "a mark of the advancement of the nursing profession" (1980, pp. 21–22). It is the author's experience and conviction that the CNS role is not only a creative answer to the challenge of improving nursing care but is essential to nursing's growth as a profession. The strategies presented to promote positive resolution represent beginning steps to strengthen CNS performance. As more is learned about the phases of role development and more experience is gained in role implementation, many of the difficulties new clinical specialists experience can be anticipated and resolved.

REFERENCES

American Nurses' Association, Congress of Nursing Practice, Description of practice: clinical nurse specialist. In ANA, Congress of Nursing Practice, *The scope of nursing practice.* Kansas City Mo: American Nurses' Association, 1976.

American Nurses' Association, Congress of Nursing Practice, *Nursing—A social policy statement.* Kansas City Mo: American Nurses' Association, 1980.

Aradine, C. R., & Denyes, M. J. Activities and pressures of clinical nurse specialists. *Nurs Res,* 1972, *21,* 411–418.

Baker, C., & Kramer, M. To define or not to define: The role of the clinical nurse specialist. *Nurs Forum,* 1970, *9,* 45–55.

Baker, V. Retrospective explorations in role development. In G. V. Padilla (Ed.), *The clinical nurse specialist and improvement of nursing practice.* Wakefield, Mass.: Nursing Resources, 1979.

Barrett, J. The nurse specialist practitioner: A study. *Nurs Outlook,* 1972, *20,* 524–527.

Georgopoulos, B. S., and Christman, L., The clinical nurse specialist: a role model, *Am J Nurs,* 1970, *70,* 1030–1039.

Fagin, C. M., The clinical specialist as supervisor, *Nurs Outlook,* 1967, *15,* 34–36.

Kramer, M. *Reality shock: Why nurses leave nursing.* St. Louis: C. V. Mosby, 1974.

Lewis, E. P. (Ed.) *The clinical nurse specialist.* New York: American Journal of Nursing, Educational Services Division, 1970.

Oda, D. Specialized role development: A three-phase process. *Nurs Outlook,* 1977, *25,* 374–377.

Padilla, G. V., & Padilla, G. J. Nursing roles to improve patient care. In G. V. Padilla (Ed.), *The clinical nurse specialist and improvement of nursing practice.* Wakefield, Mass.: Nursing Resources, 1979.

Reiter, F. The nurse-clinician. *Am J Nurs,* 1966, *66,* 274–280.

Riehl, J. P., & McVay, J. W. (Eds.). *The clinical nurse specialist: Interpretations.* New York: Appleton-Century-Crofts, 1970.

Scully, N. R. The clinical nursing specialist: Practicing nurse. *Nurs Outlook*, 1967, *13*, 28–30.

Shaefer, J. A. The satisfied clinician: Administrative support makes the difference. *J Nurs Adm*, 1973, *3*, 17–20.

Smoyak, S. A. Specialization in nursing; From then to now. *Nurs Outlook*, 1976, *24*, 676–681.

Woodrow, M., & Bell, J. Clinical specialization: conflict between reality and theory. *J Nurs Adm*, 1979, *1*, 23–27.

II. ASPECTS OF CLINICAL NURSE SPECIALIST PRACTICE

4. Direct Patient Care and Independent Practice

Lauren A. Felder

DIRECT PATIENT CARE

The clinical nurse specialist (CNS) is charged to implement a variety of subroles, those of clinician, educator, researcher, consultant, manager, patient advocate, staff advocate, liaison, and change agent. Each specialist then interprets and implements these functions uniquely. While appropriate to meet the needs of the individual environment, this variance has also served to perpetuate the debate concerning the question of "Just what does the CNS do?". Generally, the individual CNS places a major emphasis on one or two subroles, though not to the total exclusion of the others. Rather, CNS activities reflect concurrent implementation of several subroles. For example, the surgical CNS who is in a CNS–researcher position obviously has research as a major area of focus. Inherent in this position nonetheless is the specialist's regular contact with patients and staff, which results in her or his serving as educator, consultant, and patient advocate.

It is well acknowledged in nursing literature that the CNS position emerged in answer to the increasing lack of clinically skilled nurses at the bedside. This lack occurred as a result of the upward managerial movement of experienced nurses within the profession. These experienced nurses were advanced professionally but were thereby removed from administering direct patient care. The CNS role was envisioned as a reversal of this trend. Thus the provision of direct care to patients has been a major component of the definition of the nurse specialist since its origin (Kohnke, 1977, p. 14).

A 1977 survey of registered nurses with active licenses in the United States reported on the percentage of working time that nurses spent in various activites. Of 11,469 nurses returning the questionnaire, 92 CNSs addressed the issue of direct patient care activities. The average amount of time reported for these specialists in direct care was 65 percent (Moses & Roth, 1979, p. 1754), indicating that direct involvement is a major component of actual role implementation today.

Advantages of Direct Care by the CNS

The direct care activities of the CNS can have numerous beneficial effects. Patients, families, nursing staff, the health care team effort, and the CNS her- or himself may all benefit from this direct involvement. Patients and their family members comprising the specialist's case load should receive high-quality care. The CNS provides more advanced services and skills not yet available from the general nursing staff. Regarding the nursing staff, the CNS involved in direct care not only learns of but experiences the obstacles and constraints under which the staff must function, and can then better identify the need for and assist in developing reality-based nursing care methods and tools. The CNS is also in a good position to evaluate nursing care and personnel performance and identify appropriate means of strengthening both. With the CNS's help, problem solving among the staff may be based on more accurate perceptions. In addition, direct care activities increase the visibility and accessibility of the CNS, and the increased contact with staff enhances the specialist's ability to serve as a staff advocate. A key factor in promoting acceptance of the specialist role is the opportunity that such direct involvement provides for establishing and maintaining the CNS's credibility with the nursing staff.

The specialist's direct involvement may also improve and facilitate the health team's interdisciplinary effort, resulting in a heightened perception by other professionals of the validity of the nurse's role. With regard to physicians, the specialist can demonstrate clinical competence and establish collaborative, collegial relationships. The CNS–educator (joint appointment) can better provide a more reality-based classroom teaching experience for student nurses. Staff may also be less resistant to the student nurses when the instructor is perceived to be a unit member. By engaging in direct care, the specialist can pursue continued development of her or his own practice, improve skills, and remain current.

In general, direct care activities by the specialist help to assert an autonomous role for nurses, one utilizing independent judgment and defining nursing care, with nurses assuming both responsibility and accountability as professionals.

It is of major significance that the other CNS subroles are also fulfilled through the direct patient care activities of the specialist. The functions of educator, consultant, staff and patient advocate, researcher, and innovator are all directly served and improved by the clinician functions. For example, while providing direct care the CNS may realize the need for better coordination of services among the team members. As a result, the specialist can consult with the team and in doing so also serves in the advocacy role.

Problems in the Direct Care Subrole

The appropriate functions of the CNS have been defined since the mid-1960s; why, then, is direct care still a controversial subrole? Why has the course of implementing the role and utilizing the expertise of the CNS in direct care been so rugged?

While there is no question that the "select" patients cared for by the CNS receive high-quality care, only a limited number can benefit, and the care is thought to be expensive. Nursing staff do not always express satisfaction; in fact, they often vent anger and frustration at the freedom and the "right of selectivity" of the specialist. A particularly sensitive point, explored by Kohnke, is that nurses prepared at the baccalaureate level, if properly utilized, would be performing at precisely the level described in the literature as appropriate for the master's-prepared CNS.

> The literature describes the specialist as planning and giving direct care to patients and thus acting as an expert practitioner and setting practice standards for other nurses. This is exactly the role of the nurse prepared at the baccalaureate level (Kohnke, 1977, p. 31).

It is hardly surprising, therefore, that nurses with baccalaureate degrees feel resentful of CNSs. In addition to staff dissatisfaction, administrators have also expressed disappointment. When the CNS is involved so directly in patient care, broader system changes that had been anticipated may not be forthcoming. Overall, these problems can contribute to the specialist's experiencing a personal sense of failure (Everson, 1981, p. 17). This feeling may also be prompted by initial reactions of mistrust, hostility, and perception of the specialist as a threat communicated by the nursing staff. These reactions are not necessarily insurmountable, and they may subside as the CNS demonstrates her or his competence and approachability.

In a report of their own activities, Woodrow and Bell (1971, p. 23), examined care activities and utilization by nursing personnel. Of the 88 patients cared for by the medical-surgical CNS author, only 14.8 percent had been nurse-referred. For the psychiatric CNS author, of 21 patients in individual therapy, 14.3 percent had been nurse-referred. Of the 14 patients in group therapy with the same psychiatric CNS, only 7.1 percent had been nurse-referred. Although a considerable amount of time was spent in direct care activities, the authors concluded that actual utilization by nursing staff of their CNS services was minimal. Nursing was not demonstrated to be a collaborative effort between nursing and the specialist; in contrast, it was one of functioning in isolation (p. 25).

Woodrow and Bell's suggested reasons for such underutilization included staff time pressures, lack of administrative supports to effect change, and resistance to respond to role modeling. Additionally, they recognized that the degree of threat inherent in the role and the experimental nature of the role itself inhibited utilization of the CNS by the nursing staff. No single force, however, was identified as being of more significance by the authors (p. 25).

As mentioned, and commonly acknowledged in the literature, adequate time must be allowed for staff to accept the specialist first as a person, then as a professional. Woodrow and Bell project hope for the reverse to occur in the future; "acceptance of the position, acceptance as a professional, and finally acceptance as an individual" (p. 26).

The specialist's involvement in direct care activities sometimes elicits a threatened feeling from both nurses and health care professionals in other disciplines. In their discussion of inherent threat, Woodrow and Bell described a pattern of behaviors and responses on the part of the nursing staff in utilizing the specialist. When a patient care problem was unresolved, staff nurses recognized either their lack of time or lack of knowledge as causes and felt frustrated or inadequate. Action on the patient problem often terminated at this point. If referred to the specialist, though, the nurses then tended to feel guilty, as manifested by either depression or hostility toward the CNS. Nor were the nurses rewarded for calling in the specialist, since the specialist then established a bond with the patient, and staff nurses failed to experience the rewards of the patient's trust or gratitude, which resulted in even greater resentment. The authors consider the possibility that the specialist would function better if she or he served solely in the role of consultant, avoiding this nonproductive relationship (p. 26).

Nonproductive relationships and perception of the CNS as a threat also develop among other health team members. As a result of the specialist's broadly defined role, feelings of territorial threat may surface: this is particularly true in the area of social service, since there is an overlapping of roles at times. Counseling, patient advocacy, and coordination/utilization of community agencies are elements common to both the social service role and the CNS role. Doctors have also experienced cultural shock in response to the CNS's appearance on the scene (Mandell, 1978). While the nursing profession has so actively been pursuing growth as a true profession, the medical profession has resisted these changes. In expanding professionally, nurses have developed high-level skills in both care giving and decision making, and they have learned to utilize more independent judgment in practice. Nursing's increased autonomy conflicts with medicine's traditional view of the nurse as an assistant following the physician's orders (Kalisch & Kalisch, 1978, p. 642). The CNS, whose advanced practice and autonomous role is especially evident in her or his direct patient care skills, has been viewed as a threat by physicians. The medical community's poor response has also stemmed from the confusion of the CNS role with that of the nurse practitioner (NP) role, which presents more of a threat because of its focus on primary care practice.

Solutions

The CNS must evaluate the negative risks of direct care activities—that is, the fostering of competition, arousing of territorial responses, and possible isolation of the CNS. If the specialist plans to undertake direct care responsibilities, it is advisable that she or he carefully consider the individual environment and plan accordingly. Prior to implementing the direct care role, the CNS needs to examine the initial advantages and disadvantages in light of the ultimate gains.

On what basis does the CNS choose direct care activities as a modality? Initially, there are two reasons: one is to demonstrate clinical competence and the second is to function as a role model for other nurses in order to promote change. The reasons for direct care activities may change as the role evolves for the particular specialist. Initially the specialist may function as a staff nurse overtly in order to "learn the routines" but with the underlying motivation of proving competence. Proving competence in the staff nurse role, however, may not be adequate to prove capability as a CNS. It may promote initial clinical acceptance, but further demonstration of high-level functioning will be necessary in order to to gain acceptance as a specialist. There are, nevertheless, other important advantages to introducing the role by this method. The staff and CNS become acquainted, a team feeling is promoted, and the specialist can begin to realize the supports and constraints under which the staff actually function. Working in a staff nurse capacity initially, therefore, can promote both personal and professional acceptance.

A conscious decision then needs to be made concerning working as "staff" in the future and employing this role as a modality for promoting change. One can easily become caught in the trap of shortages, both of time and personnel, and while being used to "fill in the gaps" rationalize that it promotes the desired changes. Once initial acceptance for basic nursing skills competency is achieved, provision of direct care by the CNS needs to be on a higher level.

Although functioning as a specialist in a direct care role promotes gains for the select patient and for the CNS her- or himself, it is generally accepted that the specialist can make a significant contribution through role modeling. However, the effectiveness of the CNS as a role model needs to be examined. The process of role modeling requires, in addition to a role model, an appropriate opportunity or situation and a person who seeks to or is expected to emulate the model. Only one of these factors seems to consistently present itself: the presence of the CNS as a role model. If nursing staff are reacting with hostility or disregard, they will not seek to emulate the specialist. If there is no incentive, such as that provided when the CNS has formal authority or obvious support from the administration, the process will not occur. If the staff do not utilize or observe the specialist and the specialist performs high-level skills in isolation, again the process will not occur (Woodrow & Bell, p. 26). If the CNS plans to participate in direct care–giving activities for the purpose of serving as a role model, then her or his strategy needs to include an evaluation of these essentials. Perhaps such an effort can be delayed until the CNS has gained acceptance with the health care team and can be gradually incorporated later as the environment becomes more favorable.

It may also be advisable to utilize other modalities besides role modeling for serving as an "example" or "motivator" to effect change. Some CNSs have relinquished their direct care activities and now provide their services only on a consultative basis (Everson, 1981, pp. 17–18). This method encourages the process of change, since the services of the CNS are furnished upon request of the staff nurse involved. Consultation as the basis for influencing patient care, however, is often a source of frustration for the specialist. The CNS has to be able to accept the fact that patient care may not be changed, since the final choice remains with the requesting nurse.

Other specialists, instead of seeking alternatives to the role modeling process, have sought to strengthen the process by incorporating the necessary administrative supports (power) or direct reward systems to serve as incentives for behavior changes. For example, the specialist may move from a staff to a line position. This provides the authority needed to achieve change, yet the accompanying administrative responsibilities can create another set of barriers to serving in a clinical capacity. Two other methods that provide freedom from major administrative duties while still giving the CNS administrative backing are (1) obtaining obvious support from the existing authority figures and (2) functioning at times as a team leader and thus gaining direct authority to achieve changes in patient care. Requiring staff nurses to rotate the assignment of working directly with the CNS is also a useful method, as long as it has administrative support (Baker, 1973, p. 61). Also, holding nurses accountable for the quality of patient care is a form of direct reward system. This can be done most effectively by including such accountability as a part of the performance evaluation.

The direct care function as offered by the specialist role should not be devalued because it is experiencing "growing pains." Educators, the profession, and specialists need to carefully examine methods for strengthening this important subrole. Carefully defining the role of direct care in one's practice and adequately preparing the CNS to implement such activities in light of expected responses will serve to improve acceptance of direct care involvement and promote nursing's growth.

INDEPENDENT PRACTICE

Origins

For the CNS who is particularly committed to the direct care subrole, the evolving potential of private nursing practice may be a promising alternative. It may even be representative of a natural progression for the role, as an outgrowth of nursing's increased body of knowledge and ability to implement it autonomously. It is interesting to note that the specialist role is venturing forth into this new territory (with a whole new set of rewards and obstacles) when it has not yet conquered its place of origin. The CNS was originally intended to be clinically based within an institutional setting. The position, after two decades, is still actively struggling for acceptance in that setting. The move toward private, independent practice therefore stimulates a number of questions: Is this movement a statement that the role itself is not the problem but the setting? Is this truly an appropriate, natural evolution, reflecting the changing needs of the health care system and the desire of nursing to grow into roles to fill the needs? Or is it a reactive move, a response to feelings of frustration, anger, and betrayal experienced by "pioneers" impatient to receive the sanction of their own profession? Or, rather, is it a form of escape: Is it a "fight or flight" phenomenon, in which private independent practice is overtly promoted as an acceptable and even respectable movement but is covertly a flight mechanism of coping? And finally, regardless of the individual motivation, is private independent practice economically feasible? The answers to these questions remain to be answered; for purposes of this chapter, the issue of private independent practice by specialists will be explored in light of them.

Historically, the concept of independent nursing practice has evolved from the nurse practitioner (NP) movement. The role of the NP was developed in response to the rapidly growing need for primary health care (see Chapter 17). The focus of the role was not only congruent with the medical model (treatment of illness) but consistent with nursing concepts (treating the patient's response to illness). Initially the NP was tied to a physician or an agency. In the early seventies, however, practitioners realized that while they functioned interdependently with physicians, the mechanism for providing services could be in a setting not reliant on an agency or medical practice.

In the early seventies, NPs were the first nurses known to "hang out their shingles" and open private nursing practices. Today there are an estimated 5,239 nurses working on a fee-for-service basis and claiming to be self-employed. According to the 1977 National Sample Survey of Registered Nurses, 10 percent of these self-employed nurses were nurse practitioners/nurse midwives. CNSs accounted for only 4 percent of the self-employed. Among all the nurses surveyed, only five-tenths of 1 percent were self-employed (Moses & Roth, 1979, pp. 1751–1752).

Although considerably more has been written on NPs in private independent practice than on CNSs, the reasons for the movement of CNSs into this type of practice are essentially the same as for NPs. Private practice is appealing to nurses because it presents a means of upward mobility and an opportunity for experiencing greater professional fulfillment and recognition. It allows increased autonomy (in reaction to the "deep frustration at not being able to practice the full scope of nursing in an emotionally satisfying environment") (Koltz, 1979, p. 9) and greater ability to benefit patients with direct care. Such a practice offers personal benefits, such as greater potential for financial compensation, and increased scheduling freedom; the practice can be structured around personal life constraints. It has benefits for patients, since private nursing practice allows expanding health care needs to be met at less expense. Pursuit of such a practice appeal to nurses with the pioneer spirit, those interested in promoting innovation within nursing. On the other hand, it appeals to nurses who desire to channel their energies in the direction of refining the specialist role, as opposed to struggling to define the role in the traditional setting. The motivations of nurses may vary, but the incentives for movement in the private, independent direction are weighty, since they represent personal, professional, and health care system benefits.

Regardless of individual motivation, in the author's view the move to independent practice represents a natural progression in the development of the specialist role. Although the CNS role was originally hospital-based, the role has always possessed an independent element. With the increased skills in advocacy, supportive care, and counseling of a CNS, often a patient population is better served by the specialist as primary caretaker than by the physician. After medical management or concurrent with medical care, the CNS administers the nursing care required to (1) promote the patient's necessary adaptation to life-style changes, (2) provide crisis intervention, (3) furnish counsel, and (4) refer the patient to other appropriate resources. The need for this level of independent functioning exists for almost all specialty areas, from medical–surgical to psychiatric nursing. The CNS role, as originally designed, can serve a variety of populations independently as well as interdependently. Any population of patients with catastrophic, terminal, or chronic conditions presents the potential for the need of a non-hospital-based nurse specialist prepared in the appropriate medical specialty. For example, once a patient has been discharged from the hospital setting, the need for medical supervision lessens, yet the need for supportive care, patient and family education, home care recommendations, and coordination of health care resources heightens. These needs can be effectively and appropriately met by the specialist. The potential for a direct care private practice is obviously lessened, however, for the specialist who limits her or his expertise to a hospital specialty area such as intensive care or neonatal care.

A traditional distinction between CNS practice and NP practice is that those patients with generalized, short-term problems comprise the population of the NP. In actual private practice, the roles will overlap, but the areas of focus will differ. The CNS has a greater understanding of and application of nursing principles to a medical specialty area, while the practitioner serves as a generalist with greater physical assessment and medical management skills. As this author views the roles, the NP combines both physician extender and expanded nursing services, whereas the specialist role is primarily an expanded nursing role.

Currently these differences have greatly influenced the prospects for success of nurse specialists in private independent practice. NPs are evidencing a greater rate of success in opening and maintaining private practice. Practitioners are prepared to provide primary care, but at a cost less than that of physician care. The role evolved to fill in the gaps in the health care system without contributing further to the existing high costs. "Nurse practitioners, it was assumed, could alleviate the problems created by the maldistribution of health personnel, particularly physicians. Nurses trained in primary skills could provide health services in underserved areas (e.g., the elderly, poor and minorities)" (Feldbaum, 1979, p. 61). In the early seventies, nurse practitioners began the private practice movement. It was hallmarked by the national attention drawn to the opening of

M. Lucille Kinlein's private practice in 1971. Since then, the number of nurse practitioners in successful private practice has steadily increased (Kinlein, 1979).

Factors Affecting the Success of Private Practice

In contrast to the large numbers of success stories for NPs in private practice, there is a scarcity of literature regarding the success of CNSs in private independent practice. The specialty area experiencing greatest success in the private arena is psychiatric/mental health care. In the November 10, 1980, issue of the *Los Angeles Times*, psychiatric specialists with 12–14 years of private practice experience were reviewed. In 1974, alterations in the California Nurse Practice Act legalized these already existing private practices and opened the opportunity for more to be established. There were a reported 20 such psychiatric/mental health specialists in the Los Angeles area alone at the time of publication of the article. The specialists in the article attributed their success to:

1. Their ability to offer care less costly than that given by a psychologist or psychiatrist;
2. Patients' desire to avoid being labeled "sick";
3. Their effectiveness as therapists (Barnes, 1980).

Private practice is believed by some to be a natural evolutionary outcome for any mental health therapist; psychotherapy is within the accepted scope of practice for the psychiatric nurse specialist and lends itself well to a private, fee-for-service practice. Hundreds of such nurses are reported to be successfully carrying on private practices as mental health professionals (Rouslin & Clarke, 1978).

On the other hand, reported success for the clinical specialist in medical–surgical specialties in private practice is negligible. In the September 1979 issue of the *Journal of Nursing Administration*, Rothlyn P. Zahourek, R.N., M.S., describes a private practice group. The group began with a combination of clinical specialists and NPs. The practice weathered a variety of changes, including dissolving as a corporation and reforming as a partnership. A primary reason for the dissolution was financial: the psychiatric/mental health group evolved to be the main source of income, while the other specialties generated inadequate income. Eventually the practice lost all the nonpsychiatric CNSs and NPs (Zahourek, 1979). Ultimately the practice dissolved, primarily for financial reasons. The nurses had been working full-time in other positions and were hesitant to risk working only part-time in those positions to allow a greater chance for development of the private practice. Another factor leading to the termination of the practice was the lack of third-party payment for nursing services. The group was not able to generate adequate revenue on a private pay basis and from an occasional payment from a few private insurance companies or CHAMPUS (Department of Defense Health and Medical Program of the Uniformed Services) (Zahourek).

An independent private practice in oncology nursing was opened by Cheryle Van Scoy-Mosher, R.N., M.N., in the Los Angeles area in January 1976. Her description of the practice was published in *Cancer Nursing* two years later. She identified her focus as that of assisting oncology patients to physically cope with the symptoms of their disease, the treatment and its side effects, and manipulating the treatment program to minimize the disruptions experienced by the patient. "The goal of this aspect of professional nursing care is to fit the treatment program to the individual needs of the patient (not vice versa), thereby maximizing the therapeutic benefits, and to assist the patient to maintain or regain optimal physical function" (p. 22).

Van Scoy-Mosher believes that the independent nurse specialist is an appropriate partner in the care of all cancer patients. Analysis of her referrals, however, revealed that she primarily served patients and families with severe management problems (p. 28). Six months after her article was published, Van Scoy-Mosher terminated her private practice. She continues to assert the need for and validity of such practice but admits that round-the-clock responsibility for only severely ill and dysfunctional patients and their families was unmanageable on a long-term basis. Such a practice needs a population blend, rather than one of only the worst extremes (Van Scoy-Mosher, 1981). Another major barrier identified by Van Scoy-Mosher was financial. Her gross income in the first year was five thousand dollars, payment for a total of 182 visits. Although she experienced minimal difficulty in receiving payment for her services, she acknowledges the impact that third-party support would have on increasing the viability of such a practice. Physicians were often reluctant to refer patients who lacked insurance coverage, in an effort to limit expenses of an already financially depleted family. With access to billing, Van Scoy-Mosher believes that her interventions could have been initiated earlier in the course of the patients' disease; instead she primarily received referrals for patients with end-stage disease (1978, p. 28).

In addition to possessing high-level nursing skills, the CNS in private independent practice needs to be familiar with principles of business and management. The first step is to make a realistic survey of the needs of the particular community and offer appropriate services. The CNS also needs to be able to market these services and establish a referral base, in order to obtain access to clients. Fees for services need to be established; these must be realistic and encompass all expenses yet remain within the ability of clients to self-pay. In order to avoid failure, the nurse establishing such a practice needs to have business experience or obtain advice from someone with appropriate experience. Decisions on location, purchases, unplanned expenses, equipment, taxes, record keeping, and organizing are crucial for the success of a private practice venture (Edmunds, 1980).

The following are some general recommendations for the specialist considering opening a private independent practice:

1. Have at least one year's salary in savings. It is estimated to take between two and five years to become economically self-sustaining (Edmunds, p. 50).
2. Establish and utilize a support network with successful nurses in private practice and others in similar ventures. Use the network for validation, avoidance of typical pitfalls, problem solving, and support when expectations exceed the results.
3. Review the nursing literature; the number of relevant articles is rapidly increasing, primarily authored by psychiatric CNSs and NPs.
4. Maintain another position until the private practice develops sufficiently. It can be very demoralizing for a motivated nurse to be underutilized while waiting for a practice to become established.
5. Utilize the Small Business Administration (SBA). The SBA provides numerous written materials and routinely offers workshops to assist persons establishing a small business of any type. Direction provided by the SBA can strengthen the business decisions one must make to succeed in such a venture.

FUTURE PROSPECTS

Regardless of the present challenges and obstacles and the individual's motivations in choosing a setting, the future holds great promise for the nurse specialist. Health care is a primary issue at present in our society. Costs are high, the maldistribution problem remains, and the demands of the public are ever growing. Once there is a better avenue for reimbursement for nursing services, the potential will evolve for the services of the CNS to become indispensable. Two specific aspects of modern health care will also contribute to the overall need for nurse specialists. One is the growing emphasis on preventive health care and self-care. This need is not, and traditionally has not been met by the disease-oriented medical profession. The nursing profession, with its extended and expanded roles, holds the potential to effectively meet the need for these services and in a cost-efficient manner. The second force is the result of our continued scientific and medical advances. The survival rate for the elderly, the terminally ill, and the catastrophically injured is on the increase. The intense needs of these populations and the affected families has created great demand within the health care system. The specialized skills and services that the CNS can offer within both institutional and private settings are a creative and realistic solution to easing many of the strains in the existing health care system.

REFERENCES

Baker, V.E. Retrospective explorations in role development. In J.P. Riehl & J.W. McVay (Eds.), *The clinical nurse specialist: Interpretations.* New York: Appleton-Century-Crofts, 1973.

Barnes, Y. Clinical specialists: Psychiatric nurses practice on their own. *Los Angeles Times,* Nov. 20, 1980, pp. 1–11.

Edmunds, M. Financial concerns of nurse practitioners. *Nurse Pract,* 1980, *5,* 33–51.

Everson, S.J. Integration of the role of clinical nurse specialist. *J Cont Ed,* 1981, *12,* 16–19.

Feldbaum, E.G. Will nurses alleviate health service maldistribution problems. *Nurs Adm Q,* 1979, *4,* 61–66.

Kalisch, P.A., & Kalisch, B.J. *The advance of nursing.* Boston: Little, Brown, 1978.

Kinlein, L. *Independent nursing practice with clients.* Philadelphia: J.B. Lippincott, 1979.

Kohnke, M. (Ed.). *The case for consultation in nursing: Designs for professional practice.* New York: John Wiley & Sons, 1977.

Koltz, C. *Private practice in nursing.* London: Aspen Systems, 1979.

Mandell, H.N. The physician and the nurse specialist, or the tiger and the lady. *Postgrad Med,* 1978, *64,* 24–25.

Moses, E, & Roth, E. Nurse power: What do the statistics reveal about the nations' nurses. *Am J Nurs,* 1979, *79,* 1745–1756.

Rouslin, S., & Clarke, A.R. Commentary on professional parity. *Perspect Psychiatr Care,* 1978, *16,* 115–117.

Van Scoy-Mosher, C. Personal Communication, September 1981.

Van Scoy-Mosher, C. The oncology nurse in independent professional practice. *Cancer Nurs,* 1978, *1,* 21–28.

Woodrow, M. and Bell, J. Clinical specialization: conflict between reality and theory, J Nurs Adm, 1971, *1,* 23–27.

Zahourek, R.P. Personal Communication, August 1981.

Zahourek, R.P. Two management systems in a nursing private practice group. J Nurs Adm, 1979, *9,* 48–51.

5. The CNS as Researcher

Eileen Callahan Hodgman

At Boston's Beth Israel Hospital, clinical specialists operate out of the nursing education department. Although their primary responsibility is direct consultation with primary nurses about clinical problems, they are also responsible for running large-scale, formal continuing education programs on topics related to their specialties. In addition, their recently revised job description requires that they engage in nursing research. Some also try to carry a small patient case load. I remember thinking, "How can one person do all those things?" The term *clinical specialist* itself implies *clinical* expertise. How and when were the other subroles, especially research, added? Is there an educational program that can prepare for clinical excellence and competency in these other areas as well?

One thing was particularly striking as I worked with clinical specialists. When the research expectation was added to their job descriptions, I began to receive many more requests for research consultations. It became clear during our discussions that the clinical specialists believed that they were expected to "do" research; that is, to produce research. It was also clear that among this group there was a wide variation in very basic research "savvy," that is, a basic grasp of how to approach a nursing

This chapter was prepared when the author was Director of Nursing Research at Beth Israel Hospital. The original version of this chapter was presented as an address at the conference. "The Clinical Nurse Specialist Role: Current Trends and Future Directions," sponsored by the Department of Nursing, Mary Hitchcock Memorial Hospital, Hanover, New Hampshire at the Lake Morey Inn and Country Club, Fairlee, Vermont, November 1979. The author wishes to point out that although her views have not changed since that time, the interested reader would be advised to consult the growing body of literature on the subject of research in practice settings (see references following this chapter).

problem using a research framework; variations in clarity about what constituted a nursing problem amenable to systematic study; and variations in their familiarity with, or perhaps memory of, the basic steps in the research process. There also seemed to be a great deal of variation in the interest that each brought to the discussions; some seemed excited about a specific clinical problem they were hoping to solve, while others appeared to be searching for any topic related to their specialty that would be "researchable," in order to meet the research expectation in the CNS job description.

These observations raise several questions. Do clinical specialists really see research an integral as part of their role? Do programs preparing specialists see research as an integral part of the role? Do employers? Does the profession? How did this whole notion begin? If we persist in claiming that research is an integral part of the role, what was the original concept behind the claim—how and for what purpose was the clinical specialist supposed to fulfill a research function?

When I went back to early literature to answer this last question, I was truly amazed. In the fifties and early sixties, when the role first began to be formally defined, the clinical specialist seemed to be the repository of all of the profession's hitherto unfulfilled hopes and dreams. The CNS would be the truly professional practitioner; this specialist would be the one who would bring about the advances in nursing practice; the CNS would be the one who would improve and control the standards of practice (Riehl & McVay, 1973). Not only would the clinical specialist be the new hope for nursing practice, however; she or he would also be the new hope for nursing research. In particular, the CNS would be responsible for generating what the profession had failed to generate up to that point: clinical nursing research. As illustrations of the magnitude of the research hopes that were riding on the implementation of the clinical specialist role, a few excerpts from some of those early writings follow:

From the National League for Nursing, in 1958:

> The purpose of the clinical specialist in psychiatric nursing remains clear: to bring advances in the art and science of psychiatric nursing and to promote the application of new knowledge and methods in the care of patients. *Investigative* and consultant functions are implied in this purpose (cited in Riehl & McVay, 1973, p. 8, emphasis added).*

From Frances Reiter, in 1961:

> As a result of her clinical care and treatment, she would be able, to a greater degree than all other nurse practitioners, to study a situation until she has identified the essence of the nursing problem and would then search for the solution according to the nature of the problem (cited in Riehl & McVay, 1973, p. 16).*

From Hildegarde Peplau, in 1965:

Clinical specialization is also a basis for clinical nursing research—of which there is very little. . . . As the numbers of clinical specialists increase, the clinical nursing research will also increase (cited in Riehl & McVay, 1973, p. 26).*

From Luther Christman, 1965:

It seems reasonable to expect that much of the nursing literature in the next decade will be written by specialists as they attempt to apply the scientific method to clinical practice (cited in Riehl & McVay, 1973, p. 42)*

As late as 1971, which does not seem very long ago, the editor of *Nursing Research* wrote, "We believe one promising development in nursing that may help to counteract the lag in clinical research is the emerging field of clinical specialism (Notter, 1971, p. 99).

But these statements represent primarily the hopes of that era about the clinical specialist's role in research, and it is the nature of hopes to be expressed in rather broad, nonspecific terms. For the moment, let us contrast these somewhat vague injunctions with what today's clinical specialist actually brings to the position. Specifically, the CNS brings certain values, preparation, and personal proclivities that, to some extent, will have an influence on whether or not she or he makes any attempt to operation-alize a research component within the specialist's role.

First, each clinical specialist holds certain *values and beliefs* about nursing research, including its ultimate goal and purpose. These values are often assimilated through research courses offered within graduate or even undergraduate programs in nursing, and less directly, but probably with as much impact, from faculty members and nursing research journals. Some of these values and beliefs have to do with the relevance of nursing research to nursing practice. Variation in these values is understandable, since the history of research within the profession is such that even though we have evidence of a clinical focus in nursing research as early as the 1920s, most of the studies conducted between the 1930s and the 1960s were not clinical or practice-oriented.

In 1975, Gortner pointed out the distinction made by some writers between nursing research and research in nursing (1975, p. 193). She noted that the distinction lay in the subject or focus of the research, stating that nursing research "has as its subject the care process and the problems that are encountered in the practice of nursing: maintenance of hygiene, rest,

---

*Reprinted with permission from Riehl, J. P., & McVay, J. W. (Eds.). *The clinical nurse specialist: Interpretations*. New York: Appleton-Century-Crofts, 1973.

sleep, nutrition, relief from pain or discomfort, counseling, health education, and rehabilitation" (p. 193). Research in nursing, on the other hand, "has as its subject the profession itself—its practitioners and the characteristics of their practices: utilization, costs, administration, career patterns, educational levels of nurses and nurse students" (p. 193). One would expect the clinical specialist to hold values consistent with the first definition. If the specialist does not, she or he is not likely to see the connection between research activity and clinical activity. As Gortner points out, "Values are what influence human behavior, and the relative worth attached to nursing research or to research in nursing education or nursing practice or nursing administration is going to have an effect upon the amount of research activity ongoing, upon the extent to which it is supported, and upon how quickly application can be made to the practice field" (p. 193).

Clinical specialists may also leave their master's programs with values about the *techniques and methods* of research. For example, they may believe that "good" research is synonymous with large-sample, tightly controlled studies that make use of experimental or, at the least, quasi-experimental design, productive of numerical data that can be statistically manipulated. When they compare these values with what they realistically know to be possible for them to do within the structure of their positions, they may despair of trying to engage in research activity. Unfortunately, small-sample research, particularly that at the descriptive level, such as the case study, has gone out of style over the years. In the thirties, the case study began to be recognized as a worthwhile approach to the systematic study of the problems of nursing care—that is, to nursing research—as well as a valuable teaching tool (Gortner & Nahm, 1977, p. 18). But one hears very little about case study methodology today. Our failure to continue to value this approach as a legitimate research method, along with its decline in popularity as an educational technique, has in my opinion deprived us of a great deal of valuable nursing data. In addition, the fact that the case study has been devalued over time in both research and education may have something to do with the deficits in analytical and documentation skills that we tend to see in otherwise good practitioners at all levels today.

If the clinical specialist does not view such activities as the single case study, a series of case studies, or any form of systematic collection and analysis of descriptive patient data as valid research—activities that directly stem from the clinical aspects of the specialist's role—she or he may end up not doing any research whatsoever.

Clinical specialists also bring to the position the *preparation* they have had for engaging in research activities. There is a wide variation in the scope, quality, focus, and intent of the research courses required or available within the many programs preparing clinical specialists. The budding clinical specialist's exposure to nursing research may be as little as 40–60 hours of class time (the equivalent of a 14-week, 1-semester course), or it may be much more. In some cases, these have been eliminated or made optional. Offerings may be quite specific in terms of their emphasis on nursing research, or they may be conceived more broadly as an introduction to scientific method, or may focus on the methods of the non-nursing academic discipline in which the instructor was trained. Other variations have to do with the scope and intent of offerings, ranging from simply familiarizing the clinical specialist with research concepts to the expectation that the CNS will conduct a study before the course is over. These variations lead to variations in the specialist's self-confidence about engaging in research activities, not to mention in actual ability to fulfill the employer's expectations.

Other variants that will influence the degree to which the clinical specialist tries to integrate research activities into the role are the CNS's own interests, motivation, and natural abilities. When we consider the many facets of the role, it is unrealistic to expect a CNS to have the same degree of interest in all of them. I think we can safely say that of the various components of the clinical specialist role—practice, consultation, teaching, and research—the research component has been the least interesting to CNS's, not only because of the factors mentioned previously, but also because of the very practical difficulties in trying to implement it. Consequently, the research component has also been the least developed over the years. Where does that leave us in terms of the early hopes the profession had for the clinical specialist's impact on the production of clinical nursing research?

We *have* seen a change in the relative proportion of published clinical research reports in the last decade. In the annual editor's report in *Nursing Research* in 1975, for example, Elizabeth Carnegie reported a dramatic rise in the number of clinical articles appearing in the 1974 issues: nearly half were clinical (p. 3). That proportion was sustained through 1977, the journal's anniversary year, when the percentage dropped because of the large number of special articles solicited to mark the celebration.

Of even more interest is the shift in the authors' reported place of employment over those years. Whereas in 1974 and 1975 most authors still held university faculty positions (Carnegie, 1975, p. 3; 1976, p. 3), by 1976 the next largest group of authors were employed by hospitals (Carnegie, 1977, p. 3). Even in 1977, when the overall percentage of clinical articles dropped, almost 20 percent of the nurse authors of the regular articles were employed by hospitals (Carnegie, 1978, p. 3). Although the author data is not reported by positions, it is probably safe to assume that at least some of these authors were clinical specialists. If one accepts that form of logical deduction, one might well suspect an association between an increase in the numbers of clinical specialists and an increase in the production of clinical nursing research as Peplau predicted in 1965. Of course, some CNS-conducted research may be unpublished or published in journals other than *Nursing Research*. The research activities of a large number of clinical specialists are, however, unaccounted for. I believe we can propose a model that will increase the level of that activity—one that encompasses both differing levels of CNS research involvement as well as a variety of ways in which the CNS can contribute to nursing research.

I think we can speak to both a basic research expectation and advanced research expectations within the clinical specialist role. We need to make this distinction for honesty's sake alone. We have to move the research component of the role out of the realm of fantasy—a mutual fantasy that is shared by graduate programs preparing clinical specialists, by employers of clinical specialists, and by clinical specialists themselves. This fantasy consists of the notion that regardless of how much or how little the CNS has been taught about nursing research in graduate school, regardless of the amount of time consumed by other performance expectations, and regardless of the specialist's own interests and natural abilities, every clinical specialist should be conducting the equivalent of a doctoral dissertation on the job. I am not overstating a point to make my case. In my experience, these fantasies are expressed indirectly over and over again, in various ways and contexts, by all three groups. But beyond the demands of basic honesty, we have to give up these fantasies so that nursing research activities can begin to have some meaningful, practical impact on patient care.

What can we reasonably expect in terms of research activity from clinical specialists? At the very least, at the most basic level, they should be able to interpret, evaluate, and communicate to nursing staff nursing research findings pertinent to their fields of specialization. This implies that specialists keep up with the research literature in their fields, are able to judge the validity and reliability of the findings, are able to identify any conceptual difficulties in the research, and can draw the implications that the findings have for direct patient care. Specialists have the right to expect training in these activities from their educational programs. They need to plan in order to perform these activities systematically and on a regular basis, as part of both the educative and consultative components of the CNS role. Their immediate managers have not only the right to expect this of CNSs but also the responsibility to assist them in planning practical ways to fulfill the expectation and to set up mutually agreed upon methods of evaluating this aspect of their performance. This research expectation is basic, and the motivation for it, the improvement of nursing care, is quite distinct from any motivation or interest clinical specialists may have in conducting their own studies. When fulfilling this expectation, the CNS serves as a communicator of nursing research.

The next highest level of research involvement after evaluation and communication in terms of both time and energy expended, is activity associated with the testing and application of nursing research produced by others. This activity takes research findings one step beyond communication and into the realm of evaluation. In this process, valid research findings related to a specific aspect of care are translated into protocols for providing that care. Because the research findings represent new knowledge, the protocols generally represent innovations in care. The most simple evaluation design is used: the taking of baseline measurements under the prevailing system of care; implementation of the new protocols; and postimplementation measurements. Both sets of measurements should be based on the expected outcomes of the nursing practice being examined, not on outcomes that are so far removed from the practice conceptually that it becomes impossible if not meaningless to try to sort out the direct impact of the change. When protocols are confirmed as resulting in improved nursing care, they can be used within a quality assurance program to develop or refine standards of care, their consistent application can be monitored, and the stability of patient outcomes can be evaluated over time. This type of research activity constitutes an advanced performance expectation for the clinical specialist. The basic expectation— evaluation and communication of research findings—and the more advanced expectation—application and testing of research findings in practice—are different levels of *research utilization.*

In requiring that the clinical specialist perform these functions, we are indebted to two projects for their contributions to the state of the art: the CURN (Conduct and Utilization of Research in Nursing) project at the University of Michigan (Horsley, 1978; Haller, *et al.*, 1979; U. Mich., 1979), and the WICHEN (Western Interstate Council on Higher Education for Nursing) project on the application and utilization of nursing research (Krueger, 1978; Krueger *et al.*, 1978; Krueger, 1979; Lindeman & Krueger, 1977). The CURN project is providing us with standard protocols for innovations in nursing practice as well as guidelines for use in determining those research findings appropriate for development into protocols. The WICHEN project has made its own unique contribution in its emphasis on and development of practical tools for planning and managing the change process itself. Without these developments in the state of the art, it is doubtful whether the research utilization role of the clinical specialist could have moved from the realm of hope to that of realistic expectations. In order to fulfill these expectations, specialists should expect their educational programs to provide them with appropriate skills. Their employers should be prepared to provide them with support in terms of time and other resources and hold basic expectations that staff nurses will actively participate in this type of research for the improvement of patient care and opportunities for continuing education, if necessary. Clinical specialists should recognize their responsibility to actively collaborate with and use the insights of the nurse managers on whose units the research takes place and to assume the major coordination role for research utilization projects. Their performance of this research activity can be evaluated by their own managers in terms of these coordinating responsibilities. When carrying out nursing research utilization projects, the specialist acts as research *collaborator* (with staff, managers, and others who participate in the study); as research *coordinator*, in assuming the leadership and administrative responsibilities of the study; and, because research utilization is itself evaluation research, as research *generator*.

These two research expectations relate directly to the jointly held goal of the individual CNS and the nursing services: the provision of high-quality nursing care. Such expectations are therefore entirely appropriate. In my opinion neither the clinical specialist nor the employing agency nor the curriculum builders of master's programs preparing clinical specialists can claim to believe in the value of nursing research for nursing practice unless they provide evidence of a practical commitment to educating for, implementing, and evaluating on the basis of these two performance expectations.

Beyond these activities, there are other ways that clinical specialists can participate in research, depending on their own motivation, interests, and in certain instances their natural abilities and the breadth and depth of their research knowledge. These include acting as research replicator; research preceptor; research generator of original studies at all levels of inquiry; and research collaborator with other nurses and physicians. The decision to go beyond the performance expectations proposed above should be based on the potential a project has for improving nursing care within the CNS's specialty, and the degree to which the specialist can tolerate and the employing organization can justify the time and energies diverted from the other components of the role.

The nursing research performance expectations for the CNS proposed in this chapter were, in fact, listed among the core functions of the CNS in 1970 by Georgopoulos and Christman (p. 1034). Perhaps we have failed to prepare and hold the CNS accountable for performing these functions in the intervening years because the supply of valid clinical research findings has been slow in coming, or because we were not aware that a methodology for the utilization of knowledge could be seen as distinct from methodology for the discovery of new knowledge. The CURN and WICHEN projects have shown that the two processes are distinct, and the number of meaningful clinical studies is increasing. We need to act on these developments.

The performance expectations described in this chapter put the research function of the clinical specialist into a meaningful framework, consistent with the basic nature of the role and the primary mission of nursing services. Equally important, one can extrapolate from them some reasonable limits to the research activity of clinical specialists that should clarify the situation for many employers and possibly relieve the minds of many specialists. My experience with both graduate students and master's-prepared clinical specialists has shown, however, that acquiring the skills and the habits of mind involved in successfully carrying out these activities are no small matter. They need to be actively taught in graduate programs preparing clinical specialists, both in courses specifically devoted to the research utilization process and in clinical courses.

I agree with Ackerman (1976) that the emphasis in both the research training and the research practice of clinical specialists needs to be on the evaluation, communication, and utilization of new knowledge to improve practice rather than the discovery of new knowledge, but not because I believe the former activities are more basic than the latter, as Ackerman claims (p. 757). Nor do I think that evaluating, communicating, and utilizing new knowledge are less intellectually demanding than discovering new knowledge. In my opinion, however, we have done a disservice to the CNS by implying that the research component of the role is synonymous with the discovery of knowledge. Such a position ignores the absolutely critical part the CNS plays in completing the knowledge cycle within a practice discipline through her or his efforts in evaluating, communicating and utilizing nursing research findings. This is the area that, in my opinion, will allow the greatest number of clinical specialists to have the greatest impact on clinical practice through research activities.

REFERENCES

Ackerman, W.B. The place of research in the master's program. *Nurs Outlook*, 1976, *24*, 754–758.

Carnegie, E.M. Editor's report—1975. *Nurs Res*, 1975, *24*, 3.

Carnegie, E.M. Editor's report—1976. *Nurs Res*, 1976, *25*, 3.

Carnegie, E.M. Editor's report—1977. *Nurs Res*, 1977, *26*, 3.

Carnegie, E.M. Editor's report—1978. *Nurs Res*, 1978, *27*, 3.

Georgopoulos, B., & Christman, L. The clinical nurse specialist: A role model. *Am J Nurs* 1970, *70*, 1030–1039.

Gortner, S.R. Research for a practice profession. *Nurs Res*, 1975, *24*, 193–197.

Gortner, S.R., & Nahm, H. An overview of nursing research in the United States. *Nurs Res*, 1977, *26*, 10–33.

Haller, K.B. *et al.* Developing research-based innovation protocols: Process, criteria, and issues. *Res in Nurs and Health*, 1979, *2*, 45–51.

Horsley, J. *et al* Research utilization as an organizational process. *J Nurs Adm*, 1978, *8*, 4–6.

Krueger, J. Utilization of nursing research: The planning process. *J Nurs Adm* 1978, *8*, 6–9.

Krueger, J. Research utilization. *Western Journal of Nurs Res*, 1979, *1*, 148–152.

Krueger, J. Nelson, A.H. and Wolanin, M.O. *Nursing research*. Germantown, Maryland: Aspen Systems Corp., 1978.

Lindeman, C.A. & Krueger, J. Increasing the quality, quantity, and use of nursing research. *Nurs Outlook*, 1977, *25*, 450–454.

Notter, L.E. Empirical research in nursing. *Nurs Res*, 1971, *20*, 99.

Riehl, J.P., & McVay, J.W. (Eds.). *The clinical nurse specialist: Interpretations*. New York: Appleton Century Crofts, 1973.

University of Michigan. Research into practice. *Research News*, July 1979, 12–14.

6. Implementing the Research Role

Shirley Girouard

Clinical nurse specialist (CNS) definitions, job descriptions, and graduate programs clearly indicate that research is an expectation of the role. We CNSs believe that we are expected to do research. How could we possibly believe otherwise? Learning about research was an integral part of our graduate education. (Did not most of us conduct research in graduate school?) Research efforts are rewarded by the nursing profession. (Has anyone ever received a grant to *practice* for two months?) The literature discussing the clinical specialist's role is filled with references to the research component of the role. (How can *I* question such a position?) Most job descriptions refer to research expectations. (If your job description states that the CNS "investigates problems relating to clinical practice," how can you *not* think about research?) Also, in an era of increased attention to the economics of health care, CNSs must find methods of evaluating their effect on patient care. If we do not justify our role, we cannot support our continued existence.

As Hodgman has stated in Chapter 5, one option available to the CNS wishing to implement the research component of the role is to utilize rather than discover new knowledge. Others of us may wish to discover new knowledge and conduct research. When we attempt to do this, there are many factors that may stand in our way. The obstacles that the CNS commonly encounters in attempting to conduct research and some methods for overcoming them are the subjects of this chapter.

All nurses conducting research are faced with obstacles. According to Deets, nurse researchers face problems relating to methodology, definition, and theory (1980). Methodological problems include the difficulty of controlling variables and of establishing validity and reliability, and the lack of testing instruments. Definitional problems are those relating to the meaning of concepts and the subsequent operational expression of them. For example, what is quality nursing practice? Different authors and practicing nurses may define this concept from varying perspectives. Likewise, the lack of nursing theory contributes to difficulty in identifying meaningful subjects for research. Jacox gives a similar list of problems encountered by nurse researchers (1974). She notes the difficulty of obtaining appropriate samples, the complexity of clinical phenomena and their measurement, and the need to control extraneous variables. Textbooks and journal articles reflect the obstacles that all researchers face when conducting clinical research. Certainly the CNS must consider all of these problems as she or he attempts to conduct research.

Aside from these difficulties inherent in the research process, individual CNSs may feel poorly prepared for the research component of their role (Jacox, p. 383). In addition, the "ceaseless daily demands of the hospital" may prevent the CNS from conducting research (Jacox, p. 382). The demands and conflicts of the role provide additional obstacles. The need to assure quality patient care, provide staff education, and participate in policy, procedure and standard setting may have a higher priority for the CNS (and the employer) than research activities. Aradine and Denyes clearly identify the dimensions of this problem (1972).

To illustrate some of these issues, I would like to share with the reader an experience I had in attempting to conduct research in my first CNS position. After I had been employed as a CNS for two months, I was eager to fulfill the research aspect of my role by doing research. I felt that there was a need to improve the quality of preoperative teaching of patients being done on the two units for which I had clinical responsibility. Thus I decided to replicate the research I had done for my master's thesis. This study had involved the CNS's acting as change agent by using "Linker Theory" to bring about an improvement in preoperative teaching (see Chapter 2, and Girouard, 1978). An experimental pretest–post-test design was employed. The nurses in the experimental group and in the control group were studied before and after a planned intervention in order to evaluate their opinions and performance. The intervention included staff education, role modeling as patient teacher, and supervising other nurses doing preoperative teaching.

Prior to initiating data collection, I solicited the support of the director of nursing and the other clinical specialists in the hospital. Although I was not fully aware of my reasons at the time, I believe I did this to ease my nonarticulated fear that I should not spend my time doing research. My colleagues' and supervisors' interest and enthusiasm made me feel more comfortable and increased my motivation. The staff of the units, on the other hand, were aware of my interest in conducting a study but did not express much enthusiasm.

In light of the conservative nature of the medical staff, the director of nursing suggested that I request the support of key members of the department of surgery. The physicians initially presented resistance, and I found myself "presenting my case" to the entire department of surgery. As the only woman and only nurse in the room, and very new to the hospital, this was an anxiety-provoking experience. I felt threatened and very alone. Eventually they reluctantly gave their "permission" for me to proceed. Another event that occurred prior to the conduct of the study was the submission of the proposal to the Human Subjects Review Board. Since I was the first nurse to submit a proposal to them, they required much explanation before approving the study (they were most familiar with clinical drug trials). This obstacle was easily overcome by educating the board, but it slowed my progress considerably.

The obstacles mentioned above were significant enough to make me consider abandoning the research project. My initial enthusiasm was rapidly fading. But this option was not possible because of the publicity that the department (and I) had received while attempting to pave the way for the research effort. Had I abandoned the project, later nursing research proposals might have been given less than full attention. My credibility in the department and the hospital would also have suffered.

Although I was aware that I was always very busy, I did not realize how busy I was until I tried to find time to conduct my research. The typical day described below illustrates the situation:

It is 6:30 P.M.; I've been busily involved with other aspects of my role all day. The evening seems like a good time to collect data for my study, so despite my fatigue I approach the unit to begin data collection with patients. While I am in the unit, three nurses need my help immediately: (1) the nasogastric tube will not work on my primary patient, and she is vomiting; (2) one of the patients needs teaching about his newly diagnosed hypertension before he leaves for home tonight, and the nurse doesn't know what to teach; (3) the head nurse is in tears and wants to quit. One of the chief residents also demands that I tell him why nurses can't pull out central venous pressure lines. Awaiting me in my office is a 10-inch pile of mail, and I have a class to prepare for tomorrow on Total Parenteral Nutrition.

My approach to this situation, which I do not recommend, was to overextend myself. I was not aware of it at the time, but in retrospect I recognize that my willingness to become overextended resulted in fatigue and a lack of enthusiasm for my research project.

As I now analyze my first research attempt, I can easily recognize where I erred. First, the CNS role and I were both new to the units and the department of surgery. Had I taken the time to assess the climate and establish my credibility as a clinician, I probably would have received more support, both directly and indirectly. Second, I did not involve the unit staff in the project. Had I done so, their interest and assistance could have aided my efforts. Third, I did not realize how much would be required to undertake such an elaborate research project. The usual problems of clinical research have at least been discussed, if not encountered, in our graduate school experiences. Such things as trying to measure abstract concepts in an often uncontrolled environment are not totally foreign to us. We recognize the problems in developing data collection tools, establishing the reliability and validity of our tools, and obtaining an acceptable sample. Although we may be prepared to deal with these clinical research issues, we may find that when the real world is superimposed, the research task seems impossible. How do we organize our time (and ourselves) to design and carry out a research project? Who will support us? What should we know about the system before beginning a research effort?

Many of us may find that the multiplicity of demands on our time creates the greatest obstacle to our research effort. One approach would be for the CNS to do a time study of her or his own activities prior to undertaking a research project. Although many of the demands cannot be reduced, one can begin to set priorities and schedule activities so that one can remain goal-, rather than task-directed. Time can also be saved if the CNS uses a research design and methodology that she or he, or another researcher, has used previously. Replication research may therefore be a good way to begin.

Another way to overcome the obstacle of time constraints is to combine efforts. For example, the nursing staff might express a desire to develop an educational program for patients who are about to undergo gastroscopy. The CNS could fulfill her or his research obligation by studying the response of patients who are prepared for gastroscopy through the program. Standards could also be developed, thus fulfilling another aspect of the CNS role—that of setting expectations for practice. The fringe benefits of staff involvement are twofold: (1) the CNS can help the staff to learn to do research and appreciate its usefulness and (2) the specialist can save time by using the staff as research assistants. Many of the projects the clinical specialist is involved in can be evaluated through research. Research activities could also be done in collaboration with other CNSs in the setting or elsewhere. For example, a group of clinical specialists could develop a methodology for testing the effectiveness of a certain procedure or standard of practice.

Support for research activities includes money, psychological support, and freedom from day-to-day operations when required. Financial support for typing, duplicating, and other minor costs are usually obtainable through regular nursing department services. Grant money is also available from a variety of local sources. For example, the local Heart Association may have small amounts available for research. Psychological support and freedom from day-to-day operations are closely related. If the CNS is able to convince those with whom she works most closely (head nurse, staff nurses, physicians, and so forth) of the value of her or his research to their practice, the battle is half over. Clear expectations of the proposed research and regular progress reports will often enhance the interest of others in the project. Involving unit staff (and others) in the project and its publication effort is another useful tactic. CNS colleagues and nursing administrators can also provide the researcher with support and motivation. Other sources of direct and indirect support are more experienced nurse researchers and university faculty with whom the CNS has studied in graduate school.

Familiarity with the system in which one wishes to conduct research is required if these supports are to be secured. A research project of interest to others in the setting will generate psychological and other more tangible supports. Acceptance of the CNS and her or his role will establish the specialist's credibility. Generally, this acceptance will take a minimum of six months—perhaps longer if the position is a new one in the agency.

Another way the CNS can develop a supportive environment is to encourage a climate of scientific inquiry. Utilizing the results of published research to improve patient care is one way to do this. In our institution, the establishment of a Nursing Research Committee and the addition of a nurse representative to the Human Subjects Review Board contributed to the development of a climate more conducive to nursing research. Nursing research can be discussed at seminars, and the results of studies can be utilized in in-service and continuing education classes.

My involvement in a more positive research effort may serve to illustrate how the CNS can conduct research successfully. It is important to note that at the time this research effort was initiated, I had been employed in the position for three years. By this time I had established my credibility, the climate was supportive, and nursing research was not an alien concept to the leadership and staff I worked with.

The head nurse and assistant head nurse on one of the units that I worked with told me of their concern that the staff they supervised were not performing well. Specifically, they thought that many of the nurses did not use the nursing process effectively, resulting in poor nursing care. They also felt that members of the unit got little satisfaction from their jobs. The unit leaders sought my help in solving this problem. My interest in change theory and the development of a system of supervision by one of my colleagues prompted me to propose the development and testing of a system for supervision on the unit.

The unit leaders were enthusiastic about the proposal. They viewed the research as a way to test a theory of supervision that might meet the needs they had identified. Thus my research was of potential value to their practice. Frequent reports that I made to them on the progress of my research enhanced their interest and support. I also used my experience as a way to teach them about the research process.

Obviously, the second research effort overcame many of the obstacles encountered in my first effort. Of significance was the fact that this research did not overlap with the sphere of medical practice. The CNS may perhaps wish to begin with research activities that do not have implications for medical practice. This would serve to reduce the obstacles encountered when another discipline would be affected by the research process and study results.

Because the research was focused on an accepted component of the CNS role (supervision), the problem of lack of time and multiple activities was reduced. In supervising staff (the study intervention), I was performing a function that was clearly part of my practice. The difference was that I was now studying this activity in a systematic manner. Support for my research effort was spontaneous because the study was so clearly an integral part of my role.

In summary, the following suggestions may be helpful to the CNS who wishes to conduct research:

1. Establish credibility as a practitioner before initiating a research project. If the CNS has demonstrated her or his knowledge and skill in nursing practice, when a research effort is begun the nursing staff will have confidence in the CNS's ability to identify with the needs of patients and staff.
2. Identify sources of support. Know the agency in which one will be conducting research and the experience of other nurses who have been involved in research. For example, if there is a research committee, they may be able to critique proposals and find sources of funding. Potential allies can also be nurtured and may later provide motivation at difficult points in the research process.
3. Assess the "research climate" and, if necessary, try to establish a favorable one. If research has not been utilized in nursing practice and education, the CNS may wish to promote such activities. Other staff members interested in research may assist in proposing and developing a research committee.
4. Attempt to identify potential obstacles and plan strategies to overcome them. Sharing one's proposal with others and asking for their input can be very helpful in overcoming potential problems. For example, the head nurse who is most resistant to one's research idea may be able to alert the researcher to significant problems in the project design as it relates to that particular unit.

5. Involve the staff in the research effort. The interest and enthusiasm of the staff cannot be underestimated as a motivation for completing a research project. Also, if the staff anticipates results helpful to their practice they will expect a finished project.
6. Focus research on clinical problems shared by others. As mentioned above, the interest of nurses in the setting can help to maintain one's motivation. Also, the study of clinical problems shared by others demonstrates the value of research to practice.
7. Consider beginning with a simple research question. Such questions and the results of the research are often more immediately applicable to practice. Thus the CNS, the staff, and others will achieve more immediate gratification from the research activity.

The CNS can and should do research. If nursing practice is to move from practice based on tradition and ritual to practice based on knowledge, research is a critical activity. Because the CNS is in a position to encounter numerous nursing problems that lend themselves to systematic study, she or he is obligated to study such problems; the result should be significant contributions to the development of professional nursing practice.

REFERENCES

Aradine, C., & Denyes, M. Activities and pressures of clinical nurse specialists. *Nurs Res*, 1972, *21*, 411–417.
Deets, C.A. Methodological concerns in the testing of nursing interventions. *Adv Nurs Sci*, 1980, *2*, 1–11.
Girouard, S. The role of the clinical specialist as change agent: An experiment in preoperative teaching. *Int J Nurs Stud*, 1978, *15*, 57–65.
Jacox, A. Nursing research and the clinician. *Nurs Outlook*, 1974, *22*, 382–385.

7. The CNS as Consultant

Anne-Marie Barron

The role of the clinical nurse specialist (CNS) encompasses many subroles. Synthesizing and implementing these subroles presents a challenge indeed. The emphasis that the clinical specialist chooses at any particular time is generally determined by the organizational structure of the nursing department, the individual's position within that structure, the expectations of nursing administrators, the needs of the staff and patients with whom the specialist is working, as well as the expectations, needs, and goals of the CNS her- or himself. Since, as a psychiatric liaison CNS, this author's emphasis in practice has been on consultation, this chapter will explore the subrole of the CNS as consultant. The examples used are all taken from the author's experience.

CAPLAN'S THEORY OF CONSULTATION

Caplan (1970) defined the process of consultation and described the types of consultation. While Caplan's work related specifically to mental health consultation, the principles of the process he outlined are applicable to most professional consultations.

Definition of Consultation

According to Caplan consultation is a process of communication between professionals that can be systematically taught, applied, and

91

analyzed. The process and techniques will be similar from consultant to consultant and situation to situation, but the content of the consultation will vary widely depending on the specialized knowledge of the consultant and the individual needs of the consultee.

According to Caplan, consultation is an interactional process that occurs between professionals—the consultant, who is a specialist, and the consultee who seeks the assistance of a specialist in relation to a work problem that she or he has identified as problematic. The consultee identifies the problem, recognizes it as being within the realm of expertise of the consultant, and initiates the consultation process. In mental health consultation, the problem is likely to relate to the treatment or management of clients. The professional responsibility for the client remains with the consultee; the consultant accepts no responsibility for implementing intervention directly with the client. Rather, the consultant offers clarifications, diagnostic formulations, advice, and education in relation to management issues. The consultant has no administrative authority over the consultee, and the consultee is free to accept or reject the recommendations of the consultant. In fact, in general a coordinate rather than a hierarchical relationship between the consultant and consultee is fostered, because the consultant often is a member of a different profession and comes from outside the consultee's institution.

The dual goals of consultation are to improve the consultee's skill in handling a current work difficulty and to enhance her or his ability to master future problems of a similar type. Although the consultant focuses on the consultee's work performance rather than the well-being of the consultee, enhancing the consultee's mastery of a problem may well have the effect of improving her or his self-esteem. The feelings of the consultee are considered in consultation only to the degree that they affect the consultation problem. That is, the consultant respects the privacy of the feelings and personal problems of the consultee and does not focus on them overtly except as they are displaced onto or are influencing the problem under consideration.

The consultant does not enter into the consultation with a prescribed set of information to impart. Rather, she or he responds to the specific issues and concerns brought up by the consultee and does not seek to remedy other problems of the consultee's practice. Caplan made the point that consultation is generally one of the professional functions of a specialist and that it is sometimes necessary in a consultation situation to step out of the role of the consultant and back into the role of specialist. If the consultant recognizes that the consultee's actions may be endangering the client or patient being considered in the consultation, then the consultant steps aside from that role and reassumes the responsibilities of a specialist. This point is particularly important for nursing consultation. The CNS who recognizes a dangerous situation during the course of a consultation has the responsibility for intervening directly to assure the safety of the patient. That type of intervention obviously destroys the coordinate relationship and interferes with the consultation process. While the consultant rarely encounters that type of situation, she or he must be prepared for the possibility of abandoning the consultation process when patient safety is being jeopardized.

Types of Consultation

Caplan described four types of consultation. In practice consultations are often not purely of one type but rather a synthesis of types. A staff nurse who requests consultation for enhancing the care of a severely burned adolescent patient may well need assistance both with planning the patient's treatment and with the nurse's own lack of confidence in her or his ability to implement the plan effectively. The purpose of dividing consultation into discrete categories is to demonstrate the differing foci and goals for the various types of consultation. As the consultant synthesizes these types, she or he can then be aware of the specific emphases and objectives that are being combined for the specific consultation.

Client-Centered Case Consultation

In this type of consultation, the consultee seeks the specialized knowledge and skill of the consultant for assistance with the management of difficult clients or patients, or groups of clients. This is a very common type of consultation in CNS practice. For example, a staff nurse recognizes that a patient recovering from surgery for metastatic lung cancer has complex nursing needs beyond the postoperative implications for care. The staff nurse consults with the oncology nurse specialist for assistance with planning nursing care that will address the needs of the patient in relation to the ongoing implications of the disease. A primary goal for the consultant in this type of consultation is to assist the consultee to develop an effective plan so that the patient can best be helped. A secondary goal is that the consultee will be able to apply the knowledge and skill gained from this consultation interaction to future patients whose cases are similarly complex, thereby enhancing the consultee's overall practice.

Consultee-Centered Case Consultation

The work problem of the consultee in this type of consultation is also related to client or patient management, and she or he seeks consultation to improve her or his handling of the case. The consultant focuses on the nature of the consultee's problem and seeks to correct it. The consultee's problem may be caused by lack of knowledge, lack of skill, lack of confidence, or lack of professional objectivity. The primary goal of this type of consultation is to help the consultee to overcome the deficits. The main emphasis is on educating the consultee to deal more effectively with the problem at hand, rather than on emphasizing the diagnosis and treatment plan for a specific patient. This type of consultation is also commonly offered by clinical specialists. For example, if the nurse seems to be lacking professional objectivity in the situation, the CNS can assist the nurse to recognize the lack of objectivity as a problem, gently explore the underlying reasons, and together with the nurse formulate a more objective plan of care.

Program-Centered Administrative Consultation

In this type of consultation the work problem is related to planning and administration. Developing a new program or improving an existing program is often the focus of the consultation. The consultant uses her or his specialized expertise to assess the need for such programs and to offer plans for their development and evaluation. Clinical specialists are offering more and more of this type of consultation.

An example of this type of consultation occurred when a hospital administrative team and the hospital's cardiac surgeons wanted to develop a care program and a specialized intensive care unit for patients who had had open heart surgery. They consulted a cardiovascular clinical specialist on the physical layout of the unit as well as the overall programs of care for patients in the immediate postoperative phase following open heart surgery.

Consultee-Centered Administrative Consultation

The focus of this type of consultation is again planning and administration. The consultant focuses, however, on the consultee's problems or difficulties as they interfere with the objectives of the organization, rather than on the organization itself. The consultee may be lacking in knowledge, skill, confidence, or objectivity, or there may be group-related problems, such as poor leadership, disorganization, lack of clear goals, or poor communication.

The author was asked to offer this type of consultation to a group of head nurses when they felt that their group was not functioning optimally and therefore not accomplishing its administrative objectives. The primary goal of the consultation was to enhance the effectiveness of the head nurses' group functioning. With successful achievement of that goal, the group was able to offer meaningful contributions to the nursing department, thereby assisting the department to meet organizational objectives.

THE PSYCHIATRIC LIAISON NURSE: AN EXAMPLE OF THE CLINICAL SPECIALIST AS CONSULTANT

The author's position as a psychiatric liaison nurse was a joint position within the departments of nursing and psychiatry at a large rural medical center. The role of liaison psychiatry and of liaison nursing have been described (Lipowski, 1974; Lipowski, 1981; Nelson & Schilke, 1976; Robinson, 1974). In general, the liaison nurse was responsible for assisting the nursing staff and other health care professionals to enhance the quality of the psychosocial aspects of care for patients and their families in the medical and surgical in-patient units of the general hospital. This was usually accomplished through nursing consultation, direct psychiatric nursing intervention with patients or families, collaboration with the physicians and social worker on the psychiatric consultation service, and through educational programs for the staff. The author's position was as a psychiatric CNS; the concerns that she addressed through nursing consultation were therefore psychiatric. While the content or focus of nursing consultation varies widely from specialty to specialty, the process and principles of consultation and many issues related to implementing the consultative role are common to all specialties.

The Process of Consultation

The process of consultation was conceptualized by the author in terms of the nursing process—that is, in terms of the four steps of assessment, planning of care, implementation, and evaluation. This schema relates to the steps of consultation outlined by Caplan: (1) assessment of the consultation problem occurs following the consultation request; (2) the consultation report; (3) implementation of the consultant's recommendations, and (4) follow-up (p. 111–124). Conceptualizing and describing the process in terms of a model that was familiar to the nursing staff made the process more easily communicated and understood.

Most commonly, staff nurses request liaison nursing consultation because they have identified psychosocial problems with patients or families and wish assistance with them. The consultant and consultee together consider the experiences of the patient and the staff members in relation to the problem, thereby often merging the categories of client-centered case consultation and consultee-centered case consultation.

Practically speaking, the process of consultation is not always divided into discrete phases. As problems are identified during the first phase of the consultation, solutions can become readily apparent. It may be that by the time the problem is clearly understood, the nursing interventions indicated for addressing the problem are also clear. In practice, the consultee and consultant may move back and forth through the four phases of the process. While the boundaries between phases can be somewhat fluid, keeping the outline and sequences of the stages clearly in mind can give structure and direction and help to establish the objectives and the limits of the consultation process.

Assessment

This initial phase of the consultation involves clarifying with the consultee the specific nature of the problem and the major variables contributing to it. Questions to be answered initially are: What is the problem specifically?, Why is it now a problem?, What is the patient or family experiencing?, and How are the consultee and other members of the staff affected by the problem?

Understanding what the patient or family is experiencing is the crucial first step in assessing the overall consultation problem. Therefore in psychiatric consultation a psychiatric nursing assessment of the patient most often becomes the first order of business and generally forms the foundation on which the intervention is based.

Initially the consultee and consultant together consider the nursing assessment thus far completed and try to come to an understanding of the patient's experience. If, after discussing it, they recognize that their assessment is incomplete, they decide together on a plan to complete the assessment. If the consultee is not confident of her or his skills in the area of psychiatric nursing assessment, the consultant can assess the patient directly. It is often ideal to see the patient together with the consultee. Seeing the patient together can offer an opportunity for teaching and role modeling for the consultant and a sense of continuity in nursing care for the patient. If, however, the problem seems to represent significant staff–patient conflict, the consultant and consultee may decide that the consultant should see the patient alone so that the patient may talk openly about what she or he perceives to be the problem. In addition, time demands on the staff nurse consultee may make interviewing the patient together impractical.

The assessment phase of the consultation is usually initiated during individual discussion with the consultee. Sometimes, however, assessment takes place in a nursing conference with several staff members. A conference has the potential advantage of offering collective data to complete the assessment; several nurses can sometimes produce fragments of information that when put together present a complete picture. It becomes frustrating to all, though, when several staff members take the time to meet and there is not enough information about the patient to plan intervention. Certainly the point of such a conference can become a discussion of assessment skills, but it has been the author's experience that staff conferences are viewed as forums for problem solving and planning of care. When that cannot take place because of insufficient information, it can become frustrating indeed. This problem can be avoided or minimized by requesting that the staff member who requests the consultation assume responsibility for gathering information and briefly presenting the problem to the other members at the conference and for inviting other staff who are knowledgeable about the situation to come. An example of the assessment of a consultation problem follows:

A thirty-four year old woman was admitted to the oncology unit because of severe back pain. It was thought that the pain probably represented metastasis from a breast cancer that had been diagnosed three years previously. The patient had had a radical mastectomy at that time. She was aware that the pain probably represented metastasis and was understandably anxious as she was admitted to the unit. She was accompanied by her husband and mother.

Shortly after her admission she became increasingly anxious, angry, and mistrustful of the nursing staff. As nurses entered her room, she sat upright in her bed demanding to know what they planned to do with her. She stated repeatedly that she would not take "their" chemotherapy for cancer treatment. When she was to receive medication for any reason, she demanded to see the pharmacy package for the medication to be assured that the medication was actually what the nurse said it was. Attempts by the nursing staff to discuss the situation with the patient were met with angry rebuffs.

The nurses, concerned about the patient and unsure about how to proceed with her care, requested psychiatric nursing consultation from the liaison CNS. The consultant interviewed the patient and her assessment revealed the following:

The patient lived with her husband and seven-year-old daughter on a farm. They had a good family relationship and spent a lot of time together tending to the farm chores. The farm was their livelihood, and while they were just making ends meet financially, they enjoyed the self-sufficient life-style the farm offered them. The patient had a close relationship to her parents, who lived several miles away.

The patient described the diagnosis of cancer three years previously as having been traumatic for her. She had never experienced a serious illness, and there had been no family history of cancer. She was very distressed by the necessity for a radical mastectomy and agreed to it, somewhat reluctantly, because she believed it would cure her of cancer. After recuperating from her surgery, she resumed her active life-style. She continued to be troubled by the loss of her breast and found that working hard around the farm helped her to keep her mind off her feelings.

Over the course of the following three years, the patient's parents, who were retired and growing older, became increasingly dependent on her for assistance with household organization and tasks. Believing the cancer to be cured, she and her husband did not discuss the possibility of recurrence and had talked very little with their daughter about the illness. The patient was concerned about the possibility that her daughter was at high risk for the development of breast cancer but assured herself that there were many years to talk with her daughter when she was older about the importance of breast examinations and frequent medical evaluations. During that time as well, a friend of the patient's parents developed stomach cancer and, in spite of treatment with chemotherapy, subsequently died.

In general, the patient had seemed to be in reasonably good health until two weeks prior to this admission to the hospital, when she began to experience back pain. Initially she dismissed it as muscle strain and continued with her demanding daily routine. After a week had passed and the pain had worsened, she saw her family physician. Her physician referred her for an oncology consultation, fearing that the pain could be indicative of metastasis. She saw the oncologist several days later, and in spite of worsening pain told him she believed the problem to be muscle strain. She refused admission to the hospital for a complete evaluation but agreed to have x-rays taken as an outpatient. The oncologist called her the day after the x-rays were taken because he was concerned about what they revealed and persuaded her to be admitted to the hospital. She arrived at his office later that day visibly upset, angry, and in significant pain. She told him that her surgeon of three years ago had obviously lied and tricked her. After a brief discussion with the oncologist, she was admitted to the unit.

The assessment offered the consultant and the staff information about the meaning of this illness and hospitalization for the patient, about her previous experiences with cancer and surgery, and about aspects of her usual coping style. With that information they could better understand why the patient was angry and mistrustful and could more effectively plan for her care.

During the assessment phase of the consultation, it is important to consider the experience of the staff members in relation to the problem in addition to consideration of the patient's experience. Psychosocial aspects of nursing care involve the nurse–patient relationship, therefore, consideration of the meaning of the problem to both patient and nurse is crucial. To know only the experience of the patient is to know only part of the whole.

The feelings of the staff and of the consultant are important not only because of their direct effect on the consultation problem but also because those feelings may be reflective of the feelings of others in the situation. The sense of frustration, anger, and helplessness experienced by the staff may mirror the feelings of the patient, the family, or other health care providers. The emphasis on the staff's feelings in a consultation is not on delving into their personal lives and problems but rather on understanding what their feelings are in relation to the specific problem, and consideration of how these feelings may be influencing the situation. Disclosing feelings requires a great deal of trust. The consultant must consciously cultivate that trust and must be willing to examine her or his feelings in relation to the consultation problem and stand vulnerable with the staff as she or he is asking them to do.

In the example cited above, the nursing staff was feeling sad, threatened, inadequate, and angry. It was easy for them to identify with the patient because her age was close to many of their own. Their attempts to offer comfort and support had been met with anger and mistrust. Acknowledging and accepting the staff's feelings and considering with them how their feelings were affecting their interactions with the patient yielded further insight into the overall situation and more complete data on which to base the intervention.

Planning the Intervention

Once the consultee and consultant have clearly formulated the problem and completed the assessment, they decide together on the best approach for planning intervention strategies. Commonly it is at this point that they organize a nursing conference, both to increase the staff's understanding of the problem and to provide a forum for collective problem solving.

Psychiatric nursing consultation problems often are conceptualized by the author in terms of a crisis intervention model. The patient is viewed as experiencing a crisis in relation to illness and hospitalization. The challenges for the health care providers are to understand the meaning of the crisis for the patient, learn the patient's usual coping style and resources, and assist the patient with enhancing those skills and resources, thereby minimizing the negative impact of the crisis and enabling the patient to attain a higher level of functioning.

In general, it is helpful if the consultant avoids prescribing the best approach to the consultee and rather assists her or him in applying the problem-solving process. The consultant may also enhance the consultee's understanding of the situation by informally teaching principles of her or his specialty as they are specifically relevant to the problem at hand.

In addition to considering the needs of the patient, it is also important to consider the needs of the consultee and staff. Does the staff need more time to focus on their feelings about the problem, more teaching in relation to the problem, additional support for carrying out the plan, or a shift or change in patient care assignment? Planning for the staff's needs is an essential aspect of the consultation. Ideally, at the end of the planning phase of the consultation the consultee, other staff members (if involved), and the consultant will have outlined a practical, workable, mutually agreed upon plan with clear objectives and realistic long-term and short-term goals; specified who is responsible for carrying out the intervention; and established a plan for evaluating or modifying the nursing interventions.

The Intervention

The overall responsibility for carrying out the nursing intervention formulated during consultation remains with the consultee. If the consultant is to be involved directly in the intervention, her or his responsibility and role should be carefully negotiated and articulated. In the case described earlier, the intervention decided upon was as follows:

From the assessment, it had been learned that the likely recurrence of cancer was experienced by the patient as understandably threatening on many levels. It was potentially life-threatening. It immediately meant that she was unable to work, care for her family and parents, and assume the responsibilities from which she derived much satisfaction. It gave rise to fears about her daughter's future health. Her normal style of coping with difficult feelings had been to work hard on the farm to avoid thinking about these feelings and to deny or minimize in her mind threatening possibilities. Hospitalization stripped away from her the ability to work hard on the farm and served as a harsh and constant reminder of the reality of the situation. Rather than being able to take charge and assume responsibility for the care of others, she was suddenly being cared for herself by doctors and nurses whom she did not know and did not trust.

As the staff and consultant conferred to plan the intervention, they reviewed the assessment and outlined the following problems and intervention strategies: The patient's difficulty in trusting the staff was a central concern. It was decided that a primary nurse would work with her. Having one nurse relate to the patient consistently and plan her care, instead of having many different nurses interacting with her, would create a climate where a trusting relationship could more easily develop.

Another concern was the patient's sense that she was not in control of her situation. While it was recognized that important aspects of the situation were beyond being controlled, it was thought that encouraging the patient to assume control and responsibility for her care in areas where that was possible would enhance her usual coping style. The nurse would discuss with the patient her nursing care needs, as perceived by both staff and patient, and they would decide together how best to meet those needs, with emphasis placed on allowing the patient to assume significant self-care responsibilities. In order to eliminate the issue of medication as a focus for mistrust and to reinforce the patient's responsibility for her own care, the nurse would also consider with her the possibility of leaving the medications in the pharmacy packages at her bedside rather than at the nurses' station. The responsibility for the medications would be the patient's.

In terms of optimizing support, the staff would relax the usual visiting restrictions, allowing the patient's daughter and husband flexibility in visiting privileges, since they had to accommodate a busy schedule of farm work. The primary nurse would make every effort to schedule tests, examinations, and nursing care during the time when the patient did not have visitors. There also would be an attempt on the part of the staff to arrange for privacy for the patient and her family when they visited.

In addition to family support, the primary nurse would let the patient know of the cancer patient support group that met weekly and of the chaplain's and social worker's availability. The consultant would continue to see the patient directly as well, to give ongoing supportive psychotherapy. The consultant would discuss her intervention with the primary nurse and let the patient know that she would be doing so.

Preparing for the likelihood that metastasis would be confirmed, the primary nurse would discuss the patient's strong feelings about chemotherapy with her physicians. The nursing staff would reinforce the fact that decisions about accepting treatment recommendations, including chemotherapy, were the patient's. It was emphasized that it was the responsibility of the physicians and nurses to respond to the patient's specific concerns and questions and to offer her full and accurate information about treatment options and the rationale for their specific recommendations, so that she would make a truly informed decision about the treatment.

Anticipating future educational needs of the patient in relation to both her own illness and her concerns about her daughter's future health, the staff would talk to the oncology clinical specialist. They would ask this specialist to be available directly to the patient and her family, if needed, and would also seek assistance from the oncology CNS in updating their own knowledge about the patient's potential educational needs.

Evaluation and Closure

As the intervention is being planned, it is important to keep in mind a method for evaluating the effectiveness of the intervention. Outlining in advance specific strategies for measuring whether or not the objectives of care have been attained helps to ensure that these objectives will be realistic. During the planning phase the consultant and consultee decide what will represent measures of successful intervention. They then set aside a time after the intervention for consideration of those measures.

In the case being described, the objectives of intervention were to offer consistent and supportive nursing care to enhance a trusting relationship between staff and patient; to augment supportive resources available to the patient in the hospital; to optimize family availability; to enhance the patient's sense of control; and to educate the patient about treatment options and implications, so that she could make an informed decision about treatment.

In this case, the objectives of treatment were met. The patient was able to form trusting and meaningful relationships with several staff members. The patient appreciated taking control of much of her care and was eager for information about her illness and treatment considerations. Extensive metastasis was confirmed, and chemotherapy was recommended. The patient decided against chemotherapy because she was concerned that the possible side effects of the chemotherapy would diminish the quality of the time she had to live. The objective of intervention was educating the patient, rather than persuading her to accept what the staff felt was the best treatment. Discussing that objective and its implications enabled the staff to respect the decision of the patient, recognizing that they had fulfilled their responsibility in the decision-making process by thoroughly educating her and that she had fulfilled her responsibility by making an informed decision. With the support of the staff, she was able to examine the meaning of her decision not to accept chemotherapy and to plan for her ongoing needs and eventual death. She and her husband and daughter decided that she would be cared for at their farm. She subsequently had several brief hospitalizations to regulate her medications for pain management. She later died at her home with her parents, husband, daughter, and several close friends caring for her.

If the objectives of the intervention are not met, the evaluation phase offers the consultant and consultee the opportunity to consider why they were not and to modify the intervention plans accordingly.

When the consultation comes to an end, closure of the process should be acknowledged. Such open acknowledgment gives the consultee and consultant the chance to review both the consultation and the relationship that they developed during the process. Flynn (1972) eloquently discussed the importance of the relationship between consultant and consultee. Very often consultation occurs because of difficult, complex situations, and trusting, valued relationships develop as the process evolves. Recognizing and appreciating that dimension of the consultation process is important. As the consultant and consultee bring the consultation to a close, they may wish to consider possibilities for future consultations.

ISSUES IN IMPLEMENTING THE CONSULTATIVE ROLE

The CNS Consultant and the Nursing Administration

Most clinical specialists do not offer consultation as members of a profession that is different from that of their consultees, nor do they enter the institution as outsiders, for the sole purpose of responding to a specific consultation request. Most CNSs are hired by the nursing administration as permanent members of the nursing staff. This fact has several important implications for the clinical specialist wanting to function as a consultant.

First, it is essential to have the support of the nursing administration for developing the role of consultation within one's CNS practice. Whether one is a consultant primarily or secondarily, the expectations of the administrators will have significant implications for the development of the position (Blake, 1977). It is not likely that the clinical specialist will be able to legitimize taking time from her or his schedule to offer high-quality consultation (and consultation is a time-consuming process) without the support and understanding of administrators. In addition, without en-thusiastic endorsement from nursing administrators, members of the nursing staff are not likely to set aside their highly valued time to get to know the consultant and learn of what she or he is offering.

Second, CNS consultants who are members of the nursing department in which they consult cannot truly be unbiased consultants. They must keep in mind organizational and departmental priorities and goals as they make recommendations in consultation. While all consultants ideally offer recommendations based on organizational constraints and priorities, CNS consultants have an extra burden in this regard. They are likely to know well the goals and directions established by their departments—in fact, they are likely to have been involved in setting them. They must, therefore, be keenly aware of their own personal biases in relation to departmental objectives, so that they can recognize these biases as they creep into consultation activities. On the one hand, as a consultant it is possible to sabotage departmental goals with which one does not agree or promote personal goals with which the department does not agree by making recommendations that may run counter to established priorities. For example, the oncology CNS believing in primary nursing could recommend that every cancer patient she or he consults on have a primary nurse, when the CNS also knows that the departmental budget could not support that recommendation. The specialist may thereby make the consultee, who cannot provide this kind of care, feel that she or he is providing less than adequate care and may also stir feelings of dissatisfaction and anger with the administration that will not provide such support. On the other hand, the consultant must be open to the consultee who is in disagreement with departmental policies and goals. Taking the time to understand the consultee's specific concerns, rather than simply reiterating the administration's policy, is important. If the consultee perceives the consultant as simply the spokesperson for the administration's point of view, she or he is not likely to talk openly and comfortably about concerns and feelings in relation to implementing departmental policies. As in other areas of CNS practice, the consultant often serves as the representative of the administration to the staff and as the representative of the staff to the administration.

The CNS Consultant and the Nursing Staff

There are, inevitably, obstacles in every setting to effective consultation. An awareness of those obstacles, both real and potential, can help consultants to avoid them and to assess problematic relationships and unsuccessful consultations.

Polk (1980) points out some of the resistance on the part of nurses to utilizing other nurses as consultants. Nurses are commonly socialized to turn to the physician as the expert on patient care issues when problems arise. Calling on a nursing consultant as the expert, therefore, often requires a change in attitude and consciousness. Because nurses often feel responsible for meeting all of the nursing needs of their patients, asking a nursing consultant for assistance with patient care may cause nurses to doubt their skills and abilities and may imply to them failure and inadequacy. Nursing consultants often have an additional potentially threatening factor to consider—that of advanced academic preparation. In this day of hot debate about the academic preparations of nurses, the issue of education and feelings related to it are no small matter.

The significance of potential feelings of inadequacy and threat on the part of the nurse consultee must be appreciated. It is critical for the consultant to minimize the degree of that threat whenever possible. No matter how knowledgeable and sophisticated a consultant is, if the potential consultee is not comfortable with the consultant because she or he feels threatened, no consultation will take place. The most effective way to dispel the nursing staff's fear is through repeated personal contact with them. Getting to know the staff and learning their goals and values in relation to nursing is very important. Creating the opportunity for the staff to know the consultant personally and learn her or his values in relation to nursing and consultation is equally important. Most often, staff and consultant ultimately recognize that their values and goals are compatible and complementary, rather than conflicting. Emphasizing the coordinate rather than hierarchical nature of the consultant–consultee relationship and then acting on that premise can help to dispel fears about the evaluative power of the consultant.

There are many ways for the consultant to have contact with the staff as she or he is getting to know them. The consultant may wish to do staff nursing for a short period of time. She or he can attend unit conferences and patient rounds with the staff. The CNS can be available to present educational seminars and conferences in response to staff requests. Such opportunities will vary from setting to setting; in general, the more visible the consultant is, the more quickly the staff will come to know the CNS and utilize her or his skills.

Confusion about the role of the CNS consultant and the process of consultation is another significant obstacle. Because staff nurses have many different nursing resources available to them, it is important to distinguish the role of the CNS consultant from the roles of team leader, head nurse, supervisor, unit-based line CNS, and unit teacher. Clarification about what the clinical specialist will and will not do as a consultant can help to dispel confusion about the role. The consultant is not a supervisor; she or he is not going to prescribe the best approach to nursing care nor is the specialist going to take over responsibility for the patients. The CNS consultant is an expert, with specialized knowledge in relation to a relatively narrow area of nursing. The consultant will bring that knowledge to bear on a nursing problem when she or he is invited to do so. Consultation is an interactional process. The consultant will listen carefully, help to identify major variables contributing to the problem, and help to create a forum for problem solving. The consultant will combine her or his expertise and knowledge with that of the staff, and together they will formulate a plan for nursing intervention. When the consultant offers direct nursing intervention to patients and families, she or he will negotiate that role carefully with the staff. Whereas most other nursing resources available to the staff have administrative and evaluative responsibilities for the staff, the CNS does not. The staff nurse identifies the problem with which assistance is needed, initiates the consultation, is free to accept or reject the recommendations of the consultant, and remains responsible for the care of the patient. It has been the author's experience that discussing the role of the consultant with new staff nurses during their orientation has been a meaningful way of having contact with the staff and clarifying the consultant's role and the process of consultation. Another helpful method for clarifying some of the issues and implications of consultation was to draft a departmental statement regarding consultation and to make it available on each nursing unit.

The overly zealous consultant can create obstacles to effective consultation. It can be tempting, as one is trying to prove oneself as a knowledgeable consultant, to teach a great deal about the problem at hand and to formulate the "perfect" approach to the problem. In consultation, teaching should be brief, concise, and narrowly focused on the specific consultation problem. Broader educational needs are often identified in the course of consultation and frequently go on to serve as the basis for the development of departmental procedures and policies and future continuing education programs for the staff. As important as those actions are, however, they are a result of, and not part of, the consultation process and should be clearly distinguished from that process in the consultant's mind. The emphasis in consultation is on effective, practical problem solving, and too much emphasis on theoretical didactic material can obscure the purpose of the consultation.

It is the responsibility of the consultant to assist with problem solving rather than to prescribe solutions. When the consultee is involved with the problem solving, the intervention formulated is more likely to be practical, effective, and actually carried out. Carrying out someone else's ideas and prescriptions can dilute the sense of personal relevance, investment, and responsibility in the problem-solving process.

If consultants find that in the course of consultation they are teaching all that they know about a particular problem and are holding themselves personally accountable for designing and implementing the best approach to the problem, they should evaluate their motives. Whose needs are being served—the consultant's or the staff's? Insecurity on the part of the consultant can motivate long dissertations on consultation problems and highly directive problem solving. That insecurity can motivate actions that are, paradoxically, perceived by others as threatening. Insecurity on the part of the consultant is valid and understandable, especially during the beginning phases of a new role. Needs related to that insecurity can be more effectively met when they are recognized and accepted, and when direct, rather than indirect action is taken. Supervision and peer support can effectively address such needs.

Prejudices Related to the Specialty

Each specialty has certain prejudices against it. The prejudices related to the specialty of the individual CNS consultant can present obstacles to effective consultation. Hitchens (1973) discussed prejudices regarding psychiatry as one of the more difficult aspects of her role as a psychiatric CNS consultant. While the prejudices may at times represent gross exaggerations and distortions about a specialty, at other times they may reflect unfortunate previous experiences with practitioners of that specialty or patients within that specialty. They may also reflect fear and insecurity of the practitioner harboring the prejudice in relation to her or his skill in dealing with that particular specialty area.

It is important for the consultant to recognize the prejudices associated with her or his specialty. For example, many health care professionals have prejudices regarding psychiatry. Prejudices against psychiatric professionals can include the notion that these specialists always speak in jargon and psychoanalyze everyone, and that when they give advice they really do little more than state the obvious or offer esoteric, impractical solutions to problems. Prejudices against psychiatric patients include fears that they are all irrational, dangerous, and difficult, and misconceptions that the patients "make themselves sick," have "weak" characters, and will never recover from their illnesses. Other specialties contend with other prejudices. For example, the oncology CNS confronts prejudices about the hopelessness of cancer care; the neurology CNS deals with misconceptions about the rehabilitative potential of patients with spinal cord injuries; and the intensive care CNS contends with prejudices that intensive care nurses overemphasize machinery and thereby dehumanize their patients.

It is important to recognize prejudice against one's specialty and to avoid interpreting it as personal criticism. Once there is an understanding of how specific prejudices are influencing the consultation problem, the consultant can attempt to dispel the impact of the prejudices in that particular situation. At times she or he may confront the prejudice directly. More commonly, however, rather than confronting the prejudice directly the consultant attempts to dispel the impact of prejudices by carefully avoiding actions that would reinforce known ones and by focusing on the specifics of the consultation problem rather than on generalities related to it. For example, a psychiatric nursing consultant worked with the nursing staff of a medical unit as they were caring for an alcoholic woman who had been hospitalized with cirrhosis. The consultant recognized that many prejudices about alcoholism were influencing the staff's perception of the patient. Rather than confronting their prejudices directly, she acknowledged their frustration but did not respond to their general biases conveyed in statements to the effect that alcoholics are always this or always that. She instead focused the staff's attention on the specific situation and the needs of the particular patient. She also hoped to demonstrate, with education and role modeling through direct intervention with the patient, that the patient was worthy of concerted and committed effort and that alcoholism was not a hopeless disease.

Interfacing with Other Professionals

In any health care setting, there are many professionals working toward the ideal of offering quality health care, and it is inevitable that the clinical specialist consultant will complement, and at times overlap with or even contradict the efforts of others as she or he also strives toward that ideal. The individuals with whom the consultant interfaces will, of course, vary greatly from setting to setting. In almost every setting, however, the CNS consultant's role will interface with that of the physician and the head nurse.

Because roles commonly overlap, it is imperative that the CNS clarify and articulate what it is that she or he uniquely offers in the setting so that her or his services can be appropriately offered and utilized. Given the somewhat amorphous general definitions of nursing, this task can be quite difficult. Once the unique aspects of the role are defined, however, the CNS consultant can negotiate with other professionals the assumption of responsibilities in the overlapping areas of practice. The negotiating of responsibilities is a complex and ongoing process that involves the difficult arenas of professional rivalry, territoriality, and threat. It requires tact, judiciousness, flexibility, and willingness to compromise, as well as assertiveness, on the part of the consultant. While ideally the other professionals demonstrate those skills as well, the new consultant must recognize that she or he is an outsider (and often the latest comer) to a system that is established and set in its ways of operating and that therefore she or he may be required to demonstrate the greatest flexibility.

Professional rivalry is a two-sided issue, obviously, and consultants must be willing to examine their own feelings, biases, and the degree to which the gratification of their personal ego needs are playing a part in their professional role definition. Recognition of these factors can prevent the consultant from acting on these motives unconsciously.

Physicians

The CNS consultant's practice affects medical practice in many ways. For example, the oncology CNS consultant may make medication recommendations for the cancer patient with a difficult pain management problem; the cardiovascular CNS consultant may make recommendations about the teaching program necessary for a patient who has had a myocardial infarction; and the psychiatric liaison CNS may identify the fact that a medical patient is delirious and make the recommendation that possible causes for the delirium be evaluated. This level of professional interaction between physicians and nurses is relatively new in many practice settings and not without its complexities. Some physicians welcome the skill and knowledge of the CNS, appreciate the collegial interchange, and recognize the potential benefits for staff and patients when nursing consultation of high quality is available. The physicians within the CNS's specialty are often valuable allies, and developing close working relationships with them is important. Those relationships can offer the specialist ongoing professional growth and stimulation and can provide her or him with support and consultation for particularly complex situations. The CNS consultant is also often in a position to recommend physician-to-physician consultations. When the clinical specialist recognizes that the primary physician on a case needs to consult with a physician within the CNS's specialty, the CNS recommends this to the primary physician. If the CNS and physicians usually work closely together, the CNS's recommendation has enhanced credibility. If the CNS consultant and physicians within a specialty have a good working relationship, they can more easily determine patterns of practice that will be complementary and synergistic rather than competitive and redundant.

Not all physicians, however, are pleased by the presence of the clinical specialist. Indeed, some have been quite displeased by the change in nursing roles and perceive the types of recommendations described above as infringements on their areas of practice. The utmost skill and tact should, of course, be demonstrated by the clinical specialist, with the hope that repeated meaningful contact with the physician will eventually lead to the development of a good working relationship. But it is also important that the CNS be operating from a strong power base within the organization and that the nursing administration supports the changes that the clinical specialist position, staff or line, implies.

The decision of a nurse to request a nursing consultation is a nursing decision that should not require the permission of the physician. The nurse may well want to discuss the reasons for requesting such consultation with the physician as they collaborate on the care of their patients, but ideally the nurse should not need the physician's permission, per se, to initiate a nursing consultation. Again, because that level of independent decision making may represent a marked change in nurse–physician interaction, strong support and advocacy is required from an institution's nursing leadership.

There are times, unfortunately, when an impasse is reached between the CNS consultant and the physician on issues related to patient care. The consultant must then decide what action, if any, she or he ought to take. If the CNS believes that patient safety or comfort is in significant jeopardy, she or he may well decide to take definitive action. At that point the CNS is, technically, stepping out of the consultant role and into the specialist role. For example,

A psychiatric liaison nurse was consulted by the nursing staff in the coronary care unit because they were concerned about unusual behavior being displayed by a patient who had had a serious myocardial infarction two days previously. The consultant assessed the patient as delirious. Concerned about the potentially dangerous implications of delirium in this patient, she stepped aside from her consultant role and assumed responsibility for going directly to the patient's intern to stress the importance of evaluating the cause of the delirium. She explained what she was doing, and why, to the staff nurses who had consulted her. The intern minimized the significance of the patient's delirium, stating that he was convinced that the patient's confusion was a psychological consequence of adjusting to the seriousness of his medical situation. Disagreeing with the intern's assessment, the CNS went to the resident and met with the same erroneous conclusion. Explaining that she disagreed with them and that, in fact, she believed that if the cause of the delirium was not evaluated the patient's safety could be compromised, she told them she would discuss the situation with the staff psychiatrist on the psychiatric consultation service and she would request that he contact the patient's staff physician directly. She did this; a formal psychiatric consultation was initiated, the psychiatrist supported the liaison nurse's assessment, and an investigation into the possible causes of delirium ensued. It was determined that the likely cause was the patient's digitalis level, which was found to be higher than the usual therapeutic range. Clearly, a potentially dangerous and correctable condition had been identified.

The degree of responsibility for patient care assumed by clinical specialists may be met with reactions of surprise and disdain by some physicians. While the tension that results from challenging a physician's assessment can be most uncomfortable, it can be a necessary step in demonstrating the depth and scope of the specialist's practice.

In addition to having the support of the nursing administration and the physicians within her or his specialty, it is also very helpful for the CNS consultant to make contact with physicians in administrative positions or other positions of authority. Explaining to such physicians the nature and purpose of the CNS consultant role can enhance overall physician support and understanding of the role. If physicians on the staff have concerns about the CNS's activities, the understanding of their department chairperson about the role can prove to be very helpful.

Some conflict with physicians is likely to occur in any case as the CNS establishes the role in the health care setting, whether it be as a consultant or a unit-based line clinical specialist. The most effective way to minimize that conflict is through repeated personal interaction with physicians, demonstrating knowledge, skill, and confidence in relation to clinical issues; sensitivity in relation to interpersonal and professional issues; and respect for the physicians' concerns, objectives, and responsibilities.

Head Nurses

In hospital settings, no group has been asked to make more changes and more concessions in adjusting to the advent of clinical specialists than head nurses. They have been asked to share their power, authority, and status and to step down from their position as most clinically knowledgeable nurse on the unit. If they are threatened, hostile, and skeptical as the CNS is ushered in, it is no wonder. Dictums from the nursing administration to utilize CNS consultants will be meaningless without the support and understanding of the head nurse. The head nurse often is in a position to use her or his power, either consciously or unconsciously, to effectively block or encourage the utilization of CNS consultants by the nursing staff.

Establishing and maintaining good working relationships with head nurses is of critical importance. The head nurse is the most important ally and advocate on the unit. Showing respect for the head nurse's position and making every effort to minimize the degree of threat associated with the CNS position is important. Asking staff nurses to clear requests for consultation with the head nurse (particularly initially, as the role is being established); making it a point to discuss consultation requests with the head nurse; seeking her or his opinion and advice about patient care problems and inviting her or him to participate in planning conferences can be effective ways of familiarizing the head nurse with the consultant and the process of consultation. Such approaches can additionally underscore the consultant's respect for the importance of the head nurse's role. It has certainly been the experience of the author that head nurses demonstrate poignant insight in relation to consultation problems and make valuable suggestions for intervention strategies.

When head nurses resist the services of a consultant, the consultant must seek to understand the motivation behind the resistance. Very often it is related to the degree of threat being experienced by the head nurse. The CNS's position is both real and symbolic. In addition to the changes discussed above, the CNS position represents the wave of the future in nursing. Head nurses who do not feel ready for the changes of the future may well be threatened by what the consultant symbolizes. The only way to work through this type of resistance is to understand it and to be sensitive to it. This can, indeed, be a complex process. As CNSs try to create a new role, they can be blinded by their own insecurity and by the wish to prove themselves, which focuses their attention on themselves rather than on others. When the head nurse and a CNS consultant have meaningful rather than competitive contact, the relationship can be mutually beneficial. In the experience of the author, a wise and caring head nurse orchestrated several model consultations for the new, insecure, and naive CNS consultant. These consultations and the head nurse's support and advocacy probably were the two most important factors in initially establishing the credibility of the consultant with the staff. The head nurse's willingness to help establish the consultant's position and her successful strategy to create the opportunity for demonstrating the consultant's skills made unnecessary what would likely have been months of solo effort.

Rejected Recommendations

An important principle of consultation (and at times difficult to live with) is that the consultee is free to accept or reject the consultant's suggestions. As previously discussed, when patient safety is clearly at stake, the consultant steps out of the role of consultant into the role of specialist and takes whatever actions are necessary. Such occasions are unusual. More commonly, the situation is a subtle hue of gray. The consultant makes recommendations that she or he believes would benefit patient care, but for any number of reasons the recommendations may not be followed. Ideally, working closely with the consultee through every phase of the consultation process ensures the practicality and workability of the recommendations and planning. But there are inevitably times when the consultee chooses not to act on the consultant's suggestions. When that occurs, the consultant must first accept this choice as the prerogative of the consultee. While respecting the consultee's power in the situation, the consultant may wish to explore with her or him the reasons for choosing not to accept the recommendations. Were the recommendations understandable, sensible, to the point, and reasonable? Did they take into consideration the needs of both the patient and the staff? Were there constraints in the situation that the consultant did not understand? Open, honest feedback from the consultee can often help the consultant to understand why the recommendations were not followed.

It is also very helpful to be able to confide in a trusted colleague. The consultant needs the opportunity to explore what occurred during the consultation to gain additional perspective, as well as the opportunity to express the frustration and anger that can result from having invested time and effort in seeking a solution to a problem that is ultimately rejected. Other CNS consultants can offer solace and understanding. Finding a meaningful way to cope with the feelings of anger and rejection is important for the mental health of the consultant as well as for the success of future consultations. Unrecognized, unexpressed negative feelings can linger and color future relationships that develop during the consultation process.

The Line CNS as Consultant

Clinical specialists who are primarily based on units that offer the care of their specialty and are responsible for the clinical aspects of nursing care on those units have a valuable role to play as consultants outside their units. Consultation requires that the consultee be in a coordinate, rather than hierarchical position with the consultant. The consultee must be able to choose or not choose to initiate the consultation request and be free to accept or reject the consultant's recommendations. Because of the clinical, administrative, and evaluative responsibilities of the line CNS, her or his relationship to the staff is not coordinate. Certainly because of the line CNS's expertise, her or his advice is commonly sought in relation to clinical problems. However, because of the leadership relationship she or he has with the staff, consultation as discussed in this chapter cannot take place between them. The clinical interchange between the line CNS and her or his staff would be viewed as teaching or supervision rather than con-sultation, *per se.*

When the line CNS becomes a consultant to another unit, her or his focus and orientation narrow, and the power base shifts. The narrow and defined focus of consultation can balance the broad responsibilities of the line CNS position. In consultation there is a beginning, a middle, and an end, and the act of completing a process can give the CNS with broad-based responsibilities a sense of concrete accomplishment. And while relinquish-ing power can be difficult, it can also be freeing. Consultation offers staff member consultees access to the skill and knowledge of a practitioner with whom contact would otherwise be quite limited.

CONCLUSION

Consultation is a complex and highly professional aspect of the role of the CNS that challenges the practitioner to blend science with art, theory with practice, and the real with the ideal. The relationship that develops between the consultant and consultee is limited in duration and focus yet can be profoundly influential. Applying the process and principles of consultation is challenging, at times arduous. Yet it is a process that creates the opportunity for mutual and creative problem solving, identification of values, sharing of knowledge, and stimulus to growth that is so necessary for the ongoing development of nursing practice.

REFERENCES

Blake, P. The clinical specialist as nurse consultant. *J Nurs Adm*, 1977, *7*, 33–36.

Caplan, G. *The theory and practice of mental health consultation*. New York: Basic Books, 1970.

Flynn, G. The romance of consultation. In J. Busman & D. Davison (Eds.), *Practical aspects of mental health consultation*. Springfield, Ill.: Charles C Thomas, 1972.

Hitchens, E. Mental health nursing consultations: some distinctions. *J Psychiatr Nurs*, 1973, *15*, 13–16.

Lipowski, Z. J. Consultation-liaison psychiatry: an overview. *Am J Psychiatry*, 1974, *131*, 623–630.

Lipowski, Z. J. Liaison psychiatry, liaison nursing and behavior medicine. *Compr Psychiatry*, 1981, *22*, 554–561.

Nelson, J., & Schilke, D. Evolution of psychiatric liaison nursing. *Perspectives in Psychiatr Care*, 1976, *14*, 60–65.

Polk, G. The socialization and utilization of nurse consultants. *J Psychiatr Nurs*, 1980, *18*, 33–36.

Robinson, L. *Liaison nursing psychological approach to patient care*. Philadelphia: F. A. Davis, 1974.

III. NURSING SERVICE ADMINISTRATION AND THE CLINICAL NURSE SPECIALIST

8. Justifying and Structuring the CNS Role in the Nursing Department

Sally A. Sample

The 1980s promise to be a decade of change, uncertainty, and challenge for health care administrators. Caught up in social and economic turmoil, our health care delivery systems are struggling to adapt to new political, ethical, and clinical environments that are only partially understood. Nowhere are the pressures for change more strongly felt and more troublesome to deal with than in the hospital. No one feels these pressures more acutely than the nursing administrator who not only must cope with the turbulent health care environment but must also deal with the issues and concerns of the nursing profession.

The nursing profession labeled this decade as the "decade for decision" at the Annual Convention of the American Nurses' Association (ANA) in June of 1980. The association's 25th president stated in her presidential address, "The decade of the eighties represents a beginning, a new opportunity to create a better world for nursing" (ANA, 1981).

Within the parameters of uncertainty and confidence, the nursing administrator must make decisions in this changing and complex health care environment to support and advance the practice of nursing. It is in this context that the justification and placement of the clinical nurse specialist (CNS) role becomes an economic and clinical imperative that must be assessed, developed, and evaluated within the unique mission of each health care institution, whether it is the academic medical center, the community hospital, the home health agency, clinic, or nursing home.

HEALTH CARE ISSUES

Health care administrators, economists, and planners are considering the current and future issues affecting our health care delivery system in an attempt to move from problem identification toward operational success. The nurse administrator, in justifying clinical nursing roles, must be cognizant of the key issues that affect both the delivery of nursing service and the health care industry. Both the nurse administrator and the clinical specialist need to identify the implications of these issues for economic and clinical survival of their roles and services.

Competition in the Marketplace

The political climate of the eighties has introduced the concept of deregulation within the prevailing health care system. Potential consequences could reward those hospitals that can give the best services at the lowest costs. The attempt to achieve both goals simultaneously may either enhance the quality of nursing care, providing excellent models of patient care delivery systems, or lower the quality of nursing care by substitution of less-skilled and less-costly nonprofessional nursing staff. At what price will the quality of care provided by the CNS become too expensive for the hospital, and at what loss of quality nursing service to the consumer?

Ethical Issues

Productivity standards, limited financial resources, and societal mandates are all intertwined with multiple ethical issues. How can we balance the extensive resources required for sophisticated intensive care units with the need to provide desired primary care, health educational programs, or hospice services? Under what conditions do we extend life, and at what cost to individual families as well as to society as a whole? How do we justify the cost of the care given by the CNS as an essential member of the critical care team or the hospice team?

Human Resource Management

There has been a resurgence of interest in the concept of the quality of work life because of the need to increase the productivity of the American worker, blue collar or professional. In a labor-intensive industry such as health care, obtaining and retaining people to do the organization's work is crucial to the industry's survival. Currently research is under way to determine what professional work climate is most conducive to fostering job satisfaction and retention of practicing nurses. The CNS may be one of the significant forces in creating a professional work climate. If retention of practicing nurses is enhanced by the support and direction of the CNSs, decreased turnover costs becomes a strong argument in a tight budget process.

JUSTIFYING THE CNS ROLE

Professional Imperatives

The American Nurses' Association, in its publication *Nursing: A Social Policy Statement*, states that specialization in nursing is now clearly established. The ANA asserts that "specialization in nursing practice assists in clarifying, revising, and strengthening existing nursing practice. Specialization expedites production of new knowledge and its application in practice" (ANA, 1980, p. 22).

It is absolutely essential that the nurse administrator and key members of the nursing management team understand the concept of clinical nurse specialization and identify its relevance to their department. Proposed utilization of CNSs must first be discussed and debated within each nursing service organization until a reasonable consensus is reached. One approach, familiar to most nurses, is to utilize the component steps of the nursing process (assessment, planning, implementation, evaluation) to determine the need for a CNS. This approach utilizes a professional problem-solving process that can be linked with the identifiable variables of the change process within one's institution.

Assessment

Assessment of the need for a CNS within an organized nursing service requires the gathering of data concerning significant patient or client populations for which nursing services are currently being provided or for whom a lack of nursing service exists or is predicted. Assessment should also identify new clinical program goals that will enhance patient care. The assessment process is congruent with the philosophy of the nursing services and the standards of nursing practice desired.

During the assessment period, a review of the literature can assist in defining clear expectations, avoiding documented pitfalls, and in justifying either a new or expanded CNS role (Baker & Kramer, 1970; Barrett, 1971; Blake, 1977; Parkis, 1974; Schaefer, 1973; Everson, 1981). The utilization of a nursing administrator network to discuss the issue of clinical nurse specialization and the diversity of roles identified within the specialization concept needs to be considered on a more regular basis within regional and professional organizations, as well as within university communities. Peer consultation with a valued and respected colleague external to the nursing administrator's organization is an excellent process to utilize in testing ideas about the CNS role, structure, title, and expectations. This process shares expertise in an objective manner. It is especially useful for the nursing director in a rural community or small agency who is ready to promote the concept of clinical specialization and who needs an opportunity to discuss with a colleague the relevance of the literature or the determination of need.

During the assessment phase the nurse administrator uses her or his own intellectual competencies and experience to shift thoughts from dreams to reality, from desires to practicalities, from constraints to strengths. In concert with a management team of nursing leaders or with an individual administrator or physician, it is the nurse administrator who will promote and justify the concept of clinical specialization within the nursing department and the institution as a whole. After the nursing administrator and the nursing management team have reached a degree of mutual understanding about the need for a CNS, dialogue with the significant others in the total health care organization who would be affected by the role is essential. Before the CNS is on the scene, it is wise to talk with head nurses and nursing staff to determine their expectations, their feelings, their support for clinical specialization, and most important, what benefits they see for the patients/clients, for the advancement of nursing practice, and for themselves. The nursing staff are the prime care-givers. They are frequently undervalued, and their ability to consider concepts of clinical specialization, change, or organizational design is frequently not acknowledged. Today's practicing nurse wants to be a part of the decision-making process that affects her or his nursing practice.

It is equally important to communicate directly with members of the medical staff and other members of the health care team who will be interacting with the CNS. Perceptions of the nurse's role are infinite among non-nursing health care professionals as well as among nurses themselves. Assessment of the need for the CNS with those who have important roles within the institution must proceed with the utmost skill and sensitivity to promote a positive alliance between powerful groups in the setting.

Planning

If it is determined during the assessment phase that the hiring of a CNS is justified, the planning phase begins. During this phase, the financial implications and timing of the change are considered. Anticipating that cost will be an issue, the nursing administrator will identify, at this stage, monies that can be used to support the employment of the CNS. The creative nursing administrator may well need to negotiate to obtain the financial support for these new roles. As in any negotiating process, one must ask what components of the nursing service budget may be eliminated to support the new program and what modifications need to be considered to preserve all essential programs. In this era of financial constraints, compromises will have to be reached with the key financial officer. Planning to influence the budgetary process is as significant as planning to make the organizational structure responsive to the new role. It is possible to bury the funds needed to support the position within the departmental budget, and that might be the most viable option for funding the position. It is equally possible to manipulate positions, to advance new clinical roles quietly in hopes of justifying the position by persuasion, fiat, or clinical results. In the tight budgetary conditions of the 80's, nursing administrators must proceed boldly to justify and finance CNSs.

While the planning for a new role may take a great deal of time, support for this planning phase can usually be found, since it involves new clinical programs and new opportunities to improve patient care services. Philanthropic foundations often support the initial planning and implementation phases for improvement in clinical services, recognizing that it takes new money to begin new projects or programs. If grant monies are terminated or financial mandates require a reduction in gross expenditures, however, CNS positions become vulnerable within the institution, since they may be regarded as a luxury, not as an essential clinical role required to advance nursing practice.

STRUCTURING THE CNS ROLE

Institutional Imperatives

Organizations exist to meet perceived needs of society. These needs are frequently described in official statements about the mission of the organization or in a series of statements about its goals. In both profit and nonprofit health care institutions, a board of trustees is appointed or elected to manage the enterprise. The formal lines of authority and responsibility can be depicted in an organization chart that schematically displays relationships between groups, departments, and divisions in the institution.

Traditionally, hospitals have tended to be bureaucratic in their organizational design. The organization of nursing services has a comparable heritage, and it is only recently that both hospitals and nursing service departments have begun to conceptualize and implement new organizational designs. Reluctance to change has been overcome by the need to be more responsive to the consumer and to the provider. We have reached a point where both the public and the government have determined that health care cost must be controlled and reduced, and no motivator for change is more powerful than economic necessity.

The structuring of the CNS role within the nursing organization should be seen as a means to the end goals of the department and the institution, not a goal in itself. A nursing position exists to meet the organizational goals and objectives, stated or implied, of the nursing service department and of the institution. At Harborview Medical Center, in Seattle, Washington, the process by which new roles are developed within the department of nursing service was set forth in a job description summarizing the scope of the nursing supervisor/specialist:

> The development of this position is negotiated with the individual in relationship to the philosophy, goals and objectives of the Nursing Service Department. In this dynamic process role definition is incumbent upon the individual and the employer and implemented within the unique organization of the Nursing Service Department. Guidelines for the development and integration of the position within organized nursing services suggest areas of primary responsibilities without limiting the individual. It is anticipated that each role/position would be periodically reviewed as to its function in the Nursing organization.*

As part of the negotiation process, an effort should be made to assure that the individual goals of the CNS implementing the role are congruent with the goals of the institution. As the structure and goals of the nursing department change in response to the mission of the institution, the CNS and the nursing administrator need to evaluate the relevance of the role to the new demands and negotiate different options or strategies that continue the advancement of nursing practice.

There are three positions within the nursing organization in which a CNS may be employed: a line position within the management structure, a staff position within the department structure, and a shared or joint appointment between two employing departments within the overall institution or in different institutions. Each requires clarity of title, role, and of placement within the organization with regard to authority, responsibility, and accountability for nursing care. Each requires careful support and nurturing by significant persons within the organization.

While the size, complexity, and need of the institution for CNSs must be taken into account, there is a general feeling among nurse administrators and CNSs that new roles are best facilitated by introducing more than one into the organization.

---

*Reprinted with permission from job description for clinical supervisor/specialist, Department of Nursing Service, Harborview Medical Center, Seattle, Washington.

Careful handling of the selection process for the placement of a CNS is critical. There are risks in the process that need careful consideration. The situation within a given institution may influence the selection process in both positive and negative ways. There may be a positive climate of anticipation and support for a new clinical nurse leader and a readiness for effective problem solving between disciplines. There may have been a major expansion of facilities and services that has created a need for new nursing leadership. There may be a known applicant who was a former nurse on the staff, well recognized for her or his nursing skills and judgment, who would be particularly well received in the CNS role. Conversely, there may be a climate of distrust and unrest in the institution that has polarized the nursing staff on such significant issues as entry-level educational qualifications, contract negotiations, or relocation of clinical services. Pressures resulting from short-staffing may have aroused old angers concerning "too many leaders and not enough staff" to do the work. The involvement of key staff members in the interviewing process may confuse the candidates by giving them conflicting perceptions of the role and desired outcomes.

During the selection process, attitudes toward the role of the CNS will be heightened. The people whom the nurse administrator has selected to conduct the interviews should represent major groups within the institution that will have a significant effect on the outcome of the CNS role; these representatives should also be trusted as advisors within their respective groups. The nurse administrator should conduct the final interview, in order to clarify the issues and negotiate the terms for each candidate, and should also make the final decision to hire. It is not unusual to have different terms for each candidate, dependent upon their individual needs and goals and how the candidate will fit in as perceived by the nurse administrator.

Line Positions

The premise supporting the placement of the CNS in a line position extends beyond the need to have formal authority to enhance nurse practice. It values the management process and supports the belief that management of a clinical nursing unit or service by a clinically competent, master's-prepared nursing leader will advance the standards of nursing care and nursing practice in that institution. CNSs can and do perform well in these roles.

Placement of the clinical specialist in a line position usurps the roles traditionally held by head nurses or supervisory staff, where the primary focus was to meet the management goal of coordinating patient care services throughout the hospital. The CNS/manager facilitates these management goals by directing the optimal utilization of human and material resources in the most cost-effective manner to meet an achievable, defined *standard of nursing care*. The determination of standards for high-quality care, development of a systematic approach to achieving them, and justification of the financial base needed to support such care are the hallmarks of the functioning of the CNS/manager.

The CNS in a line position faces the daily problems and pressures that have affected nursing leaders since the development of departments of nursing services at the end of World War II. The degree of support for non-nursing departments within the institution and the effectiveness of their services influences the degree to which the CNS manager will be able to focus on clinical development of nursing practice. The nurse administrator must assume the leadership with other members of the hospital administrative team to foster a climate favorable to professional nursing practice. Recent testimony submitted before the National Commission of Nursing addressed the need for creative and effective organizational structures in hospitals to optimize nursing resources (National Commission on Nursing, 1981).

Additionally, the CNS is expected to face the continuous challenge of new techology and its relevance to nursing practice. The development of the nursing staff requires teaching and coaching skills and a clear set of expectations for performance by the staff under the CNS's direction. The mandate for increased productivity of the staff in the care-giving process to control the rising costs within hospital budgets or to respond to the federal price controls that affect the community health care system requires new skills and understanding as a responsible fiscal manager.

The CNS in a line position assists in the management of the nursing department and determines its future direction for professional nursing. The combination of a CNS with clinical competency and leadership skills and an organizational climate that values individual creativity within bureaucratic constraints is critical to the successful implementation of the role of clinical specialist/manager.

Staff Positions

The development of the role of the CNS in a staff position to manage a clinical case load of patients/clients and to serve as a consultant or liaison nurse was an attempt to assure full utilization of clinical expertise without concomitant management responsibilities. The staff position exists, however, within the overall organizational system of the nursing department and the health care system of the institution. The CNS in a staff position must have knowledge and develop an understanding of organizational system in which she or he functions.

Placement of the clinical specialist in an advisory, consultant staff role endorses and actualizes the professional status of nursing. It is expected that the incumbent will assess and diagnose clinical nursing problems with patients and staff, develop a series of interventions for patients or families with nursing and other health professionals, and monitor effectiveness and evaluate outcomes with the patient and the team. There is an implied or explicit expectation that the CNS will utilize research findings as well as contribute to clinical research. Examples of a CNS in a staff position include the psychiatric CNS who develops a psychiatric consultation service for both patient and staff behavior problems, the enterostomal therapist functioning in both inpatient and outpatient settings, the cardiac rehabilitation nurse consultant, and the primary practitioner on a hospice team. In each case, the CNS role was structured to meet an organizational goal and a clinical nursing service need that would directly benefit patient care.

As financial constraints squeeze the nursing budget, nurse administrators are beginning to shift clinical specialists from staff positions into the line, eliminating a traditional head nurse or supervisory role. It is too early to detect the impact of this beginning trend, but one must be concerned that the CNS' clinical and research efforts could be limited by the addition of primary management responsibilities.

Joint or Shared Appointment

Within academic medical centers, joint appointments between nursing education and nursing service have proved a successful way of funding the development of the CNS role. Such appointments must be congruent with the philosophy and mission of each institution, as well as with the career direction of the individual CNS. It is absolutely essential that the dean of the school of nursing and the director of nursing service have compatible goals and objectives within the personnel rules and regulations of the academic and health care institutions. The clinical specialist, as a member of both the faculty and the nursing service organization of the institution, must be able to work effectively within these systems to achieve mutually agreed upon goals of quality nursing education and nursing service. Within clinics and critical care units, where the need to be a part of the health care team and to be an effective teacher are equally significant, joint or shared appointments are especially valuable for both agencies.

It is also possible for an assertive CNS to negotiate shared appointments between two service agencies. In the author's agency, a resourceful CNS, when faced with termination of grant funds, sought and negotiated two half-time positions within the city in her specialty of epilepsy/neurosurgical clinical services. She functions in the clinical management role in the epilepsy center in one agency and in a consultant role in the second agency. This arrangement affords two institutions the opportunity to have a clinical specialist focus in a subspecialty field, with effective outcomes to date.

Positions in Community Health Care Systems or Extended Care Facilities

Since the patient/client is discharged as rapidly as possible from the tertiary care settings into the community health care system, the need for the CNS is beginning to become more evident in settings external to the hospital. The same process is utilized to consider placement of the CNS within the home health agency to meet clinical needs of clients or in the nursing home system to serve as the primary practitioner. Opportunities are arising for the CNS in the hospice movement organized within community home health agencies, as well as in the field of gerontology. Nurses in community agencies must be skilled members of interdisciplinary teams of health care professionals striving to meet the needs of client and family in the home or extended care facility. They represent the professional component of nursing in the total patient care plan and intervene on an individual and often independent basis.

EVALUATION

Once the role of the CNS has been established, no CNS should be allowed to float free within the organization without any responsibility for justifying the effectiveness of the role within the clinical setting. The CNS can be the best advocate for the role by systematically gathering data that describe the scope of clinical responsibilities and client contacts that illustrate the need for the CNS.

For example, the psychiatric CNS in the author's institution provides the author with both written and oral reports of her activities on a monthly basis. Since this role was designed to serve as a resource to the medical/surgical services for both staff and patient consultations, the author learns where the need is for psychiatric support throughout the department. A comparison of total staff consultation and patient consultation is maintained on a monthly and yearly basis. As we have watched the data over the past two years, patient census peaks correlate with the increased need for staff consultation. The units that have moved into primary care have increased patient consultation requests from the primary nurse. This composite of data on a monthly basis is rich in patient care anecdotes needed to describe and justify the effectiveness of clinical nursing consultation. It is also appropriate for the board of trustees report.

Another aspect of the evaluation process is the review of data to determine if the role needs to be changed or modified in relation to the department's objectives or changing client population. An orthopaedic CNS, whose initial role expectation was to work with traumatic amputees in the younger age group, discovered that over 50 percent of her clientele were over the age of 50. Breakdown of a year's data demonstrated that 141 amputations were the result of trauma and affected patients under the age of 30; 179 amputations were the result of peripheral vascular disease and the patients were elderly. This data required reordering of priorities but also facilitated the justification of the CNS role, who was needed not only to promote the new senior health care program but to collaborate in meeting unmet needs of the elderly who had had amputations due to chronic vascular disease.

For the evaluation of the effectiveness of the CNS [in a line position] both clinical and management variables are considered. Data that address retention of nursing staff, participation of staff at educational forums, quality assurance, and documentation of care is useful in monitoring clinical leadership skills. A balanced budget and evidence of interdepartmental problem solving addresses management skills. Reduction in the length of stay of patients may correlate with a more sophisticated nursing process that has been advanced by the CNS. It is the combination of data that justifies the effectiveness of the role. Until more research on the nursing care system and the role of the CNS is readily available, the nurse administrator and the CNS must evaluate the results.

The essence of sophisticated justification of the credibility of the CNS role is to provide systematic data that show not only positive clinical outcomes resulting from the activities of the CNS but also negative ones due to insufficient nursing care. One can then prospectively negotiate for appropriate resources or a modification of the unit environment. In this process the nursing administrator and the CNS combine their efforts and expertise in advocating improvements in patient care.

SUMMARY

It is evident that the justification and structuring of the CNS role within nursing service organizations requires negotiation and mutual support between the nurse administrator and the CNS. The decade of the 80's will see changes in the health care delivery system. The nurse administrator and the clinical specialist will need to assess and evaluate these trends continually and to judge their implications to assure the continued advance of clinical specialization in organized nursing services.

REFERENCES

American Nurses' Association. *Nursing: A social policy statement.* Kansas City: American Nurses' Association, 1980.

American Nurses' Association. *Summary of proceedings, report of the president.* Kansas City: American Nurses' Association, 1981.

Baker, C., & Kramer, M. To define or not to define: The role of the clinical specialist. *Nurs Forum*, 1970, *4*, 41–55.

Barrett, J. "Administrative factors in development of new nursing practice roles." *J Nurs Adm*, 1971, *1*, 25–30.

Blake, P. The clinical specialist as nurse consultant. *J Nurs Adm*, 1977, *7*, 33–36.

Everson, S.J. Integration of the role of clinical nurse specialist. *Journal of Continuing Education in Nursing*, 1981, *12*, 16–19.

National Commission on Nursing. *National Commission on Nursing Summary of public hearings.* Chicago: Hospital Research and Education Trust, 1981.

Parkis, E.W. The management role of the clinical specialist. Pt. 1. *Superv Nurse*, 1974, *5*, 44–51; Pt. 2, 1974, *5*, 24–35.

Schaefer, J.A. The satisfied clinician: Administrative support makes the difference. *J Nurs Adm*, 1973, *3*, 17–20.

9. Joint Appointments

Mary L. Gresham

The clinical nurse specialist (CNS) with a joint appointment is a nurse with a master's degree, in either a staff or line position, who has formal lines of responsibility to both the dean of a school of nursing and the director of nursing service in some health care delivery system. Such an individual has been given many titles, various responsibilities, and numerous positions within organizational structures. The basic characteristic of the joint-appointment CNS (JACNS), however, that of dual responsibility to both a nursing service organization and a school of nursing, has not changed. Amounts of time allocated and activities involved in each arena vary, but the dual responsibility and accountability remain.

HISTORICAL DEVELOPMENT

Joint appointments for CNSs evolved out of the clinical specialist movement that occurred in the late 1960s and early 1970s. The CNS with a joint appointment was one of the organizational models attempted early in the development of the CNS role. Campbell (1973) described one of the first "joint appointees," who functioned at the University of Wisconsin during 1965–1966. The individual was to be a faculty member and supervisor in the hospital, responsible to the dean of the college of nursing

The author would like to thank Joan LeSage, Ph.D., R.N., and Carol Dall, M.S.N., R.N., for their constructive criticism and suggestions in the preparation of this chapter.

and the director of nursing service at the hospital. The JACNS was in a line position, with responsibilities for patient care, staff development, and student learning experiences on a clinical unit. The JACNS participated in long-range planning with the unit head nurse who managed day-to-day affairs on the unit. There is no published data on the success of this endeavor or on how other early joint appointees have fared.

Christman (1973), Cooper (1973), and Sutton (1973) focused more attention on the CNS with a joint or dual appointment by describing organizational models necessary for implementation, and guidelines for success within the position. The development of nursing as a profession based in clinical practice and incorporating education and research provided the impetus for creation of joint appointments for the CNS. A second outcome expected from creating joint appointments was a narrowing of the gap between theory and practice. This would occur because those faculty teaching students would also be involved in current nursing practice.

The practitioner/teacher model was described by Christman (1980) as an additional refinement in the development of the JACNS role, because it was not merely a new position within an existing structure but "an organizational device that is constructed to enable a professional practitioner to play the full professional role" (p. 5). Table 9-1 shows the position description for a practitioner/teacher at Rush University, with components of the role clearly delineated. Salaries for practitioner/teachers are shared by the college of nursing and the hospital unit on which the individual practices. Sharing of salaries distributes the cost of highly skilled practicing faculty and allows a greater number of full-time faculty to be employed. Other benefits of this arrangement include lower student–faculty ratios, lower patient–nurse ratios, and a larger pool of qualified individuals to develop and implement clinical research.

Since the mid-seventies, the number of JACNS positions has not increased significantly or even shown gradual consistent growth except in a few areas of the country. The number will not increase unless and until faculty see the importance of clinical practice to professional role behavior. Widespread acceptance of the need for faculty to participate in delivery of nursing care will result in creative development of organizational models necessary to support professional activity in the areas of education, clinical practice, and research. Even in institutions where the joint appointment model exists, recruitment of faculty willing to practice, in addition to carrying education and research responsibilities, is difficult (Sovie, 1981b). That some of this reluctance to practice on the part of faculty is based on insufficient or inaccurate information is an underlying assumption of this chapter. Through a specific and honest presentation of the role as interpreted by one JACNS, it is hoped that others will use the information

Table 9-1

Practitioner/Teacher* Position Description (Rush University)

Clinical	Administration	Education	Research
Functions as a clinical practitioner in area(s) of expertise.	Participates in the operational management of the department, college of nursing, and division of nursing.	Directs the learning of students in the clinical setting.	Applies research findings in one's own practice and teaching.
Assists in planning and implementing health education programs for patients and families with the primary nurse.	Participates in the unit and departmental decision making.	Facilitates the learning of students in the classroom setting.	Interprets research projects and/or findings to nursing staff and students.
Collaborates with the health care team to assess, plan, direct, and evaluate the treatment approach.	Participates in the management of a unit as negotiated with the head nurse/unit leader and departmental leadership.	Interprets the Rush University programs to patients, staff, and others.	Collaborates with members of related disciplines in research activities.
Serves as a resource person to the nursing personnel in the evaluation of nursing care.	Participates in the professional development and evaluation of students, staff, and peers.	Participates in unit and department educational efforts.	Assists with the development and implementation of nursing and health-related studies.
Serves as a consultant in patient care situations/settings.		Participates in the development and implementation of continuing education/electives.	Plans, implements, and publishes studies and projects as negotiated.

Reprinted with permission from the College of Nursing, Rush University, Chicago, Ill., internal document.

*Practitioner/teachers are faculty members who actively effect quality patient care in the clinical and classroom settings through an integrated role as clinician, educator, consultant, and researcher. The practitioner/teacher (PT) role is highly individualized; each PT contracts with the departmental chairperson a balance of the components of the role that may vary on a quarterly basis.

to their advantage in implementing joint appointment positions in a variety of settings.

The remainder of this chapter will speak specifically to the experiences, observations, and opinions of one JACNS who has been in a joint appointment position for more than five years. The author has had experience with a variety of clinical specialists, including that as a student taught by faculty both with and without joint appointments, as a staff nurse providing care to patients on units with and without a JACNS, and as a head nurse on a clinical unit to which a JACNS was assigned (Gresham, 1976). This varied experience with the JACNS role provides the basis for a primarily positive presentation of the actual and potential contributions of this model.

DESCRIPTION OF THE ROLE

According to Christman (1979), there are four components to the professional role of the JACNS, whom he calls the practitioner/teacher: clinical practice, education, research, and consultation. Administrative duties are related specifically to each of the four areas, rather than being separate from these professional activities. Organizationally, all are unit-based, whether the CNS has a line or staff appointment. This provides a clinical focus, geographical limits, and thus structure for most activities. The one exception to the unit-based model is the psychiatric/liaison CNS who may have a clinical consultative practice with several units. Teaching involvement for these JACNSs may be more appropriate for graduate than undergraduate students because of the nature of the practice and the broad clinical base. It is important to the success and satisfaction of all that a JACNS be responsible for no more than 35–40 clients. The clinical practice and educational and administrative responsibilities involved with clients and staff on a unit larger than this become overwhelming and imprac- tical.

The number and type of administrative duties vary among individuals, based primarily on whether one is in a staff or line position. A JACNS in a line position will spend more time and direct more activity to clinically related administrative responsibilities. Examples of such activities include committee work related to patient care, supervision and evaluation of staff, and long-range planning for patient care programs. It is imperative that there be organizational support for the day-to-day administrative activities such as scheduling of staff, maintenance of staff records, and problem solving with non-nursing, patient-support services. Such administrative support can be in the form of secretarial help, head nurses or assistant head nurses, or strong leadership in clinical support service departments (such as dietetics or pharmacy).

A JACNS in a staff position will have less time and activity in clinical administration but more in education or research-related endeavors. Administrative duties in these areas could include membership in academic or research committes, student counselling and advising, academic administration of a specific course, program, or section, or preparing grant applications and research reports. Again, as with clinical administrative functions, it is crucial to have adequate support in such areas as secretarial help, budgetary consultation, and preparation of teaching aids.

Conceptually and practically, clinical practice is the basis for everything else that is done within the framework of the role. Faculty must be committed to participating in clinical practice and be convinced that their advanced knowledge and skills will make a positive impact on patient care programs and the quality of student learning (Sovie, 1981a). Without such a philosophy and commitment, the benefits will not be obtained, even in the most supportive organizational structure.

The first and most crucial step for a new JACNS is to establish clinical credibility. The thought of having to do this may be threatening or insulting to an expert clinician. It is, however, absolutely imperative that staff, students, and significant others (physicians, other professionals) see for themselves that a person who professes to be a clinical expert actually is one (Anderson, 1976; Gresham, 1967; Hamory, 1976). A strong clinical base will also facilitate other components of the role. Establishing clinical credibility is particularly important to the JACSN in a staff position (Cooper, 1973). A clinical specialist with a line position has built-in authority, whereas one in a staff position must obtain authority from demonstrated professional competence. A minimum of three months of primary clinical practice is needed to lay the foundation for clinical credibility.

What does the JACNS do when active in clinical practice? A majority of time is best spent providing direct, "hands on" care of clients/patients and their families. The choice of which clients/patients to care for may be based on a number of factors, discussed elsewhere in this book. The cases chosen, however, should be ones that will allow clinical expertise and sophisticated problem-solving ability to emerge. A dangerous attitude, too frequently revealed by clinical specialists when it is suggested that they provide regular, direct patient care, is expressed by the comment "I didn't get my master's degree to be a staff nurse." This attitude, however it is expressed, discredits staff nurses and their work. The way in which clinical expertise is demonstrated is critical, since respect for staff competencies must be clearly conveyed (Gordon, 1973).

The JACNS with either a line or staff position may participate in similar clinical administrative activities, such as orienting or precepting new staff, including development and evaluation of the new staff member; planning and coordinating staff development and in-serice programs once needs have been identified; and maintaining or improving the standard of care by reinforcing (or changing as needed) policies and procedures. A major difference, as mentioned earlier in this chapter, is the amount of time spent in clinical administrative functions. Another major difference is that the JACNS in a line position has delegated authority and responsibility for all the patient care, educational, and nursing research activities on a particular unit. Some of these responsibilities may be delegated, but the CNS has ultimate accountability.

The staff JACNS, on the other hand, has some administrative expectations built into the clinical aspect of the role (see Table 9-1), but the specific activities will be negotiated with other nursing administrative personnel on the unit (for example, head nurses, assistant head nurses, another CNS with a line position) (Hamory, 1976).

The educational component or faculty aspect of the role becomes integrated into many of the activities associated with clinical practice. Once a firm clinical base has been established, the JACNS can more easily focus on teaching, both formally and informally. Participation in clinical or classroom teaching requires familarity with the course objectives, content, clinical evaluation tools, and the relationship of a course to the overall curriculum. This information is more easily learned when one is not simultaneously learning how to deliver care on a clinical unit. Relationships between a course and clinical practice are more readily learned when the faculty member is familiar with the clinical area. The JACNS is best prepared for teaching if she or he also has some formal preparation in teaching methods and strategies. Clinical expertise alone does not ensure that one can teach others effectively.

Clinical teaching of students in a patient care area will be made easier by assigning students to care for patients who are in the JACNS's case load. An obvious advantage of having a unit-based JACNS is that the specialist knows all of the patients on the unit to some degree, though some better than others. Extensive time is not spent reviewing medical records and discussing patients with staff. Since the faculty member is familiar with the patients, more time can be spent with the students in providing care and integrating course content. As Peplau (1973) emphasized, any teacher who does not give care regularly becomes rusty, which increases her or his own felt inadequacy and interferes with teaching effectiveness (p. 26). Familiarity with the usual type of patient on the unit also allows the JACNS more opportunity for creative teaching when the content of a course is particularly difficult. For example, a gerontological CNS who was a clinical instructor in a biological concepts course in an undergraduate integrated curriculum was to teach a unit in the course on reproductive physiology. The faculty member was teaching her group of students on the unit to which she was assigned, which was in a hospital for the elderly. Because of her extensive experience with elderly patients, the CNS was easily able to interpret for the students changes in the reproductive system and sexual behavior that are common in the aged.

The gap between theory and practice fades when the clinical specialist both practices and teaches on the same patient care unit (Christman, 1973; Cooper, 1973; Sutton, 1973). Integration of students into a unit is also easier if the way has been paved with staff—that is, if the JACNS has developed positive relationships with the staff and has interpreted the various components of the JACNS role to them. The quickest and most effective way to do this is to spend time working beside the staff nurses as the JACNS provides direct care to her or his own patients. Staff can be notified ahead of time that responsibilities (and, therefore, time commitments) will shift as the JACNS develops her or his plans to teach students clinically.

Classroom teaching can also be enhanced by clinical practice. Clinical examples make theory and concepts come alive and enhance integration of theory and practice. Students, particularly undergraduate students, are most interested to hear about the personal clinical experiences of the CNS; such examples make lectures more interesting and meaningful. The CNS's own clinical experiences can also be used effectively to vary teaching strategies. For example, using a case study from one's own practice can provide excellent seminar discussion of a concept or process that needs reinforcement.

Implementing the research component of the professional nurse's role is frequently a major concern (some methods for achieving this goal are suggested in Chapter 6). Maintaining research-based clinical practice is one way of being active in this area of professional activity. One must allow some time periodically to read research material applicable to one's specialty and also in the area of education. Sound research data can be used by the JACNS in the following ways: to reinforce or change current patient care practices and policies; as reference material for staff development; as reference material for students practicing in a specific clinical area.

To stimulate interest and increase the use of research findings in practice, one JACNS organized a departmental journal club. The group of faculty met monthly to discuss current research on selected clinical topics. Others have developed research questions and projects out of their own clinical practice. Clearly, implementing a project of one's own or facilitating another's research on one's own unit is made much easier when the researcher knows the unit's strengths and weaknesses as a result of being an integral part of it.

The CNS consultant subrole, a highly valued aspect of the role, is discussed in detail in Chapter 7. This component is often the one clinical specialists wish to develop first. However, a sound consultative practice is often the last aspect of one's role to evolve. It is worth waiting and working for. To be sought out as a consultant by one's own staff or peers, by staff or peers elsewhere in the institution, or by persons or organizations outside one's place of employment implies an earned reputation for expertise. Such a reputation must be individually developed. Evidence of clinical expertise evolves out of the patient care–related activities of the CNS delineated earlier.

How does one person manage to do all these things? It must be clearly understood that no one does them all at the same time. One moves in and out of major activities over a period of time. It is essential to set priorities daily, weekly, monthly, and yearly. While establishing a clinical basis for practice and development of the role, a JACNS would not also be engaged in major teaching activities. While actively involved in direct teaching of students, the amount of time spent in delivering patient care is less. As time and activity in one aspect of the role increase, they are decreased or adjusted proportionally in other aspects. It is unrealistic, in fact impossible, to consistently participate 100 percent in all components of the professional role at once.

OPINIONS ABOUT THE JOINT APPOINTMENT MODEL

The joint appointment model is either liked or disliked, supported or not supported (both philosophically and practically) by CNSs and nurse educators. Rarely is there a person who, if they understand it, feels neutral. Those who do not support the model provide very specific reasons why it does not work. They say that frequent requests to justify one's existence are draining; personal and professional gratification are delayed and indirect; the joint appointment creates role confusion, not just for the CNS but for staff as well; the demands on one's time to be CNS to staff, teacher to students, and part-time nursing administrator are exhausting; unrealistic expectations in two areas—education and practice—result in guilt and frustration; overlapping responsibilities with other leadership personnel cause conflicts; job descriptions are vague; there is lack of organizational support; and finally, the JACNS does not receive adequate reimbursement for faculty practice (Anderson, 1976; Hamory, 1976; Holm, 1981; Sutton, 1973). Additionally, many faculty members openly admit that they fear clinical practice. Enough time has elapsed so that they have "forgotten how," are rusty, and feel inadequate in clinical practice. Their honesty is admirable and can help explain their anxiety and why many of them would not be willing to become directly involved in patient care. Teaching may have become safe and secure. Another perspective on why faculty may not like dual responsibilities was suggested by Simms (1973). If a nurse leaves patient care and chooses to teach in a school of nursing, it may be because she or he decries the standard of nursing practice in the hospital. Unfortunately, however, this puts the CNS in a position where she or he cannot improve nursing practice because she or he is no longer associated with it (p. 149).

Those who support the joint appointment model in concept and practice do so because of its potential for integrating theory and practice and its potential for allowing expression of the full professional role for nurses. There are other numerous advantages of a joint appointment for a CNS. Patient care is often improved because of the direct involvement of the CNS. Student learning is enhanced because the faculty are an integral part of the patient care unit, familiar with staff, policies and procedures, and regularly give direct patient care. The JACNS's own clinical skills are maintained, and her or his knowledge is kept current. Self-direction of the JACNS is enhanced because time commitments are flexible. A joint appointment promotes trust between staff, the JACNS, and students (Sutton, 1973, p. 231). The mutual distrust that often exists between a school of nursing and its related hospital can be minimized, if not eliminated entirely, because of built-in organizational and structural links that enhance communication. Problems arising in either service or education can be studied with more objectivity because the JACNS has sources of information and firsthand knowledge from both areas. Finally, a recent argument in favor of the joint appointment model is that it may be economically beneficial to schools of nursing to share faculty salaries with health care institutions (Holm, 1981).

IMPLEMENTING THE ROLE

There are six keys to the successful implementation of the JACNS role:

1. A supportive organizational structure,
2. A balance between personal and organizational goals,
3. Communication,
4. Regular clinical practice,
5. Economy of effort,
6. Defining realistic expectations.

Because of the author's personal experience with it, the practitioner/teacher model will be used as an example throughout this discussion.

Supportive Organizational Structure

The following structural or organizational factors are necessary for successful implementation of the JACNS role: the dean of the school of nursing should also be the director of nursing service, the school of nursing must be geographically close to the setting where patient care is given and should be located in a university medical center where related educational programs are ongoing, and other CNSs should be employed in similar positions in the institution (Sutton, 1973, p. 223). Christman (1980, p. 5) describes the matrix organizational format in which the practitioner/teacher functions. Doctorally prepared nurses called chairpersons have overall responsibility for clinical practice, education, and research activities for one clinical nursing department. All faculty within a department are assigned to a clinical area. Once a year each faculty member negotiates a contract with the chairperson of her or his respective clinical department, and the percentage of time each CNS will spend in the areas of clinical practice, education, and research over the ensuing year is outlined. Since the chairpersons of clinical departments are responsible ultimately to the dean of the college of nursing, who is also director of nursing services, the goals of both service and education are included in planning. Participation in educational programs and patient care is expected of all faculty. The department chairperson meets yearly goals by balancing time allocations within individual contracts of her or his faculty (Christman, 1980, p. 7).

Individual faculty contracts are a significant part of the structure supporting a joint appointment role. Table 9-2 shows the time allocation specified in a typical 12-month contract for a JACNS practitioner/teacher. Guidelines exist for the types of activities included in each category to which time is allocated. For example, educational activities over the course of a year for the individual with this sample contract might include both instruction (acting as clinical instructor for undergraduate students for two quarters of an academic year) and administration (attending regular faculty meetings; counselling and advising students). Research activities might focus on projects such as spending four to five hours each week for six months doing literature review and developing a research proposal for implementation the following contract year. Patient care activities might be both direct (providing patient care one to two days each week for five to six months) and indirect (consultative services; supervising students giving direct care; developing or revising patient care policies). Administrative activities might include participating in committee meetings directly related to patient care. This is just one model of organizational structure that

Table 9-2
Sample 12-Month Contract for a JACNS

Type of Activity	Percentage of Time Allocated to Each Activity
Academic	
Educational	
Instruction	30
Administration	5
Research	
Projects	10
Administration	0
Nonacademic	
Patient Care	
Direct	30
Indirect	20
Administration	5

Adapted from *Employment contract for members of Rush University faculty.*

facilitates implementation of the JACNS role. Others exist and should be examined for adaptation to individual settings (Blazeck, Selekman, Timpe, & Wolfe, 1982; Sovie, 1981).

Balancing Personal and Organizational Goals

It is possible for both an individual and the organization to obtain satisfaction from joint appointment positions. To achieve this satisfaction, individual and organizational goals must both be met, at least to some degree. JACNSs must have their own individual set of personal and professional goals. They must also be aware of the goals of the college of nursing and the clinical units to which they belong. Once the goals and responsibilities of all involved are known, the fine art of negotiating an individual faculty contract begins. Specific activities and the percentage of time allocated to various areas (clinical practice, education, research) determine the configuration of one's professional life for the duration of the contract. CNSs should understand the organization's responsibilities for patient care and student education. On the basis of these, they should determine what is negotiable and what is not. It is important to clarify these areas, for they can affect the goals and expectations one has for oneself as well as anticipated time frames for their achievement.

For example, because of departmental responsibilities to students, a JACNS may be directed to allocate 50 percent of her or his time to education. Based on needs of the clinical area, she or he may be directed to allocate much of the remaining time to clinical practice (from which research and consultation activities will evolve, as has been discussed). To be given direction in allocating time to practice and education should not upset or offend the JACNS. Anyone accepting a joint appointment must expect to practice and teach professional nursing. Understanding of and support for the goals of the organization will assist in identifying the individual professional goals and activities that can be accomplished.

This is the secret to balancing individual with organizational goals. Within the broad role description for the JACNS, the specialist must develop specific goals. A plan of action (which translates into specific activities) for attaining goals must also be developed. These individual goals and activities must be carefully planned. It is in their development that "economy of effort" is so crucial (Christman, 1979, 1980). Table 9-2, with the related interpretation, is an example of how planning and balancing of goals come together in an individual faculty contract. Discriminating between the various options and activities available, bearing in mind the potential of each to be used in a variety of ways, then implementing the role on the basis of these decisions will enhance the potential for success and satisfaction.

What may appear to be nonnegotiable areas within the joint appointment position can offer multiple opportunities for professional growth and satisfaction. For example, teaching, whether in the classroom or at the bedside, provides the JACNS many chances to present her- or himself to students, patients, and peers as an expert clinician. Clinical practice, on the other hand, supplies a wealth of experiences that can be used in teaching, staff development, professional writing, developing research proposals, and consultation.

Once goals and activities have been identified and agreed upon by those involved (on the basis of organizational structure), a contract is drawn up. Communication of these elements of the contract must be ongoing with staff, students, and (when appropriate) patients. Provided all necessary considerations were made prior to signing the contract, the contract should provide direction for implementation of the role.

Communication

Even Holm, who critically analyzed the joint appointment position that she held for five years, emphasized the importance of communication in role success or failure (1981). Once a contract has been signed, the JACNS must frequently clarify her or his multiple responsibilities and activities. This must be a continuing effort, since even within one contract year activities and time involvements may shift several times. As education commitments shift during an academic year, the JACNS will have more or less time for her or his own practice. Staff, patients, and faculty to whom one is accountable must be kept aware when responsibilities and time commitments have changed. Such communication need not be interpreted by the JACNS as "reporting to" staff or others. Instead, it indicates mutual respect for those whose primary or only focus is the clinical unit. The JACNS will be missed when other commitments limit her or his time on the unit. Staff and unit leadership personnel must understand and respect the different, equally important responsibility a JACNS has for educating students. The JACNS must keep others aware of her or his varying activities (Gresham, 1976).

One useful tactic is for the JACNS to post her or his weekly schedule on the clinical unit. All regular meetings and activities should be listed, including contact time with students (teaching, advising, office hours), class hours, clinical practice, and lecture preparation time. In this way staff and others on the unit can easily see the types of activities the JACNS engages in when away from the clinical area. It is wise to maintain daily contact with the unit staff and patients during those times when the CNS is less involved there, in order to convey concern, interest, and support. Additionally, there may be a priority need or problem that the JACNS can be helpful with even if time is limited.

Regular Clinical Practice

Success and satisfaction with the joint appointment position results from regular clinical practice in which the CNS can demonstrate her or his clinical expertise. Clinical practice is also the source for research questions, which, when explored, can improve the quality of care provided. The way the JACNS intervenes with patients serves as a model for the nurses caring for other patients. Sutton has clearly summarized other benefits of clinical practice for the JACNS. Giving direct care provides an opportunity for the JACNS to observe staff delivering care, facilitating identification of their strengths and weaknesses, so that staff development programs can be planned. The JACNS is also available to staff when she or he is on the clinical unit with students. Because of the JACNS's link with the clinical unit, she or he is in a position to make changes in the environment that will enhance student learning. The JACNS will also be aware of resources available to students on the unit and may therefore facilitate the students' use of those resources and improve patient care. Student ideas for improving patient care are more acceptable to staff for inclusion in nursing care plans because staff share with the CNS a common goal, providing high quality patient care. Staff can often assist in evaluation of students when they are familiarized with evaluation criteria by the JACNS. (Sutton,

1973). With time and well-established, unit-based clinical credibility, the JACNS should find that the clinical consultation area of practice begins to expand, as unit personnel and even practitioners in other clinical disciplines learn what the JACNS has to offer.

Economy of Effort

Christman suggests that economy of effort is basic to successful implementation of the complete professional nursing role, which he has described in terms of the practitioner/teacher model (Christman, 1979, 1980). The concept of economy of effort, simply stated, means making the most out of every professional activity. Any CNS may find the concept useful, but it is extremely helpful to the JACNS, who, because of the nature of the role, must constantly juggle activities and make decisions about priorities. The JACNS must look at everything she or he does or contemplates doing with this question in mind: How can I make the most out of this activity? While delivering nursing care, the JACNS should ask

1. What can be learned from each clinical situation?
2. What can the CNS bring to the situation that is different?
3. How can students and staff or patients and their families learn from the situation?
4. Can the situation be used again? If so, how and for whom?
5. In significantly rewarding or disappointing clinical situations, the JACNS can analyze facts and their relationships, determine cause and effect; write down the facts and an evaluation of the event; use the event as a case study for education of staff, students, and peers, as basis for a research question, or save for possible use in consultation.

Other questions to ask about all current or prospective activities that can economize efforts and maximize their effects include

1. Is it publishable?
2. Would it serve as an alternate teaching/learning strategy for staff, students, peers?
3. Can it be adapted for patient teaching? How?
4. Could the JACNS contribute to the development of staff, students, or peers by involving them in or delegating to them the activity, instead of doing it oneself?
5. Could it be used for continuing education inside or outside one's place of employment? How?
6. Could it help to develop or strengthen one's own professional consultation? How?

Certain personal characteristics can facilitate economizing one's efforts. These include initiative, self-direction, ability to analyze and organize people and events, patience, flexibility, skill in setting priorities, and respect for the competencies of others (Baker, 1973; Campbell, 1973; Christman, 1979; Flatter, 1976; Gordon, 1973; Hamory, 1976; Johnson, Wilcox, & Moidel, 1970).

Defining Realistic Expectations

The JACNS frequently is the one in the institution who expects the most of her- or himself. The author's conclusion, based on personal experience and observation, is that many JACNSs do not give themselves a chance to succeed because they expect to fulfill all aspects of their role right from the beginning. It takes a minimum of one full year to experience the interaction among all components of the role and begin to feel comfortable with them. Clinical specialists who will be providing direct patient care should allow themselves a reasonable length of time to become familiar with patient care delivery systems and other health team members. For those who teach, becoming familiar with the educational system, admission and progression criteria, curriculum, individual courses, and faculty/ student resources takes time as well. CNSs who will be teaching for the first time, or for the first time in a new system, will need more time at first to develop lectures, examinations, and teaching plans. At the end of 9 months, the JACNS can be reasonably comfortable with both education and practice. At this point, a noticeable increase in satisfaction is usually experienced. Change in the self and others takes time and is not always pleasant when in progress.

During the first year, the JACNS will probably need (and should seek out and accept) assistance in setting priorities. Some trade-offs should be anticipated. This becomes most evident in the process of contracting, when the balance between personal and organizational goals must be reached. Several of the JACNS's own goals may have to be changed to become closer to what is possible within the organization, or the time frame for accomplishing a goal may have be altered. It is very important, however, for the JACNS to plan ways of achieving success for her- or himself. This means planning some goals that are easily achievable and planning intermediate steps to be used in reaching longer-term or more complex goals. Individual priorities and interests need to be communicated to the appropriate people within the organization (one must take time to find out who these are). Specific activities and suggestions can then be offered.

For example, a new JACNS had as a long-term goal to effectively lecture to a large group of students. In preparation for this, and because lecturers for most major courses had already been decided for the next four months, she felt that presenting several staff development sessions would be helpful. She would have practice organizing a brief presentation, preparing for discussion, and becoming familiar with some of the educational resources available. She discussed her short-term goal with the unit leadership group, which had developed a list of staff development needs. The CNS was able to meet one of her own goals, meet a need of the staff (which had been identified by them), and participate in meeting one of the goals of the clinical unit leadership. All these goals were accomplished in two staff development sessions.

Closely associated with making reasonable expectations of oneself is identifying sources of support. The CNS should anticipate some ambiguity and frustration initially but plan to deal with these. As expert clinicians, we all know the value of anticipatory planning for potential problems. We teach this to clients/patients and to students, and we should practice it more on ourselves. Peers, counselling services if available in one's place of employment, nursing administrative personnel, and others outside the place of work, (such as spouse or friends) can all be sources of support.

Satisfactions and Frustrations

Even if the JACNS does everything "right" and has good organizational support, she or he will experience frustrations with the role. It is hoped, however, that with some anticipatory planning, organizational support, and specific suggestions such as discussed in this chapter, many of these frustrations can be eliminated or at least minimized.

One common problem that can cause anxiety for the JACNS, besides unrealistic expectations of oneself, is unrealistic expectations by others. Because one's time is divided between faculty duties, clinical responsibilities, and research activity, others often expect 100 percent of the JACNS's time and effort to be given to one aspect of the role. One suggestion for dealing with this problem is easier to say than it is to implement, but it is also the most practical approach. When, for example, someone demands 100 percent of one's time for educational activities and less than this is allocated, the individual should be reminded of the percentage of time planned for academic work. When one's supervisor is making significantly different demands on one's time than were negotiated and contracted for, perhaps a new contract would be in order.

After five years of working in the role, the author continues to have periodic guilt about not doing more in one area or another of the CNS role. The personal growth seen in this area is that the guilt is episodic, and much less frequent and intense than during the first 12–18 months as a JACNS. Another frustration is that committee responsibilities grow as one's length of time with an institution grows. One must learn to graciously decline an appointment or at least put off a decision about joining another committee until it is clear where it falls in personal and organizational priorities. One must also learn to ask the reason for being chosen and whether there is another faculty member equally qualified and interested. These approaches are gradually introduced as one becomes comfortable and reasonably credible in the position. It takes time, practice, observation, and many mistakes to develop comfort and skill in using these strategies.

The last major frustration is the difficulty of obtaining evaluation data regarding professional performance, because of the different components of the role. When time and activities are split between service and education, it is often difficult for any one person (other than oneself) to know what one does or how well it is done. Two previously discussed strategies can help: communication and economy of effort. By discriminating and planning carefully, some control can be obtained over the number of others one interacts with. This will limit the number of individuals who must be communicated to about goals and activities. It is important, then, to be sure to keep key people informed of goals and activities and periodically, to seek feedback on the quality of one's performance. It is important that for each of the major time and activity commitments the JACNS makes she or he identify one person to keep informed and to provide feedback. This will more safely ensure that adequate evaluation is made of total role performance. For example, an assistant head nurse could help to evaluate clinical contributions. A faculty colleague could provide feedback on teaching skill and effectiveness.

What are the satisfactions of the JACNS position? These have been enumerated in the literature and include assisting staff to become better nurses (Campbell, 1973); being perceived as a clinically competent practitioner by staff, who then accept the JACNS's authority as an expert and allow her or his decisions to influence their behavior (Hamory, 1976); seeing staff and students expand and refine the scientific basis of their practice because of the role modeling behavior of the JACNS (Christman, 1973); improvement in the quality of care delivered to patients/clients; ability to change standards of care on the unit because one is an integral part of it; maintenance of one's own clinical competence; ease of exchange between one's students and staff; putting theory into practice and keeping theory practical; strengthening communication between service and education, thus reducing mutual distrust and hostility; facilitating teaching of students by providing a realistic learning environment in which students can actively participate (Sutton, 1973).

While it is difficult to add to this list, the author has personally experienced other satisfactions that are directly related to the specific institution where she works and the length of time she has spent as a

JACNS. There may be merit in mentioning them because they can be generalized to other settings.

The entire division of nursing in the author's institution operates under the practitioner/teacher model described by Christman (1980). All college of nursing faculty have both educational and clinical practice expectations, regardless of their position in the organization. One's peers and supervisors are all involved in efforts to improve patient care through planning, negotiating, communicating, balancing goals, economizing efforts, and determining what is feasible; being part of this common effort with one's colleagues gives great satisfaction.

Other satisfactions for the author include the opportunities for professional writing and publication afforded by clinical practice and educational activities; continuing relationships with former patients and their families; increasing opportunities both inside and outside the institution for consultation within a clinical specialty; increased interest and involvement in nursing research; ongoing positive relationships with staff; and increased interest on the part of students in the specialty of the JACNS; in this case high-qualilty health care for older adults. A variety of rewarding professional activities are possible for the creative JACNS in a supportive organization.

Viability for the Future

If for no other reason than economics, the joint appointment role is a viable one for the future. As so aptly put by Holm (1981), nursing education programs are caught between increasing operating costs and shrinking government funds, so that "sharing the burden of faculty salaries with health care institutions is an attractive option and a good reason to interest faculty in practice" (p. 655). Health care financing will become a larger issue in the future, and hospitals will be looking for ways to maintain quality while cutting costs. Sharing faculty salaries will also allow health care institutions to benefit from the expertise of advanced practitioners.

Other reasons for continued development of the joint appointment role relate specifically to the reasons for which the JACNS role was initially developed. JACNS positions are a necessity if nursing education is to be relevant, up-to-date, challenging, and alive for students in the future. Faculty must practice what they teach students to do: deliver skillful, scientifically based nursing care. Through practice and education the joint appointment offers the CNS a means of sharing clinical knowledge and skill to benefit students, staff, and patients and their families.

SUMMARY

This chapter has described how one model of the joint appointment can work. Clearly there are organizational and individual factors that facilitate or inhibit effective implementation of the role. The attitude and orientation of an individual to the role is also crucial to one's success with it. CNSs choosing any model of the joint appointment position must approach it realistically. Time must be taken to plan an approach to the opportunities and challenges the role offers. One must be flexible and change one's approaches if they are not initially effective. Most of all, JACNS's must give themselves and others time to get oriented to the role, develop it, and then make changes necessary to improve the health care delivered within one's scope of responsibility.

REFERENCES

Anderson, M. The clinical nurse specialist in a staff position: Sources of authority. In P. Chamings & R. Markel (Eds.), *Symposium on the clinical nurse specialist.* Indianapolis: Sigma Theta Tau, 1976.

Baker, V. E. Retrospective explorations in role development. In J. P. Riehl & J. W. McVay (Eds.), *The clinical nurse specialist: Interpretations.* New York: Appleton-Century-Crofts, 1973.

Blazeck, A. M., Selekman, J., Timpe, M., & Wolf, Z. R. Unification: Nursing education and nursing practice. *Nursing and Health Care,* 1982, *3,* 18–24.

Campbell, E. B. The clinical nurse specialist: Joint appointee. In E. P. Lewis (Ed.), *The clinical nurse specialist.* New York: Merideth, 1973.

Christman, L. Influence of specialization on the nursing profession. In J. P. Riehl & J. W. McVay (Eds.), *The clinical nurse specialist: Interpretations.* New York: Appleton-Century-Crofts, 1973.

Christman, L. The practitioner–teacher. *Nurse Educator,* 1979, *4,* 8–11.

Christman, L. The practitioner–teacher. In L. Machan (Ed.), *The practitioner–teacher role: Practice what you teach.* Wakefield, Mass.: Nursing Resources, 1980.

Cooper, E. Organizational problems and the clinical specialist. In J. P. Riehl & J. W. McVay (Eds.), *The clinical nurse specialist: Interpretations.* New York: Appleton-Century-Crofts, 1973.

Flatter, P. Facilitating and inhibiting factors influencing the role of the clinical nurse specialist. In P. Chamings and R. Markel (Eds.), *Symposium on the clinical nurse specialist.* Indianapolis: Sigma Theta Tau, 1976.

Gordon, M. Clinical specialist as change agent. In J. P. Riehl and J. W. McVay (Eds.), *The clinical nurse specialist: Interpretations.* New York: Appleton-Century-Crofts, 1973.

Gresham, M. L. Conflict or collaboration: A head nurse's view. In P. Chamings and

R. Markel (Eds.), *Symposium on the clinical nurse specialist*. Indianapolis: Sigma Theta Tau, 1976.

Hamory, A. F. The clinical specialist role: Experience in two diverse situations. In P. Chamings & R. Markel (Eds.), *Symposium on the clinical nurse specialist*. Indianapolis: Sigma Theta Tau, 1976.

Holm, K. Faculty practice—Noble intentions gone awry? *Nurs Outlook*, 1981, *29*, 655–657.

Johnson, D., Wilcox, J., & Moidel, H. The clinical nurse specialist as practitioner. In E. P. Lewis (Ed.), *The clinical nurse specialist*. New York: American Journal of Nursing, 1970.

Peplau, H. Specialization in professional nursing. In J. P. Riehl & J. W. McVay (Eds.), *The clinical nurse specialist: Interpretations*. New York: Appleton-Century-Crofts, 1973.

Simms, L. The clinical nurse specialist: An approach to nursing practice in the hospital. In J. P. Riehl & J. W. McVay (Eds.), *The clinical nurse specialist: Interpretations*. New York: Appleton-Century-Crofts, 1973.

Sovie, M. D. Unifying education and practice: One medical center's design. Pt. 1. *J Nurs Adm*, 1981, *11*, 41–49. (a)

Sovie, M. D. Unifying education and practice: One medical center's design. Pt. 2. *J Nurs Adm*, 1981, *11*, 30–32.

Sutton, L. The clinical nurse specialist in a dual role. In J. P. Riehl & J. W. McVay (Eds.), *The clinical nurse specialist: Interpretations*. New York: Appleton-Century-Crofts, 1973.

10. Administrative Support

Sarah Jo Brown

THEORETICAL FOUNDATIONS

Clinical nurse specialists (CNSs) often indicate in study surveys, in informal professional dialogue, and in accounts in the nursing literature that *administrative support* is a key element contributing to successful role implementation, to ongoing efficacy in the role, and to individual job satisfaction (Shaefer, 1973; Woodrow & Bell, 1971). In nursing literature, the term appears almost exclusively in articles written about the CNS role. Interestingly, in general management literature one gets the distinct impression that subordinates are either "managed" or, if they are considered intelligent, educated, or sophisticated, they are "developed." These terms portray a managed system in which the administrator is a social engineer of some sort who directs people for organizational purposes. Admittedly, directing, managing, and coordinating are essential administistative functions in hierarchical organizations, but the dearth of discussion about supporting and collaborating functions is distressing. Fortunately, collaborative attitudes and milieus do exist in work settings; there are departments and organizations in which cooperative human endeavors take place among people with varied role titles and different areas of expertise.

Two individuals who work at different levels of an organization may pull together in mutuality of purpose without much thought about their difference in hierarchical status. Each recognizes the need for the other's assistance; the activities of one supplement and augment the activities of the other. Such a relationship is characterized by mutual support. *Support* is primarily an interpersonal process in which one person seeks or desires assistance, guidance, recognition, or encouragement in a particular endeavor from another. When the other person responds in a way that is viewed as helpful or valuable by the first person, support has been given and received. Essentially, one person infers support from the behavior, words, or actions of another. Sometimes in a relationship one person is predominantly the support provider and the other person the support receiver, but often over a period of time the support roles are reciprocal.

The term *administrative support* implies that there is a purposeful person in the middle strata of an organization who is looking "upwards" to those with executive power and is asking for collaboration in her or his endeavors. Collaborative relationships between persons in administrative roles and those in middle-management or operational-level roles are very appealing to a person who does not want a position with administrative responsibilities, but is willing to invest much time and energy in organizational activities. Sadly, very little has been written in the field of management about supporting or collaborating with the highly motivated practicing professional who works within the framework of a multifaceted organization. Perhaps such an approach turns over too much control to the operational level of the organization; perhaps it concedes that "the front office" does not always know best. In failing to recognize the presence of intelligent, motivated individuals at the operational levels of an organization, however, an administrator loses the opportunity to truly weld the realities of daily operations to the planning and development operations that take place at the top level.

The concept of administrative support has important implications for the CNS role. As an approach to exploring those implications, let us examine some selected concepts concerning administrative support, particularly those that pertain to working with motivated, self-directed professionals, and then consider how these theories apply to the CNS.

Achievement Motivation

The original work on levels of achievement motivation was done by David C. McClelland of Harvard University (1953). He contrasted individuals who were strongly motivated by the need to achieve to those who are strongly motivated by power needs or by affiliation needs (the need to be liked and to be part of a group). Recognizing that all persons have some of each need, McClelland defined the achievement need as the desire to compete against a standard of excellence. Achievement-motivated individuals constantly set difficult but potentially achievable goals for themselves. Heckhauser, who also studied the subject, asserts that individuals with personalities including high achievement motivation find satisfaction in activities such as identifying and solving problems, thinking about better ways to do things, using skills and capabilities toward a goal, tackling challenging problems, and stretching their intellectual or inter-personal abilities (1963, pp. 4–5). Seeing the results of their work and successfully completing a job are very important to them. According to Davis, achievement-motivated persons are not afraid of responsibility but rather thrive on it, because it is the vehicle by which they achieve (1967, p. 99). These individuals want to be involved; they want to be fully utilized.

The Achievement-Motivated Individual in an Organization

A thoughtful book by Hinrichs entitled *High Talent Personnel, Managing a Critical Resource* contains valuable perspectives and suggestions for working with individuals who have high achievement motivation (1966). Hinrichs describes the highly talented man (one assumes the same description can be applied to women) as the kind of person who possesses a mixture of intelligence, creativity, and personal skills. This person also possesses skills built on knowledge and insights gained through formal education and previous experience. Such an individual is motivated to apply his abilities and skills to achieve results. "He sees a parallel between the attainment of his personal goals and the achievement of organizational objectives; that is, he is motivated to obtain personal success within the framework of the company's operations" (p. 12).

Achievement-motivated persons are unique and varied individuals, but they have in common the fact that they work diligently toward reaching personal goals. When their goals can be integrated with those of an organization, the potential benefit to both the organization and the individual is tremendous. Hinrichs believes that these persons are in-valuable to an organization in an era of change, since they are important sources of vitality, innovation, and power (p. 13). A forward-looking organization must consider how to create an organizational environment that will attract and utilize such individuals. In the nursing profession, CNSs represent a large proportion of nursing's high-talent personnel. We must maximize the impact of this important resource.

Supportive Supervision

Achievement-motivated individuals are responsible and self-moti-vated; excellence is always their aim. As a result, they work best in an environment in which they are trusted and given freedom. They value and need considerable dialogue with their supervisors to assure that their goals are synchronized with those of the organization, but once set toward goals they require relatively little close supervision; periodic guidance, yes, but over-the-shoulder direction, no.

Rensis Likert refined a theory of organizational behavior known as the Supportive Theory of Organization Behavior. He holds the view that employees will be responsible, motivated, and creative if the work environment provides relationships and processes that build and maintain their sense of personal worth and importance (1961, pp. 102–103). Putting his theory into practice requires supervisors who

1.   Have confidence and trust in subordinates;
2.   Are concerned about how the work experience feels to the employee;
3.   Value employees' ideas;
4.   Are aware of problems faced by those on the operational line; and
5.   Involve a broad spectrum of employees in decision making, goal setting, and problem solving (1967, p. 44).

While it may be debated at length whether most workers will respond to such supervision with responsible, creative, and motivated performance, it may safely be assumed that there are significant numbers of individuals and even categories of workers who function well with this type of supervision. Most clinical specialists are persons who are very productive and satisfied with supportive supervision. Thus Likert's concept of supportive supervision provides the basis for the administrative/supervisory strategies advocated in this chapter.

Terminology

"Developing and utilizing talented persons" requires the same administrative strategies and actions that CNSs ask for when they seek support. "Developing talent" describes the process from the management perspective, whereas "receiving administrative support" is the term used by those who are not in the upper level of the administrative structure but who recognize the necessity of bringing executive power, resources, and processes to bear on their particular role functions and goals. A "developed" employee is presumably one who is accomplishing things. She or he can only be productive when her or his activities are synchronized and integrated with those of the whole organization. Such an employee can be maximally productive only when all the resources and influences of the total organization are available to her or him, not necessarily directly but through the hierarchical structure of the organization. If the supervisor is comprehensively "developing" her or his subordinate, the subordinate will feel supported. The cement that binds development to support is shared goals—goals that further the organization's objectives while meeting the needs and fulfilling the personal and professional goals of the individual. This matching of organization needs and objectives to those of the individual is an intricate process involving candid dialogue, trustful negotiation and priority-based thinking. Although such a matching is demanding, it may be crucial to organizational success and to individual job satisfaction. Achieving a match is a major goal of the recruitment/job selection dialogue. While initial exploration of the potential for mutuality is important, an ongoing dialogue is equally important if the individual and the organization are to remain satisfied with one another.

The term *supervisor*, which will be used in this chapter to connote the person in the organization to whom the CNS reports, is unsatisfactory because of its authoritarian implications. It is difficult to find a word that conveys the idea of an administrative role that, even though it has ultimate organization authority over other roles, emphasizes the responsibilities of being coordinator, advocate, and advisor for persons in nonadministrative roles. *Supervisor*, because of its acceptance in everyday parlance, is the more useful term, but a more precise one might be *mentor/advocate*, which conveys both the function of guiding another and that of representing another's cause. Pilette (1980) has explored mentoring in the nursing profession in a particularly humane manner. She describes the nursing mentor as a skilled guide. Mentors give positive feedback, affirm nursing actions that are creative, innovative, or just plain right, and foster dreams and visions that nurses have about nursing (p. 23). Pilette's emphasis on mentoring as a function of the supervisor is valuable because it stresses the relatedness of two human beings in common endeavor. As a further point of definition, the word *supervisor* also refers to the role that is superior in authority and broader in responsibility than that of another who is known as the *subordinate*. This dyad exists at all levels in a hierarchical organization; thus the meaning of supervisor is not restricted only to the first-line management role.

A Conceptual Framework for Supervision of CNSs

By integrating the three concepts of achievement motivation, supportive supervision, and the mutuality of personal goals and organizational objectives, a simple conceptual framework for supervision of CNSs can be synthesized. It states that most CNSs are highly achievement-motivated; by seeking CNS positions they seek to achieve personal and professional goals within the framework of the nursing department's activities. If the CNS's personal and professional goals can be integrated with those of the particular nursing department and if supportive supervision is provided, the CNS will be a productive and satisfied member of the department. This productivity will be evidenced by enhancement of nursing activities in the department and by positive impacts on many aspects of patient care. A model of this framework is diagrammed in Figure 10-1.

PRACTICAL CONSIDERATIONS

The CNS's Unique Need for Support

The CNS role has gained considerable acceptance and recognition for its impact on the quality of nursing care in acute and intermediate care settings. In some nursing departments the role is well established, while others are only beginning to introduce the role. Regardless of the length of time the role has been established in a particular setting, the need for administrative support exists. The specific nature of the support changes as the role becomes integrated with other roles in the health care facility. For example, the CNS in a department where the role is well established will require fewer demonstrations of administrative sanction of her or his authority than will the CNS in a newly established role. Certain characteristics of the CNS role, however, point to a continued need for administrative support.

Three of these characteristics exist primarily because the role is relatively new within nursing. First, the role is still in the experimental stage and is not defined in the same way from setting to setting or even by all incumbents within a setting. This lack of uniformity creates an ambiguity in the minds of role counterparts about the CNS that does not exist with more established roles (e.g., head nurse). Second, the role responsibilities of the CNS include activities that other nurses have for years viewed as their responsibility. In moving into these areas with greater depth, the CNS may walk on what others have felt is their turf (e.g., staff development, clinical supervision, improvement of patient care), causing conflict. Third, at this time, most CNSs are women—often well-educated, articulate, confident women, who have well-formulated ideas about patient care and the role of nursing in the delivery of care. Some physicians and hospital administrators may not be at ease with nurses (or women) who are skilled in presenting their ideas. This changing profile of the female nurse may in some settings produce resistance to the CNS role or to the CNS's ideas.

Three other characteristics of the CNS role which relate to administrative support reflect inherent characteristics of the role. The CNS is often charged with responsibility for affecting nursing care. To accomplish this, the CNS must be involved in operational activities (i.e. participation in on-the-unit interactions with patient and staff). Involvement in the

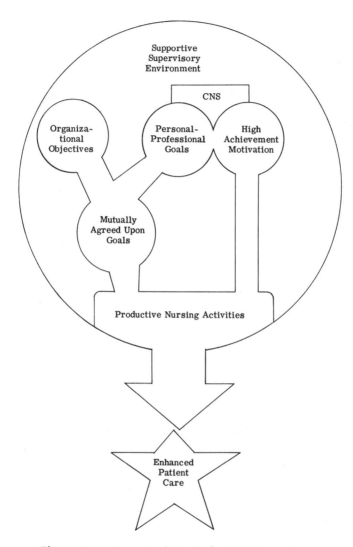

Figure 10-1. Conceptual Model for CNS Supervision.

operational sphere intrinsically excludes much involvement in administrative activities, thus, the CNS is dependent on nursing administrators for power and influence in broad organizational matters. Second, the role hinges to a great extent on patient advocacy. This necessitates activities that cross interdisciplinary boundaries in seeking clarification and coordination of patient care goals. As the CNS does this, she or he is bound to encounter differences of opinion and the obstacle of role territoriality, both of which make the role prone to conflict. Lastly, the role is dynamic and flexible, in that a broad scope of activities may be utilized in the pursuit of quality nursing care. At any point of time, the CNS chooses the strategies that seem to be most effective in meeting the goals at hand (e.g., interdisciplinary dialogue, role model practice, clinical supervision, or staff development offerings of some kind). This lack of clear-cut, circumscribed functions can produce confusion in the minds of others as to what the CNS does.

Because of these ambiguities in the role and the difficulty of implementing it, persons in the CNS role are in particular need of administrative support.

Interdependence of the CNS and the Nursing Administrator

In 1973, Shaefer queried 208 nurses who functioned as clinical specialists regarding factors contributing to job satisfaction (1973, p. 18). Items pertaining to administrative support were included to elicit CNSs' perceptions about it. Administrative support was defined as "aid given the clinician by nursing and hospital administrators and included advice, encouragement, and sanctions to her role as indicated by the salary she received, the authority vested in her, and the willingness of administrators to support her ideas and projects" (p. 18).

This is a useful, pragmatic definition, but it overlooks the collaborative aspect of support. Support is primarily an interpersonal process that takes place between the clinician and nursing or hospital administrators. Shaefer's definition implies that the clinician seeks, needs, or desires something from the administrative person. This is true: the CNS does need guidance, recognition, feedback, active acts of advocacy for her or his goals, and, at times, emotional sustenance. The other reality of this relationship, however, is that the administrator is dependent on the CNS in several ways. The administrator needs productivity from the CNS to meet departmental goals in patient care delivery; input and collaborative assistance in planning broadly for the department; and the vital clinical expertise and involvement that are at the heart of the CNS role. In fact, the relationship is an interdependent one; it should be viewed and operationalized as truly collegial and collaborative, rather than hierarchical. Even though the relationship has hierarchical aspects, they should be minimized in day-to-day dialogue. By following Likert's suggestions (described earlier) for supportive behavior by supervisors, a nursing or hospital administrator can establish a collegial relationship with the CNSs who report to her or him. It is extremely important, however, that this supportive style of leadership (participative management style, if you prefer) be utilized consistently—not just when it is convenient or when it is to the supervisor's advantage. Going back and forth between a collegial style and a hierarchical one can be confusing and frustrating to the CNS, since she or he never knows what the "style du jour" is.

It is important to be quite clear about what CNSs expect from nursing administrators. Many specific expectations will be suggested in subsequent sections of this chapter, but the essence or key element of the support that CNSs are looking for is comradeship—that is, a sense of mutual purpose and a working together toward that purpose. For most CNSs and nursing administrators, that purpose is to provide the very best nursing care possible and to continue to strive for even better care. Since the nursing care is given in a complex organizational setting, clinical expertise in a department is not sufficient. Clinical expertise, the special province of the CNS, must be united with administrative expertise if a nursing department is to bring together the many variables that are prerequisite to quality nursing care.

The value the department places on quality nursing care should be evidenced by its willingness to devote considerable fiscal resources toward providing clinicians who have the expertise and background to develop the staff's capacity for quality nursing care. It should be evidenced by the existence of strong clinical programs, including both those in which nurses function independently and those in which they collaborate with professionals from other health care disciplines. It is important that this desire for quality nursing care be evidenced by well-formulated clinical goals for the department. If these contingencies exist or are evolving, the CNS feels supported; she or he knows that the nursing administration and probably the hospital administration truly value quality care and the role of nursing in caring for people.

The CNS needs to know that not all of the work toward a particular goal needs to be done by her or him. This may mean, for example, that the specialist knows that the nursing administrator is working to increase the number of registered nurses or that the associate director is striving for clarification of the resuscitation policy, or that the staff development department is working to improve the orientation program. In short, the CNS needs to know that she or he is not going it alone and that a problem is being approached from several angles. Indeed, many problems require a pluralistic approach to resolution; an on-the-unit action, an interdepartmental change, an interprofessional clarification, a departmental procedural change, a special in—service offering, or a long-range administrative plan may be required to completely resolve a problematic situation. The CNS is usually willing to undertake those aspects of a problem that pertain to her or his area of responsibility but looks to others to render assistance with the broader, specialized, or allied aspects. If the CNS finds that her or his concerns and ideas are frequently met with responsiveness by those in nursing and hospital administration, she or he will feel supported.

Perceptions of Support

As stated earlier, support involves a perception by one person of another's activities and attitudes; one person infers support from the behavior, words, and actions of another. As in any interpersonal process, the backgrounds, personalities, values, goals, and expectations of both parties affect their perceptions of what is occurring between them as well as determining their behaviors in the process. In any group of peers reporting to the same supervisor, some members may feel that the supervisor is supportive while others do not perceive the person as such. This difference in perception occurs because the specific words, manner, or actions that *feel like* support to one person do not necessarily feel like support to another. If the supervisor listens well and offers a few helpful suggestions, one person may come away from a meeting feeling supported, while another may say, "That was a waste of time. Nothing is different. We still have the problem." For some persons, a relationship that is characterized by authentic concern, respect, trust, and mutuality of purpose will encourage and uphold them in an endeavor, while other persons need to see concrete plans and actions in order to feel upheld.

Thus, a helpful consideration for a person in the position of offering support is to know the person or persons being guided. This knowing comes through regular, planned sessions as well as through spontaneous encounters in which the person "sounds off" about a problem that has just happened or is evolving. While some individuals can delay discussing most problems until a regular session, other persons have a need to discuss them at the time they occur. Furthermore, some persons can state very clearly what they expect from their supervisors, while with others intuition must guide the supervisor in knowing how to help. In some dialogues, the supervisor may need to ask directly, "What would you like me to do to help you in this situation?" The frequency of encounters needed, both planned and spontaneous, will vary with the personality makeup and maturity of the CNS. Generally, younger CNSs who are new to the role benefit from more frequent dialogue with their supervisors. The role can be frustrating, however, and experienced as well as beginning CNSs benefit from free, open access to the supervisor. The supervisor must be careful that her or his days do not become so tightly scheduled that it becomes impossible to fit in time for a short talk or schedule an appointment with a CNS with one or two day's notice. If this happens, the supervisor should look at her or his activities, prioritize them, and possibly put some goal on "hold" so as to improve the CNS's access to the supervisor.

As the relationship between two people develops, the other person's words, style of expression, and expectations from the relationship become clearer to each. The supervisor who has several CNSs reporting to her or him will quickly learn that people are different and require different kinds of guidance from their supervisor. The supervisor must develop the ability to relate to each CNS individually and to look at the uniqueness of each situation discussed while at the same time maintaining consistency in overall approaches. This balance of flexibility and consistency is necessary if the CNSs are to know what their supervisor expects of them. Once again, the balance is easier to find if the department has a good, operationally defined philosophy and annual goals, and if the supervisor has a defined philosophy of supervision.

The interpersonal quality of being "present" to another person is a challenging part of leadership; it can, however, be emotionally draining. It is important to remember that one cannot hit the bull's-eye of support with every person every time. Sometimes one just cannot get attuned to how the other person is experiencing a situation, or maybe the person comes with unrealistic expectations of support. And then there are those times when one's attempts to assist or "run interference" for the other person just do not get anywhere because of organizational obstacles such as lack of resources, or resistant individuals, or a conflict of interest among the principals involved. These are the realities of pressured service organizations, but the supervisor can, nevertheless, aspire to be an advocate for those who report to her or him.

Organizational Placement

The organizational placement of the CNS has great influence on her or his ability to obtain administrative support. The nursing literature offers accounts of success and difficulty with quite a few different approaches to organizational placement of the CNS. Generally, no particular structure or placement has a corner on effectiveness (Crabtree, 1979). Ehrenreich and Stewart studied the Veterans Administration Hospital system and concluded that CNSs who are placed within the educational component of the nursing service experienced less satisfaction than those in other organizational placements (1979, p. 267). Barrett advocates an organizational structure that separates management responsibilities from nursing care responsibilities (1971). There is also the two-decade-old issue of how staff as opposed to line placement affects the CNS's influence and job satisfaction. Advocates and incumbents of both approaches have ably described the advantages and disadvantages of each (Crabtree, 1979; McGann, 1975; Odello, 1973).

There has been considerable debate as to whether a CNS's influence should come primarily from expertise or from legitimatized organizational authority. Most effective CNS's, regardless of whether the role has formal organizational authority, derive their influence from their clinical expertise and informal leadership skills. Padilla and Padilla (1979) proposed that in many settings, particularly those in which much change is required, the CNS will be more effective if she or he is perceived as a leader who has the authority to elicit behavioral changes from nurses. This admonition should be carefully considered when deliberating the matter of organizational placement and how the role is to be defined, since it is a recurrent theme in the literature and is clearly a determinant of success with the role. If the CNS does not possess vested positional authority, it becomes very important that the specialist have a channel to authority through the person to whom she or he reports. This means very clearly that persons in consultative roles should report to persons with some legitimate organizational authority—that is, line authority. Frequently, major organizational obstacles to practice do exist and must be moved aside so that the consultative process can occur and influence patient care. Organizational authority or access to it are essential to bringing about these kinds of change.

There are numerous organizational placement possibilities for the CNS, as described in Chapter 8. Cutting across all placements, however, is the constant that all CNSs must have someone to whom they are accountable and who presumably is to be a support person to them. Whatever the title of the person, it is essential that she or he be effective at a higher level of the organization in which the CNS has little involvement and influence. The CNS needs an influential supervisor if she or he is to be maximally effective. If the CNS's immediate supervisor is not a person in top-level nursing administration, a whole series of relays must occur to influence the upper level of the organization where decisions regarding expenditure or future programs are made. Too often, much is lost in these relays, and the importance or intent of the CNS's concern is dissipated as it is relayed. It is best, therefore, if the CNS reports to one of the top persons in nursing administration rather than to a middle manager or to someone several steps below the director of nursing. Nothing is more frustrating to the CNS than reporting to a powerless supervisor who cannot influence major adminstrative decisions. Conversely, the CNS whose superior conveys the specialist's concerns accurately and effectively in hospital administration forums will experience smoother pathways to attaining her or his goals.

The administrative skill and personal qualities of a CNS's superior are equally as important determinants of support as the organizational structure. Persons to whom CNSs report should be carefully chosen. The author's many interactions with clinical specialists suggest that they want their superiors to be persons who are not content with the status quo and who are open to new ideas. At the same time, they expect their superiors to appreciate the persons who are providing direct care, to understand the tremendous demands made on nurses while rendering care to the sick, and to be concerned about the frustrations nurses experience in providing that care. In short, CNSs want superiors who are familiar with the activities of bedside nursing and who attempt to facilitate the care-giving process and enhance the care-giving environment.

If an organization can procure several individuals who possess administrative skills and the personal qualities just mentioned, a decentralized structure with one or several CNSs reporting to each assistant director may be a wise choice for the nursing department. If, however, the director of nursing knows that the organization cannot attract several such assistant directors, a structure in which one qualified person is vested with responsibility for all the CNSs would be best. This would certainly be preferable to having educated and experienced CNSs reporting to less well-prepared and less able individuals just because of a bias toward a particular organizational design. CNSs are pivotal persons in determining the quality of care provided in a particular setting. For this reason, when designing or redesigning an organizational structure one must give much thought to who will be their supervisor/advocate and what channels to administrative power will be available to the specialists.

Scope of Responsibility

Closely related to the issue of organizational placement of the CNS is the matter of scope of responsibility. CNSs have indicated that their effectiveness and job satisfaction are greatly diminished when their scope of responsibility is too great (Woodrow & Bell, 1971, p. 27). When they have too large a patient population for whom to care or when they have too many units for which they are responsible, CNSs experience frustration and feel as though they are skimming the surface of things. While no magic number for the correct patient load or number of beds can be set because of the varying ways the role is defined, it can surely be stated that careful consideration should be given to this matter. The ideal scope of responsibility may be smaller than people estimate it to be. In a recent experience with CNSs who had line authority for nursing care functions, the specialists subjectively found that their impact was greater when they had only one 50-bed unit. CNSs functioning with two 50-bed units or three 20-bed units felt that they had less impact on care and experienced frustration trying to keep up with what was going on. They found that their decreased visibility and availability detracted from the extent to which staff sought them out and thus resulted in fewer spontaneous, direct patient care involvements. Activities that systematically brought the specialist into the care-planning and care-giving interfaces had to be arranged. Having responsibility for two or three units also increased the number of relationships that had to be developed and decreased the time the CNS was available to help each staff member evaluate the care individual patients received. Similar guidelines probably exist for case loads of CNSs in consultative and direct care roles.

The scope of responsibility for each CNS should be kept small enough to allow considerable involvement in the activities of her or his assigned units. If the CNS is a member of a consultative or multidisciplinary care team, the case load must be of a size that allows time for follow-through, literature review, and some extemporaneous contact with staff. This limiting of the scope of responsibility may mean that some units or patient groups do not have the benefit of CNS influence; this is unfortunate, and further positions should be sought, but it is a sounder approach than stretching the CNS's scope of responsibility just so that each unit or each patient group is "covered" by CNS service. In overextending the CNS's scope of responsibility, the credibility of the role is decreased, its impact is diluted, and the frustrations of the CNS are heightened. The staff will bring problems to the CNS or the specialist will see them her- or himself, but the CNS will be unable to truly address the problems because of conflicting demands for her or his time. This lack of ability to respond to staff requests and the small amount of time the specialist is available to the staff can seriously undermine the credibility and effectiveness of the role.

Even when the scope of responsibility is appropriate, CNSs may become overextended if they are unable to limit their involvements. Many hospital and nursing department endeavors clamor for the specialist's expertise; the CNS must learn when to say no to a request that she or he be involved in some work group, committee, or new service. Such decisions should be discussed with the supervisor, since the latter may have ideas as to how the department can either free the particular CNS for the involvement or find someone else to represent the department. The ability to pick and choose the most worthwhile involvement is a delicate matter but is absolutely crucial if the specialist is to avoid the endemic burnout syndrome.

Interaction between the CNS and the Supervisor

The relationship between the supervisor and the CNS should reflect the individual CNS's experience and competence. The CNS who has demonstrated competence and responsibility should be viewed as a partner or associate. The CNS should be consulted whenever major decisions affecting her or his area of responsibility are to be made and should have considerable influence on these decisions. She or he should be granted much self determination in fulfilling job responsibilities. On the other hand, the CNS with little experience or the CNS who has demonstrated difficulties in meeting her or his responsibilities will require considerable guidance.

It is widely recognized in the literature on organizational theory that recognition and rewards from an employee's supervisor can be a strong motivation for the employee and a source of good feelings about the work situation (Herzberg, 1959, pp. 59–60). Recognition from a superior undoubtedly contributes to one's sense of personal worth, a basic need that often is not sufficiently met in work settings. The activities and role relationships in complex, busy health care facilities often fail to consistently recognize the efforts, accomplishments, and overall worth of individuals to the working of the organization. This lack of recognition should not and cannot go on indefinitely. While some persons can remain productive employees with very little acknowledgment and support, others need such responses in goodly amounts and frequently. The employee who does not receive her or his perceived due portion of recognition will eventually cease to feel good about working in the organization and will seek employment elsewhere.

CNSs, as achievement-motivated persons, place a high value on objective feedback about their performance. The subject of performance evaluation is addressed in detail in the chapters on evaluation (Part IV), but it should be noted here that an ongoing dialogue between the CNS and her or his supervisor is especially useful. It is of immense value for these two persons to agree on goals for the CNS's activity and to then regularly assess progress towards these goals. To fully accomplish this, it is very helpful if the nursing department has a written philosophy with clearly stated values, as well as yearly objectives that broadly set priorities.

While the department's objectives are important considerations in the goal planning of the individual CNS, the work unit of which the specialist is a member—whether it is a nursing care unit, a consultation team, or a multidisciplinary patient care team—may identify objectives that are unique to its situation and stand apart from broad departmental objectives. This is appropriate and necessary to success in daily operations. The CNS's objectives may therefore be determined in part by the department's objectives and in part by the objectives of the particular unit or work group of which she or he is a member. If the CNS, head nurse, assistant head nurse, and even staff of a unit agree on yearly objectives, the CNS can define her or his contributions within that context. The staff should be made aware that the CNS also has goals that extend beyond the unit's objectives or else emanate from outside that scope of activity, so that the staff's expectations of the specialist will be realistic. The supervisor should respect the objectives of the work group of which the specialist is a part and incorporate them when discussing the CNS's individual goals, since the effectiveness and credibility of the specialist are greatly affected by her or his ability to contribute relevantly to the operational work group.

Planning goals together may well be the heart of the relationship between the clinical specialist and the supervisor. Through such discussions the organization and the individual professional find the mutuality of purpose that binds them together. In this dialogue, the CNS and the supervisor agree that "of all the problems that we face and of all the goals you could pursue, these are the appropriate ones for you to address." This assures that the CNS is pursuing goals that are sanctioned by the department and releases the specialist from any guilt she or he may feel because of problems that she or he is not addressing.

The goal-setting approach requires that the specialist and the supervisor also discuss the methods to be used in obtaining the goals. This is a crucial aspect of the dialogue, because there are often several possible strategies. Further, the CNS's activities may need to be preceded or augmented by someone else's involvement. For example, the CNS who has a goal of reducing the unnecessary taking of vital signs by nurses on her or his units may find that departmental policy regarding this procedure must be rewritten to authorize nurses to use their own judgment in determining when to take vital signs. Such a policy undoubtedly will need to be accepted by the medical governing board, since the frequency of taking vital signs is tradionally "ordered" by physicians. This troublesome but legally delicate issue may therefore require considerable prepatory work by the supervisor.

The CNS and the supervisor should discuss each proposed goal, consider its appropriateness, and chart a course of action that identifies all the major steps on the road to that goal. The new CNS, particularly, will benefit from this kind of exchange and through it can be helped to learn to take into account organizational factors that either impede or facilitate change.

The use of the goal-oriented approach may seem overly confining to some CNSs, and they may rebel at the structure it seems to impose. To be sure, in a complex, changing, and unpredictable health care setting, only a limited portion of one's activities can be dictated by goals. Flexibility is needed, so that one can respond to problems of the present. Without a goal orientation, however, a CNS can easily be busy all the time in extemporaneous involvements that will not be productive in the long run. Immediate problems must be dealt with, but an organization and the persons in it must also have goals that will assure that today's problems will not continue to be issues in the future. A balance must be struck in which the CNS is available to staff for situation-specific guidance but is also engaged in activities that lead toward sanctioned goals. The specialist and the supervisor must be both future-oriented and present-oriented. To help in striking this balance, the number of goals that require change should be limited so as to allow time for impromptu, supportive involvements. The overly zealous CNS will be tempted to have many future- or change-oriented goals and will need to be reminded that time must be kept available for guiding and supporting the daily activities of staff and patients. Activities such as discussing the care of a particular patient with the nurses on the unit is an invaluable involvement. Granted, no momumental change is in process, but some insight or understanding may be added to a staff nurses's perspective so that the care that this nurse gives in the future will be a little bit better than it was in the past. The balance the CNS must reach is much like the building of a stone wall: the little stones are absolutely necessary to keep the bigger ones in place.

A goal-oriented approach to CNS activity has many advantages: it offers a framework in which the specialist can obtain feedback regarding her or his performance; it assures the compatibility of organizational and personal goals; it fosters purposeful activity and good planning for change. Significantly, evaluation of the degree to which the CNS has achieved the stated goals, provides a relatively objective assessment of the extent to which the CNS is succeeding in the role. If the results are positive, this feedback is a form of support, providing encouragement for continued growth and development.

Fostering Additional Supporting Relationships

Important as the relationship between the CNS and the immediate supervisor is, it is not the only source of support available. Support for the CNS may come from relationships with peers, head nurses, physicians, and other health care professionals, hospital administrators, or department directors. Involvement in patient care is an important source of support. In the course of working with patients, the specialist's belief in her or his goals is strengthened as patients learn about how to take care of themselves better or as they are comforted or assisted in returning to a healthy state. Likewise, as the CNS works with staff nurses and sees their use of knowledge become more honed and their nursing actions become more skilled, the specialist's commitment to her or his activities is nourished. The supervisor should recognize the value of these other relationships for the CNS and foster them.

A peer group made up of all the CNSs or even all the masters-prepared clinicians in an agency can be a particularly valuable link in the support system. It is quite likely that informal, supportive relationships will develop among those in this group. Beyond that, there is a need for an organizationally sanctioned forum in which CNSs can discuss issues, activities, and problems or plan endeavors of mutual concern. Such a group can be a wellspring of ideas, encouragement, and stimulation for its members.

Experience with such groups suggests that the group should try from the beginning to clarify its purposes. A certain amount of meeting time may need to be devoted to information passing, for example, but this should be restricted to those things that cannot be passed along in written communications. The group should also decide whether or not it wants members to share problems and frustrations. While such sharing can be a source of help to the CNS in a highly problematic situation, it may be redundant for those who have worked through similar problems or who feel they have enough problems and do not want to hear about someone else's. Most likely the difficulties which the individual CNS encounters are best discussed within the supervisor–CNS relationship and informally between select affiliates in the peer group.

What, then, should be the purpose of the meetings? If the group feels that broadening of clinical knowledge and exploration of professional issues are important purposes, a portion of each meeting could be devoted to such matters as reporting on a recently completed research study; group exploration of a professional issue, with a resulting position paper that presents the group's stand on the matter; presentation of a newly offered clinical program or service; or planning of a group endeavor such as initiating dialogue within a department about the use of the consultative process. These topics are broad enough to be of interest to CNSs in various stages of role development and should encourage meaningful dialogue among group members.

In hospitals where only one or two CNSs are employed, either because of size or because implementation of the role is just being initiated, special arrangements to provide peer support may need to be made. Contact with other CNSs is an important nutrient for the lone or new CNS and should be encouraged. Such contacts may take place at professional conferences and educational offerings. Or, the director of nursing in a rural hospital may know of another hospital relatively nearby which also employs a CNS and could encourage the two persons to get together for lunch and an afternoon of exchange—even better if the two directors of nursing join the CNSs on occasion. The state nurses' association might develop an interest group made up of CNSs that could develop into a valuable peer group. In all cases, the department of nursing should support the CNS in obtaining peer support by allowing her or him the time and paying whatever expenses are necessary; it is bound to be a worthwhile investment.

Involvement in Decision Making

Another source of encouragement besides the peer group is for CNSs to be involved in one or several areas of broad decision making within the department and the hospital, particularly those pertaining directly to patient care and those that involve setting departmental goals. Through such involvement, the CNS can influence patient care issues of particular interest to her or him and provide input on how various patient care services should be developed (for example, quality assurance or patient education programs).

The CNS who belongs to at least one departmental and one institutional committee or work group will enter into dialogue with others to solve operational problems and plan for new services. Through this dialogue, the CNS will be exposed to new ideas and will gain appreciation for the contributions of others. Furthermore, the involvement of specialists in the decision-making forums of the nursing department and the hospital enhances the likelihood that credible nursing perspectives will be incorporated into new or changing programs.

Introducing the CNS Role

Thoughtful planning and good groundwork are important forms of support for the persons who will fill the first CNS positions of a department. Barrett (1971) offers excellent suggestions to guide the director of nursing who is considering introducing the CNS role. Barrett advises that in the planning stages the nursing leadership think quite carefully about why they think the department should introduce the CNS and be explicit about what they want them to do. The role should not be initiated as an easy panacea for a multitude of problems or as trendy evidence of the department's progressive attitudes. It should be introduced because many members of the department have arrived at the point where they agree that nursing care could be improved if the department had master's-prepared specialists to take an active role in direct patient care and in clinical supervision.

Before a CNS is actually appointed, discussions should be held with the persons whose responsibilities will be most affected by the introduction of the specialist. A written job description can serve as a framework for these discussions. This description should define the main responsibilities of the position and be specific about expected outcomes, but it should allow the CNS discretion in selecting priorities and activities within that scope.

While the job description may be a helpful document when used as a basis for discussion about the CNS role within the nursing department, it will have limited value when explaining the role to physicians and other department heads. Most of them simply will not take time to read the description; thus, the nursing administrator and others who are responsible for introducing the role should have in mind a succinct, practical statement that describes the role's purpose and activities as well as how it fits into the existing structure. In spite of the frequent unwillingness of physicians and staff members in other departments to learn about the role prior to actually meeting and working with a CNS, these personnel should at least be informed of the specialist's arrival; her or his scope of responsiblity and authority should be clearly sanctioned by the top nursing administrator.

Even with a good job description, clear sanctioning of the role's authority by nursing administrators, and ongoing discussion sessions, role conflict may still exist for several years because inevitably some people are resistant to change. To some extent, time must do its work. Slowly the role will carve its place among others in the department. It is important that the first incumbent(s) be chosen for their clinical knowledge and skills, their interpersonal aptitude, their ability to articulate nursing purposes, and their ability to persevere against resistance.

The temptation to introduce the CNS role and fill it initially with a person with outstanding clinical skills but without the educational credentials of a master's degree must be avoided. This has often been attempted, but most such attempts have failed miserably; master's speciality education develops a whole set of abilities that are prerequisite to success in the role. Talented young persons who do not have the conceptual background or the awareness of professional issues that are acquired during graduate education simply are not CNSs in knowledge or perspective and cannot be made into them through on-the-job development.

CONCLUSIONS

CNSs are highly motivated to address issues in health care and to enhance nursing's role in health care. As well-educated clinicians who have a vision for nursing practice, they are a vital force in nursing today. They ask for support from nursing administrators in order to meet clinical objectives.

The central support person for most CNSs is the immediate supervisor. This relationship is extremely important, since within it ideas are developed and refined, goals are validated, and encouragement and recognition are bestowed. Certain organizational variables, such as the CNS's ability to influence administrative thinking and the scope of responsibility assigned to the CNS, also greatly augment or detract from the specialist's experience of support. In addition, each CNS will find informal support among peers and other health care professionals as she or he goes about her activities. These informal, sometimes quasisocial sources of support should not be disparaged, since an individual needs to have a system of support persons, each with a slightly different perspective and contribution.

As nursing's best-prepared acute care clinicians, CNSs play an important role in improving and maintaining the quality of nursing care, but they cannot do it in isolation. The plurality of interests and complexity of relationships in health care centers require that nursing administrators represent the concerns and interests of CNSs in administrative decision-making processes. The CNS needs an advocate if she or he is to significantly enhance nursing care and the nursing administrator is that advocate. Together the skilled clinician and the skilled administrator can accomplish a great deal.

REFERENCES

Barrett, J. Administrative factors in development of new nursing practice roles. *J Nurs Adm*, 1971, *1*, 25–29.

Crabtree, M. S. Effective utilization of clinical nurse specialists within the organizational framework of hospital nursing service. *Nurs Adm Q*, 1979, *4*, 1–10.

Ehrenreich, D., & Stewart, P. Clinical nurse specialists' perceptions of role facilitators and inhibitors in the practice setting. A.N.A. Kansas City, Mo: Division on Practice, Clinical and Scientific Sessions, 1979. (N.P. #59)

Heckhauser, H. *The anatomy of achievement motivation.* New York: Academic Press, 1963.

Herzberg, F. *The motivation to work.* New York: John Wiley & Sons, 1959.

Hinrichs, J. *High talent personnel: Managing a critical resource.* New York: American Management Association, 1966.

Davis, K. *Human Relations at work: The dynamics of Organizational Behavior* New York: McGraw-Hill, 1967.

Likert, R. *New patterns of management.* New York: McGraw-Hill, 1961.

Likert, R. *The human organization.* New York: McGraw-Hill, 1967.

McClelland, D. C., Atkinson, J., Clark, R. et al: *The achievement motive.* New York: Appleton-Century-Crofts, 1953.

McGann, M. The clinical specialist: From hospital to clinic, to community. *J Nurs Adm*, 1975, *5*, 33–35.

Odello, E. J. The clinical specialist in a line position. *Superv Nurs*, 1973, *4*, 36–41.

Padilla, G. V., & Padilla, G. Nursing roles to improve patient care. In G. V. Padilla

(Ed.), The clinical nurse specialist and improvement of patient care, *Nurs Digest*, 1979, *6*, 1–13.

Pilette, P. C. Mentoring: An encounter of the leadership kind. *Nurs Leadership*, 1980, *3*, 22–26.

Shaefer, J. A. The satisfied clinician: Administrative support makes the difference. *J Nurs Adm*, 1973, *3*, 17–20.

Woodrow, M., & Bell, J. Clinical specialization: Conflict between reality and theory. *J Nurs Adm*, 1971, *1*, 25.

11. Contributions and Organizational Role of the CNS: An Administrator's Viewpoint

Marilyn P. Prouty

ESTABLISHING THE CNS ROLE

Becoming the administrator for nursing of the Mary Hitchcock Memorial Hospital in Hanover, New Hampshire, in the fall of 1972 offered a special challenge to me, because plans were being made to make the hospital a component of a developing medical center. In response to the increasing health care needs of people in the Dartmouth area, the hospital had been enlarged; by 1969 there were 420 beds and multiple specialty units to treat patients with a variety of illnesses. The Dartmouth Medical School had also resumed its M.D. program, and in July of 1973 a confederation composed of the Mary Hitchcock Memorial Hospital, the nearby Veterans Administration Hospital, the Hitchcock Clinic (a large physican group practice), and the Dartmouth Medical School was created. This confederation made a commitment to provide highly skilled medical care to its client population.

The Dartmouth-Hitchcock Medical Center did not magically become a center just because it was labeled as such in July of 1973; rather, the formation of the confederation represented a commitment to a plan. By 1975 the delivery of medical and nursing care had become complex and difficult indeed. The hospital admitted fewer ambulatory patients for diagnostic workups or for minor surgery than formerly, and more patients with serious trauma or multiple system problems, in keeping with the profile of a medical center–a complex delivery system dealing with patients who present serious illnesses involving multiple body systems. Literally on

171

a daily basis, nurses described to me their overwhelmingly complex patient loads, and, literally weekly, new medical department chairmen told me of their plans for new programs (a misnomer, because their "plans" were the realities the nurses were already describing to me daily).

Meeting my own responsibilities in this setting was a challenge. I first took part in the budgetary process in late 1973 when I presented the nursing department's budget for fiscal year 1974–1975. Even though I had participated in planning for the formation of new and demanding specialty units and community outreach programs, I was less than successful in convincing members of hospital administration that the nursing budget had to reflect an increase in the number of staff nurses as well as nurses with advanced education in clinical nursing speciality areas of practice. We had also requested a position for a nurse researcher, one who could assist us in evaluating the effectiveness of change as we built and altered the nursing organization to meet the changing needs of a medical center. This position was granted, but only by a "fluke." (The neophyte nurse administrator should note that on rare occasions a "fluke" happens that defies all that one has learned or read. One should just be happy about it—rather than attempting to analyze it.) It may come as no surprise to the reader that we were unable to recruit a qualified nurse researcher. We retained the position, however, suspecting that we might be able to "trade" it for some critical position in the future.

The dominant reason for requesting clinical nurse specialists (CNSs) was to assist our staff nurses to understand how to provide nursing care to a whole new population of patients with complex medical problems. It was expected that CNSs would

1. Impart knowledge to head nurses and staff nurses;
2. Enhance the new staff nurse's seeking, inquiring, motivated start on her or his professional career;
3. Ease reality shock for the neophyte staff nurse;
4. Serve as clinically knowledgeable nurses to work with other disciplines in planning and implementing new clinical programs that would affect nursing practice;
5. Augment the quality of nursing care by giving direct care to selected patients and thus serving as role models for other nurses.

Actually, three major nursing department problems confronted us. First, there were too few nurses to care for the numbers of patients who were coming through our doors; second, there were no nurses with advanced clinical expertise to provide care or advise others on how to give care; and third, there were no nurses with advanced education in nursing administration, other than myself, to assist *me* to problem-solve organizationally or to assist the head nurses to meet management complexities with skill and confidence. Because of budget limitations, it was impossible to request enough dollars to address all three problems, so I decided to begin by investigating the best avenue to follow in adding clinical strength. It seemed that the best way to accomplish this would be through the addition of staff nurse positions and clinical nurse specialists. At first I sacrificed obtaining staff nurse positions in order to add clinical strength.

While I was preparing the nursing department budget for fiscal year 1974–1975, the chairman of the department of psychiatry told me of a grant proposal submitted by members of his department. Recognizing the need of many patients in the general medical and surgical areas for mental health assistance, his department had become interested in the psychiatric liaison model, which provided a team of one or two psychiatrists and a nurse with master's preparation in psychiatric nursing. This plan was fortuitous, arriving at a time when I had been unsuccessful in budgeting for CNS positions during fiscal year 1974–1975. It also indicated that a physican group recognized the potential contribution of a nurse with advanced preparation. If one such position was successfully added, other CNSs could probably follow. Thus the first specialist became a member of the nursing department within six months after the grant was funded.

The first CNS to enter a nursing organization is important for reasons that are no more significant than those for the introduction of the second, third, and all later CNSs, but the reasons are special. I had not planned to introduce the first specialist as a psychiatric liaison nurse within medical–surgical patient units; I would have preferred to assign a medical–surgical or cardiovascular specialist to a specific unit, since nurses unfamiliar with the role of a CNS adjust more quickly and with less suspicion to this "new" person when the assistance they receive is related to a definitive body-system problem. Psychiatry or a psychiatric focus still elicits fantasies and apprehensions from nurses in medical–surgical settings. They have difficulty conceptualizing the potential value of such a person and tend to think that they themselves are going to be studied and analyzed. An administrator, however, must seize opportunities and then make them work for the organization. Members of a nursing department such as ours, who have never experienced a professional relationship with master's-prepared nurses, find it most difficult to conceptualize the value of a specialist. I attempted to prepare the staff for what I was determined would be the inevitable—the acquisition of CNSs—by "giving sensitizing doses." In meetings with head nurses, when complex patient care problems were addressed, I seized the opportunity to briefly explain the role of the CNS. When supervisors in various states of anger and frustration brought problems to me, I expressed understanding about their difficult jobs and pointed out that a new breed on the nurse market could be of assistance. I planned night staff nurse breakfasts, day nurse lunches, and evening nurse suppers once every month and responded in a similar way to their protestations of jumbled feelings about the complex patient care that had seemed to descend upon them. Occasionally I followed up these conversations with articles that addressed the characteristics and contributions of CNSs in other nursing departments. When I was unsuccessful in budgeting for specialists in the 1974–1975 budget, I rationalized that I just had that much more time to "give sensitizing doses."

When our first unplanned-for psychiatric CNS arrived in May of 1975, I was therefore unsure of how she would be accepted. I was, however, most careful in making the selection. In selecting candidates, I am less concerned about the knowledge the candidates have than about their personalities. If they have graduated successfully, the chances are favorable that they are sound clinically. The individual's personality profile is critical. This is particularly true when introducing the first specialist. When interviewing a candidate, the director of nursing needs to be honest about telling the CNS where the organization is in its development. This openness usually elicits from the candidate comments that indicate whether or not her or his sensitivity to an organization and understanding of how to make change in an orderly and therapeutic manner is part of this specialist's modus operandi. It is always important to have candidates meet with other members of the department, including staff nurses. It is unwise for an administrator to attend these interview sessions, but a well-planned luncheon with the candidate with other members of the staff gives the director of nursing an opportunity to determine how questions are fielded by the candidate, a sense of her or his attitudes, and a feeling of whether or not there is general acceptance of the candidate by the staff. We have eight CNSs now, and the staff have become experts in the interviewing process. My profile is much lower now, and I am comfortable with this.

Some detail concerning the organizational placement of our CNSs may be useful. Because the first specialist was a psychiatric one, she was placed in a staff position. The role of this particular specialist required consultation to all of the adult medical–surgical patient care units. She was confronted with the difficult challenge of establishing rapport and credibility with the nursing staff with every encounter. I was concerned that the mobility of her work would make it more difficult for her to succeed as the first CNS. Her work was so dispersed that repeat encounters were few. However, the psychiatric CNS "made it" in our organization and made it grandly. Her quiet, patient way with nurses was the reason and much time was the price.

Our nursing staff had to learn how to use the CNS in a consultant role. A nursing staff must be quite sophisticated to utilize a consultant; consulting with colleagues about a care problem or with peers to ask for information does not yet seem to be a natural way of thinking for nurses. It is as though nurses have been imbued with the idea that either they should know what they are doing or else should surreptitiously go to the literature to find the answers. This attitude seems to be changing, but until using nurse colleagues as resources becomes an integrated, natural process, and a way of thinking, for the nurse, the first CNS should ideally not be placed in a consultative staff role but on a specific patient care unit, where the opportunity exists for frequent and consistent nurse–CNS interaction. In this way, rapport develops more quickly, and the CNS's credibility is more easily established. Another positive result of assigning the first CNS to a single patient care unit might be called "organizational jealousy." Nursing personnel on other units feel that the unit that has the specialist is being treated as "special"; they want to be special too. It is wise for a director to look for signs of this negative organizational behavior, capitalize on it and convert it to positive organizational behavior.

If the administrator has selected the first CNS skillfully, acceptance in the entire organization will move rapidly, and the administrator will be able to place as many CNSs successfully as the budget allows. Once the role is in place, CNSs themselves enhance the development of the "consultative think." Because they are comfortable consulting colleagues, they serve as role models and thereby assist other nurses to integrate consultation into their everyday practice.

When the nursing budget for fiscal year 1975–1976 was presented, we were able to obtain three CNS positions. The next year we requested and were permitted to add three more. My persistence in articulating the importance of these positions, coupled with excellent detailed reports from the specialists, enabled us to obtain these additional positions. Nursing administrators should call upon the specialists for support and information. CNSs are convinced that they are important and indeed are committed to this value. In addition, they are articulate, have writing skills, and are therefore able to translate with ease the real environment of their practice into the verbal and written word that can serve as evidence for the value of their positions at the time of budget review.

ORGANIZATIONAL DESIGN

Prior to the submission of the nursing budget for fiscal year 1975–1976, I had presented a plan for the organizational placement of the CNSs to influential members of the nursing staff. The design of this organization had been part of my thinking long before I was able to include more specialists in the department. An integral part of the challenge and excitement of being a director of nursing is being in a position to engineer a plan of one's own design. The plan, idea, and design must, however, be shared and explained to members of the nursing staff in order to stand any change of being successfully launched. There are influential nurses in every nursing department. We had our share, and I brought these people into a group discussion task force for the purpose of selling my organizational design. One other member of this task force was a master's-prepared nurse whom I had employed as an associate director in the department. Her education, combined with her sensitivity, provided the devil's advocate role during our deliberations of the recommended design. This was important, because it assured that I would not be pushing a plan that others did not understand or approve.

Traditionally, nurses with clinical expertise have been rewarded with administrative responsibilities. The pressure of administrative duties, however, make it difficult for such nurses to retain their clinical skills. Insidiously, the clinical knowledge and skill of supervisors became diluted, and heavy reliance for clinical expertise was placed on the head nurse. Since administrative and clinical skills are equally important, it seemed desirable to design an organizational structure within our nursing department that would give equal weight to both of these nursing functions.

The new design called for two associated directors of nursing—one for administrative affairs and the other for clinical affairs. The administrative supervisors were to be responsible to the associate for administrative affairs and the CNSs were to be responsible for the associate for clinical affairs. Since the specialists employed were prepared on the master's level with a specialty track, their unit assignment would correspond to their specialty. Both the administrative supervisors responsible for administrative affairs and the CNS in charge of clinical matters were placed in line positions. Simplistically expressed, the head nurses were responsible to the CNSs for clinical matters and to the administrative supervisors for administrative matters. This structure symbolizes our belief that the clinical component of nursing is truly as important and significant as the administrative. Administrative knowledge is a specialty that is not reserved for the director of a nursing department alone. Understanding personnel scheduling and developing innovative schedules; dealing with human behavior problems and responding to them, rather than allowing unions to; determining how to diagnose organizational change and the most effective way to go about it; having the skill to select or tap potential leaders in the organization—such issues as these are all-consuming activities for the administrative supervisor. Placing the CNSs in line positions says something about the department's hopes for the role and sets the stage for action. It says that the department believes that the clinical aspect of care delivery is important. It says that the CNS is there on the unit to be listened to, to ask questions of, to be included in patient care challenges. Indirectly, it says that the specialist is not there so that the staff can accept her or his clinical direction only if it suits their fancy.

The "doing" component of the specialist in a line position is up to the CNS. The way in which she or he establishes rapport, the technique used to impart knowledge, the methods devised to enhance the quality of patient care all depend on the skill of the specialist. One cannot overemphasize the importance of looking for these characteristics during the interviewing process of the CNS. If this seems difficult at first, one should not stumble, or be fearful of missing the mark but should call on a skillful interviewer for assistance or consult a colleague in another hospital; directors should also utilize the consultative process.

Many question the soundness of an arrangement whereby a head nurse is directly responsible to two people. The question most frequently asked is "How does the head nurse know whom to ask what of?" The explanation is as follows. The head nurse is provided with two resource people, rather than two "bosses." We were realistic enough to realize that problems are not always clearly administrative or clinical, and herein lies the substance of the functioning of the roles of all three—the head nurse, the administrative supervisor, and the CNS. Dialogue is an essential ingredient for the participants in these roles. Some problems presented by the head nurse are clearly appropriate for the specialist to respond to. An example at our institution was the hint a head nurse had received that a patient was going to the operating room the following day for a radical surgical procedure new to our hospital. The head nurse informed the CNS, and the CNS moved quickly to verify this information and to explore the nursing care implications. Other problems are not as clear and demand conversation among the three. Frequently the end result is a role for them all. An example of this kind of problem occurred when hyperalimentation hit the patients in our department with great suddenness. Pump equipment was needed for a patient, and no physician had communicated this new need to the head nurse. The head nurse realized that the supervisor and CNS could help her to solve this problem quickly. The head nurse defined and stated the problem. The CNS assisted the staff to understand how to manage the pump and observe the patient. The supervisor had obtained the pump and had also anticipated the need for more. She set the wheels in motion for monies to purchase more and to expedite the action. This was not easy to accomplish: she had to present a sound proposal that convincingly and knowledgeably substantiated the need to purchase five more pumps, at $900 each in the middle of the fiscal year. If the CNS had had to do this, there probably would have been little time left for her to instruct the nurses and to set up a procedure that included safety measures.

There are naturally some problems with this kind of structure, as there are with any structure in which a group of people work closely together. Despite this, our organization has worked well; the key is that talking together and problem solving are the modus operandi. Very few "orders," per se, are issued in our department. (This appears to be true in most organizations today.) If an impasse is reached on the unit, the associate directors are appealed to. Usually their problem-solving skills and their ability to ask meaningful questions open new avenues for thinking that clear away the obstacles. There are times (though rare) when I have to become involved. It is usually not too difficult for me because so much thinking has been brought to bear on the problem that I am able to be quite objective, and a reasonable and agreeable solution can be determined together quite quickly.

The problem-solving process that occurs when the head nurse is responsible to a CNS as well as an administrative supervisor is in some ways analogous to problem-solving within the organization of the family unit. The head nurse is not, of course, truly in the position of a child, but the CNS and supervisor are somewhat in the position of parents, who must make decisions together even if they do not at first agree on how to solve a problem affecting the family. Wise parents dialogue with one another, problem solve, and frequently arrive at a decision with the child's input or make collective suggestions to the child. The two parents accountable for their actions and directions must have dialogue with one another and the third participant in order for the organization of the family unit to work with harmony. It is not problems in a home or in a nursing department that cause disharmony; rather it is whether or not the problems are addressed. It is true that from the frame of reference of most people, a line position means that one is the "boss." Our organizational structure, including the relevant job descriptions, clearly elaborates the responsibilities of the specialists as well as the supervisors. In the real world of the patient unit where nurses interact, however, this organizational placement is difficult to discern. Staff nurses ask more questions today; they challenge decisions with which they do not agree and force dialogue with their head nurses, CNSs, and supervisors, with little heed to the fact that these positions are higher on the organizational chart than their own. An organization today moves forward, is dynamic, and meets everyday challenges not because certain people are in staff or line positions but because a climate is established that provides expert nurses and the right and expectation that these experts will be utilized. The line position sets the stage, and indeed it says something about limits, but it is the role participants and the interactions that take place that determine the outcomes.

THE ORGANIZATIONAL CLIMATE NECESSARY FOR THE EVOLVING CNS ROLE

The CNS needs considerable freedom; the nature and substance of the role demands flexibility in its performance. There are variables in the practice setting that specialists must be free to respond to as they occur. CNSs understand that her or his guidance and assistance are needed on evening and night shifts as well as day shifts, and that working hours may change. In addition, their sense of responsibility to the growth of nursing as a profession occasionally takes their time away from the patient unit. If there are times when a director is concerned that the CNS's professional organizational commitments are disproportionate to their unit commitments, such a concern must be discussed and negotiated openly. To impose a rigid structure for their practice is to dilute the potential effectiveness of their role. Provision of such freedom is difficult, particularly if one is a leader with remnants of the autocrat remaining within. Risks are involved, and as director one must be willing to take them. The knowledge of the CNS in clinical matters, for example, in many instances is close to that of the physician. In addition, CNSs are usually able to preserve their sensitivity to the patient and to the nurse caring for that patient. They are generally persistent and do not shy away from shallow reasoning, aggressive putdowns, or procrastination from others in the health care team. For the director of nursing, this can mean visits from vexed physicians who wonder what the new role encompasses, or administrators who do not want the boat rocked, or the head of housekeeping who wonders why her or his work is being challenged. The director of nursing and her or his associates must support these people, while also assisting the CNS to make necessary changes. Occasionally one may need to help the specialist to change or alter her or his approach, but more often the CNS is identifying and facing problems or situations in the organization that should have surfaced long ago. Multiple problems in an organization that surface too quickly can precipitate anger and anxiety within the organization. There may be times when the CNS needs support and appreciation for exposing problems, but she or he may also need assistance in prioritizing and pacing the solutions.

EVALUATION

In evaluating the performance of a CNS, the administrator seeks to determine the CNS's impact on (1) the practice of nursing, (2) the nursing department, and (3) the administrator for nursing. Such an evaluation is not a scientific measurement of the impact of the role but is formulated on the basis of impressions, supported by examples.

Impact on Practice

The impact of the CNS on nursing practice becomes evident in many ways, among them the development of standard care plans, implementation of preoperative teaching, and development of such programs as an ongoing cancer patient support group. This impact is elusive at first, but within a year the effect of such activity becomes tangible. The type of patient unit and the individual style of the CNS influence the characteristics of this impact. For example, the cardiovascular CNS was the first CNS in our center to be assigned to a specific unit—the cardiology unit. This unit had been dedicated as a 32-bed unit shortly before the CNS arrived. Because so many new programs were being developed within the medical center, some departments were more successful in realizing appropriate dollars for their particular program than others. The cardiac exercise program received low priority for funding during the first four years of the center's rapid growth. Our cardiac exercise program (which now includes the post–open heart surgery patients as well as the post–myocardial infarction patients) would not be a reality today if it were not for this specialist and her persistence in repeatedly demonstrating the need for such a program. Although she assisted with the development of ever more complex acute care of the coronary patient, her specialty was cardiac rehabilitation. Nursing allowed her to move ahead both with assisting the nursing staff and planning with the physicians. Gradually the cardiac exercise program took shape, however, and as it progressed the nursing staff were well challenged and committed to the program. The CNS brought expert knowledge to this program, as well as writing skills, visual arts skills and a sense of how to make change. Her expert communication with me assisted me in playing an important role in supporting the program at budget sessions.

The style of each of our CNS's is quite different, but they all accomplish much. Our specialist for the neurological unit works in a quiet, steady way, demonstrating much skill as a role model. She spots problem areas with ease and moves in and out, teaching, demonstrating, and supporting nurses. She has a patience that is in rhythm with the kind of nurse who selects neurological nursing.

The oncology CNS, in conjunction with the psychiatric liaison specialist, has enhanced the staff's ability to deal effectively with the dying patient, his or her family and, very importantly, with the CNS herself. She reinforces their skills in providing basic nursing care (which is so needed by these patients) but she also leads them a step further and introduces them to a skillful assessment level with a research bent. Her question, "Have you noticed any particular comfort measure that is helpful to this particular patient with this particular kind of cancer?" assists them to stretch their minds and apply this knowledge in delivering holistic patient care.

The medical–surgical specialist quickly perceives new surgical procedures, asks pertinent questions of the surgeons, and leads the staff nurse to the logical development of a postoperative plan of nursing care.

These kinds of activities, these ways of relating to nursing staff, these examples of affecting the quality of patient care continue in our organization. Such behaviors, with their resultant positive outcomes, are reasonable and appropriate expectations nursing directors may have of the CNS.

Impact on the Nursing Department

The impact the specialists had on the nursing department as a whole became recognizable after several CNSs had been working for about two years. One could see that they had infused excitement into the process of setting professional goals for the department. Setting goals and establishing ways to achieve them seems to attract staff nurses more if this approach emanates from others in the organization besides the director of nursing. The CNSs have also drawn other members of the center into programs and activities that have affected patient care both directly and indirectly. For example, physicians and physical therapists involved in the formulation of our arthritis program consulted the medical–surgical CNS to assist them in describing the role of the nurse when applying for grant monies. And, very important, the CNSs have moved out beyond the walls of the hospital to make contributions to the state of New Hampshire, as well as to our profession, by publishing and by their activities in various professional associations. Indeed, by virtue of the way our organization is structured, the CNSs have focused narrowly on their specific units but have also shown their sense of responsibility to the organization as a whole, to the community, the state, and to their profession in the broad sense, showing themselves to be true nursing professionals.

Our CNSs have designed investigations, which in our setting was a challenging undertaking. That a nurse would embark on research in our institution was a shocker, as traditionally this was regarded as the purview of the physician. Nevertheless, the CNSs have persisted through some difficult obstacles and have achieved a great deal. They have assisted us to set standards of practice and to shape policy. They are persistent, never allowing important issues vital to the integrity of the organization to drop between organizational cracks. They are patient, yet they store issues in their memories and check back or follow up to determine if they are being acted upon. A special kind of stress is placed upon the organization because of these qualities that generate progressive and purposeful action. We surely know the CNSs exist; they are busy, they make their presence known. They are universal, rather than local; they are usually in orbit.

Impact on the Administrator

My dialogues with colleague nurse administrators on the role of the CNS focus on the specialists' contributions to the quality of patient care and their contribution to the new graduate. That the CNS might also have an impact on the nursing administrator is a thought that does not come about naturally to administrators, but this aspect is important and significant. All of us in this position need "organizational nourishment." We require intellectual stimulation about our organization: how does it work? How does it facilitate or impede the attainment of our goals? What ideas exist for change? We need to hear when all is going well and not so well, and further we need to learn from other nurses in the department why they think things are going well or not. It is vital for us, as directors, to have this input.

Without exception, in my experience, CNSs are articulate. They speak freely and demonstrate orderly thought. They provide a real link between the activity on the patient unit and the leader of the entire department.

In order to meet with the CNSs on a regular basis, I try to schedule an individual appointment with one of them every two weeks. Of course, this rotation has meant that as the number of specialists has increased we see each other less often. Our meetings are not structured; the dialogue is free-flowing. The CNSs always manage to present an assessment of where they are in their work. This assessment approach appears to be an integral part of them—their modus operandi—and it is one of their strengths. It explains, perhaps, why they are never standing still. Through these meetings I glean much information about my department. Talking with the CNSs helps the director to keep her or his finger on the clinical pulse of the organization.

The CNSs stimulate me; frequently revive me; *and* encourage me to "keep reaching." In these ways and more they contribute to the nursing administrator. It is a wise director who keeps in touch with them.

RECOMMENDATIONS

Though I have had a considerable amount of experience introducing the CNS into our organization, I still find it difficult to explain to physicians, some hospital administrators, trustees, and colleagues from other hospitals how important specialists are and what their potential contributions could be to other institutions. There is still apparently a hiatus between what these groups perceive the level of nursing care to be and the level it could potentially achieve. Physicians and some hospital administrators perceive the nurse with advanced education as a superfluous addition to the profession. Once the physician has worked with the CNS, however, the specialist's value is usually accepted. The CNS's focus on patient care gains support from the physician. If a director is able to find a way to obtain the first specialist and utilizes her or him appropriately, then the chances are excellent that the CNS will have sold the role and paved the way for the acceptance of more. Any documentation that provides specific proof that the quality of patient care has improved will also be of great value at budget time. Are letters from patients praising their care on the increase? Are the nurses more enthused about their work, more challenged? Has morale taken an upward turn? These indicators are positive evidence and well worth documenting.

It is not always possible (or even desirable) for all organizations to have an associate director for clinical affairs to whom the CNS reports. It would be useful, however, if some mechanism could be created permitting the specialist to have periodic dialogue with a nurse who has current clinical expertise as well as experience in the dynamics of an organization. For the small hospital, this may mean establishing a relationship with a hospital that does have such a resource person. This experience is essential, for the CNS needs a perspective concerning the totality of her or his practice. No matter where the setting—a large medical center or a small community hospital—the specialist has a contribution to make.

Another careful consideration to be made, is the size of the patient caseload carried by the CNS. I consider an assignment to a patient population of more than 50 beds to be the point at which dilution of the specialist's contribution occurs. The larger the patient population, the smaller the impact of the CNS. Considering that nursing staff are inextricably linked to the patients and considering that there are physicians and significant others relating to patient care, one is fairly accurate in estimating that in one 50-bed unit the specialist potentially comes in contact with over 100 people. The cost of such a nurse prohibits a lesser ratio that would enrich and even hasten the process of their effectiveness. One CNS, however, is better than none, in any setting. It is important that the one not be expected to have the same impact as two or more. Small hospitals eager to have a CNS on their staff frequently assign one to the entire nursing and hospital population, whether it be a 60-, 80-, or 100-bed hospital. Such a move sets up the CNS for frustration and even failure. Under today's economic stress, a director may have to search for trade-offs in the department in order to employ the first or additional specialists. Motivation brings forth creativity in most of us. Chances are that if one CNS practices in a unit or units of reasonable size, her or his effectiveness will be well recognized.

I have yet to develop a sophisticated method of monitoring the effect of the CNS. Our CNSs present overviews of their activities every year. Several of them write up detailed case studies that clearly describe how essential their presence is. I read these carefully, and so at the right moment I am able to elaborate to administrators or other colleagues on the specialists' worth and their influence on quality patient care. As cost-containment pressures mount, I must assume responsibility for proving the CNSs' worth. A director of nursing introducing the CNS role should make a study of their effectiveness early on. To be in an offensive rather than a defensive position, to establish the value of the specialists, is a far more comfortable and, organizationally, a healthier posture for a director and the department of nursing.

In closing, I hope that those organizations that are contemplating introducing the CNS will feel more courageous about such a plunge, and I trust that those who do have them will have been provided a new perspective. Clinical specialists have been essential to our department and will probably prove to be even more so in the future. Although there are more difficult challenges ahead for all of us, the CNS must be with us.

IV. EVALUATION

12.   A Model for Developing Evaluation Strategies

Ann B. Hamric

Evaluation of quality nursing care and of the practitioners who deliver that care is currently one of the most important issues in the nursing profession. Nowhere is this concern more evident than among clinical nurse specialists (CNSs), whose numbers and influence are being threatened by cost-containment pressures and limited budgets. The CNS was conceived as a self-directed practitioner capable of determining and evaluating her or his own performance. These independent characteristics and a resulting lack of consensus regarding performance criteria have undoubtedly delayed the development of sound evaluation procedures. It is certainly true that few attempts to evaluate either the effectiveness of the CNS role or the practice of an individual CNS have been reported. Both of these aspects of CNS evaluation need further development if the worth of this nursing role is to be demonstrated.

Adequate evaluation of the role's general impact—that is, of whether the CNS as a prototype is effective in improving nursing care—requires careful research methodology. There are few sound studies that clearly document the effectiveness of the CNS. Such evaluation is necessary for a number of reasons.

First, current health care economics emphasizing fiscal restraint cause administrators to be reluctant to experiment with untried roles. The CNS is a relatively new role on the health care scene and thus is more vulnerable to budget cuts. Additionally, the CNS is an expensive nurse. It is realistic and legitimate for hospital and nursing administrators to question the impact of the CNS on quality of care. It is equally legitimate for them to expect some positive effect after a reasonable length of time. Although this point is generally agreed upon, problems arise when one attempts to define what is a "positive effect" and what length of time is "reasonable."

Administrators are requesting evidence that the CNS's impact extends beyond that of a traditional staff nurse or head nurse. Again, this is a reasonable request. Evaluation is complicated, however, by the fact that the CNS is not only a care provider. Rather, the CNS is charged with effecting change for two particular groups: patients in the CNS's specialty area and the nursing staff caring for those patients. The CNS cannot simply be evaluated on the quality of patient care she or he gives but is also accountable for a multitude of indirect patient care functions, such as consulting, teaching, and researching. In addition, there is a third level of expectation that includes the CNS's contribution to the nursing profession as a whole and impact on other health care professionals.

Another reason evaluation is such a pressing need is the continued confusion among nurses and other health care providers regarding CNS role functions. Too often, other caregivers' judgments of the worth of the role are based on one CNS's personality and achievement (or lack of achievement) rather than established standards. This confusion may negatively influence the perceptions of other caregivers and lead to inadequate utilization of the CNS.

The second aspect of CNS evaluation focuses on appraisal of individual performance—that is, whether a given CNS is effective in her or his position. Although apparently an easier task than studying the impact of the role, there are few documented procedures or instruments for evaluating an individual CNS, and many CNSs feel that performance evaluation is the most problematic area of their practice. There are important reasons why adequate individual evaluation methods must be developed. Annual salary reviews and promotions should take into account the quality of performance. The important first steps of evaluation—establishing realistic goals and planning how they may be achieved—should become an integral expectation for both the CNS and her or his employer.

Experimentation with tools for evaluating the individual CNS can lead to greater consensus regarding the functions of the role. As noted above, such standardized expectations can lead, in turn, to greater role stability and less role confusion.

DONABEDIAN'S MODEL FOR PATIENT CARE EVALUATION

Donabedian (1966) identified three areas of patient care that can be used as foci for evaluation: structure, process, and outcome. Bloch

discussed these same categories in relation to nursing care in particular
(1975). Donabedian's model and Bloch's adaptation of it are diagrammed
in Figure 12-1. The first of Donabedian's categories, structural evaluation,
focuses on the setting or system in which care occurs and the attributes of
care-providers in the system. Such factors as the characteristics of an
institution's physical plant and the numbers, qualifications, and utilization
of caregivers (e.g., nurse–patient ratios; numbers of RNs, LPNs, and aides
on staff) are structural variables. Interest in structural variables is based
upon the assumption that proper settings and instrumentalities will result
in quality health care (Donabedian p. 170). The second facet of evaluation,
process evaluation, focuses on the care provided. It examines the processes
of care delivery, such as coordination of care, technical competence, and the
appropriateness and completeness of assessment. In nursing, care delivery
can be evaluated by studying each phase of the nursing process. The final
facet, outcome evaluation, focuses on the care recipient, or the patient. In
most studies of medical care, outcome has been measured in terms of
patient recovery, restoration of function, and survival (Donabedian, p. 167).
Bloch referred to these parameters as measuring the patient's "health state"
and identified others that could be used to measure outcomes. These
additional parameters are (1) cognitive outcome (the patient's knowledge of
the disease and treatment); (2) psychosocial outcome (the patient's attitudes
toward care, motivation, family participation in treatment); and (3)
behavioral outcome (the patient's compliance with recommended health
practices and other observable health-related behaviors).

> There should be no question that cognitive, psychosocial, and behavioral
> variables are indeed outcome variables, and it is unfortunate that measure-
> ment of these variables as outcome indicators is sometimes not considered
> worthwhile, because of their, admittedly, tenuous relationship to health state
> (p. 258).

Donabedian's framework is a useful guideline for CNS evaluation for
several reasons. These categories are widely used as a frame of reference for
studying patient care (Bailit, Lewis, Hochheiser, et al., 1975; Given, Given,
& Simoni, 1979; Hegyvary & Haussmann, 1976; Luker, 1981). Although
there are differences of opinion concerning whether structure, process, or
outcome are most useful, Donabedian's model remains the accepted
"language" of health care evaluation, and most existing evaluation tools are
based on these categories. In addition, the framework keeps the focus on
what is being evaluated—that is, it prescribes the content of the evaluation—
rather than focusing on who is doing the evaluation, an issue frequently
debated in relation to CNS evaluation. Discussions of who is qualified to
evaluate the CNS can obscure the central issue of identifying relevant
criteria of effectiveness. Third, the model allows one to examine the

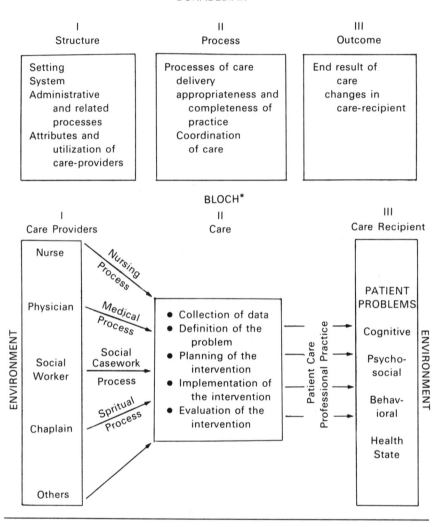

DONABEDIAN

| I | II | III |
| Structure | Process | Outcome |

Setting	Processes of care	End result of
System	delivery	care
Administrative	appropriateness and	changes in
and related	completeness of	care-recipient
processes	practice	
Attributes and	Coordination	
utilization of	of care	
care-providers		

BLOCH*

| I | II | III |
| Care Providers | Care | Care Recipient |

*Reprinted with permission from Bloch, D. Evaluation of nursing care in terms of process and outcome: Issues in research and quality assurance. Copyright 1975, American Journal of Nursing company. *Nurs Res*, 1975, *24*, p. 257.

Figure 12-1. Donabedian's model for patient care evaluation as applied to nursing by Bloch.

problems presented by a particular evaluation in an orderly manner, helping to indicate which method(s) would yield relevant data. In some situations an evaluator would need process methods and related standards, while in other situations outcome standards should be weighted more heavily. The model allows one to select the proper method(s), depending on which aspect of care is being examined. Finally, this model, as adapted by Bloch, focuses on the delivery of nursing care, the central function of the CNS toward which all her or his direct and indirect patient care activities should be directed.

CNS functions such as contribution to the nursing profession or impact on attitudes of other care-providers about nursing are beyond the scope of this model. Such activities should be evaluated secondarily to how well the CNS performs her or his central function, the improvement of nursing care. Some of the indirect care functions of the CNS (such as the liaison function) cannot be evaluated according to Donabedian's categories, and no attempt is being made to assert that this framework is all-encompassing for CNS evaluation. However, the effect of the CNS on patient care has historically been the major concern and problem of anyone attempting to evaluate the impact of the CNS role or of the performance of any individual CNS. This model offers a valid structure within which to develop sound methods of evaluation for both concerns.

Table 12-1 outlines strategies for evaluating various aspects of CNS performance according to Donabedian's framework. The three basic evaluation categories (structure, process, and outcome) are correlated in the table with aspects of CNS performance that one may wish to evaluate. The strategies suggested for studying each aspect of CNS performance can be used for appraisal of individual performance as well as for studying the impact of the role. Some strategies, such as "staff evaluation," are discrete tools for appraisal of individual performance that have been previously identified and reported in the literature (Hamric, Gresham, & Eccard, 1978). (A modification of the staff evaluation method is detailed in Chapter 13.) Other strategies listed in Table 12-1, such as studying outcome in terms of the "achievement of patient-oriented objectives," are not specific strategies, but rather general directions for selecting criteria for evaluation. For example, a CNS developing a cardiac rehabilitation program could select cognitive and behavioral patient outcome objectives specific to her or his patient population to use in evaluating the program's success. Such a strategy would assess the CNS's impact on patient care outcomes directly, if the CNS were the primary caregiver, or indirectly if the CNS were teaching others to implement the program. Finally, it should be noted that some evaluation methods, such as "staff evaluation," combine both structural and process elements and are therefore listed under both categories.

Table 12-1
Strategies for Evaluating the CNS

Evaluation Categories	Aspects of CNS Performance	Evaluation Strategies
Structure	CNS effect on selected institutional practices (A, B, C) CNS level of professional activity (A, B, D, E) Utilization of caregivers; setting, and system within which CNS practices (C, E)	A. Staff evaluation B. Dual-purpose framework C. Review of hospital records for such data as turnover rates, RN–patient ratio D. CNS self-evaluation: time study of activities E. CNS job description, position, committee activity
Process	CNS ability to perform aspects of role (A, B, D, E) • Direct care functions: skill as clinician, patient advocate, role model • Indirect care functions: change agent, consultant, clinical teacher, supervisor, researcher (some aspects) CNS impact on attitudes of other nurses and other caregivers (A, C) CNS impact on ability of nursing staff to perform aspects of nursing process (E) CNS evaluation of own professional growth (F)	A. Staff evaluation B. Administrative review, including review of • Objectives and goals • Job description (e.g., dual purpose framework) C. Consumer or other health care professional evaluation D. Peer review E. Nursing process audit— improvements in various aspects of nursing process (data collection, problem definition, etc.) F. Self-evaluation— according to objectives and goals, or job description
Outcome	CNS impact on patient care outcomes (A) • directly—role as clinician • indirectly—role as change agent, innovator	A. Outcome objectives • Achievement of optimal patient health status objectives • Achievement of

192

Table 12.1 *(continued)*
Strategies for Evaluating the CNS

Evaluation Categories	Aspects of CNS Performance	Evaluation Strategies
		patient-oriented objectives: cognitive outcomes behavioral outcomes psychosocial outcomes

STRUCTURAL EVALUATION

Structural evaluation focuses on the system, examining administrative factors within the institution and characteristics of caregivers. Examples of structural variables relative to the institution would include numbers of registered nurses (RNs) and other staff members; patient–nurse ratios on unit(s) where the CNS practices; number of committees to which a CNS belongs; the CNS job description and position within the organziation. Structural variables related to characteristics of the caregiver would include such items as qualifications of the CNS, CNS's attendance at continuing education programs, and style of supervision utilized. Structural evaluation gives information about the environment in which the CNS practices, her or his level of professional activity, and some information on the CNS's effect upon the institution and other caregivers.

The advantage of this form of evaluation is that data are concrete and relatively easy to obtain. One example is a time study of a CNS's activities, a written record of time spent on different tasks. A time study is a quantitative measure that can yield helpful data regarding the appropriateness and amount of a CNS's activities. One cannot consider a time study to be sufficient for evaluation, but rather a beginning step that demonstrates whether the CNS has structured her or his role to include appropriate functions. Structural variables may point out the constraints on CNS practice (such as excessive requirements for administrative duties) and may identify factors that facilitate or hamper CNS effectiveness. As one can see from the above examples, however, structural variables alone are minimally helpful in evaluating CNS effectiveness, since they are not directly related to quality of performance. The assumption underlying structural evaluation, that provision of a proper setting will result in high-quality care, is particularly tenuous when examining an environment as complex as the one in which most CNSs practice. For example, one cannot determine the number, qualifications, and job descriptions of the CNSs in a given institution and tell by this whether they are functioning effectively.

Some structural variables, as mentioned above, may yield helpful data.

Presence of administrative support has been shown to be an important factor contributing to CNS job satisfaction (Shaefer, 1973). It is commonly assumed that increased job satisfaction results in increased effectiveness, so that one may hypothesize that administrative support improves CNS performance. A second structural variable that may have some bearing on CNS effectiveness is the specialist's style of supervision. The superiority of the democratic style of supervision in enhancing leadership behavior has been clearly demonstrated. Staff nurse satisfaction and staff nurse turnover are two other structural variables that may indirectly relate to CNS effectiveness, although factors other than the CNS certainly influence staff nurses. Finally, structural components such as number and type of caregivers on the CNS' unit(s) and accessibility of other health team members for patient needs have a bearing on the milieu in which a CNS functions and thus may influence her or his impact. Analysis of these and other structural variables, however, cannot stand alone as an evaluation method.

PROCESS EVALUATION

Process evaluation, or the study of what the caregiver does, yields data regarding the CNS's ability to perform such aspects of the role as role modeling, functioning as a change agent, and consulting. Most studies examining individual CNS effectiveness have concentrated on process variables. Examples of strategies for making process evaluations include "staff evaluation," in which members of a nursing staff who observe the CNS evaluate her or his performance, using behavioral criteria (Hamric, Gresham, & Eccard, 1978). As previously mentioned, evaluation by the staff includes both process standards (e.g., "She performs patient activities with a high degree of clinical competence") and structural standards (e.g., "She regularly schedules in-service programs and is responsive to our ideas for topics").

Administrative review is a widely used process strategy. In this design, the CNS and her or his superior mutually establish goals and objectives and evaluate them together at regular intervals. (This method is discussed in Chapter 10.) Administrative review can also use the CNS's job description as an evaluative guideline; an example of such use is found in the "dual purpose framework" described by Colerick, Mason, and Proulx (1980). The dual purpose framework uses both structural and process criteria to formulate a job description, and divides them into four major categories: service, education, consultation, and research. The authors believe this paradigm can be used not only as guide to formulating a job description for the CNS but also as a guide for the nurse administrator in evaluating the role.

A third type of process evaluation is that undertaken by other health care professionals or consumers. In this instance, individuals are questioned regarding processes of care, as a means of evaluating the effectiveness of the caregiver. Examples of this method of evaluating the CNS appear in three different published reports. Two of these examined an individual CNS. Barrett (1972) questioned physicians regarding the quality of one CNS's performance, and Simms (1965) surveyed patients and family members concerning her own activities as a CNS. Both authors received favorable responses from those questioned. The third report was a more scientific attempt to determine patients' perceptions regarding the quality of care they received. Hardy (1977) surveyed patients on units that had CNSs and units without them but found no significant differences between the patients' perceptions of care.

A fourth type of process evaluation focuses on improvements in various components of nursing process. Most formal research on the effectiveness of the CNS role has utilized this method. Examples in the literature include the work of Georgopoulos and Jackson (1970) and Georgopoulos and Sana (1971), who examined nursing Kardex behavior and content of intershift report, respectively, as measures of the quality of nursing process. Ayers (1979) studied the "clinical insight" of nursing staff on units with CNSs. Little and Carnevali (1967) looked at nurse behaviors of CNSs as compared to behaviors of staff nurses. Girouard (1978) studied the preoperative teaching and documentation activities of nurses on two units, one of which had a CNS. Each of these studies showed positive correlation between the introduction of the CNS role and the improvement of the nursing staff's ability to perform some aspect of nursing process, according to the measures studied. These studies are methodologically the most sound and have yielded the most positive findings. Taken as a group, they constitute the strongest support for the impact of the CNS role in improving nursing practice.

A fifth type of process evaluation is that of peer review. Although Colerick et al. stated that peer review is "often utilized by CNSs," (1980, p. 29), only one effort has been reported in the literature. It involved a group of CNSs who attempted a group interactional review, in which a CNS submitted her or his self-evaluation to a peer review committee composed of CNS colleagues. The CNS then met with this committee to discuss, amplify and clarify the written statement. This program was not successful because individuals felt insecure and the group lacked criteria for measuring clinical effectiveness (Gold, Jackson, Sachs, et al. 1973). A more recent and more successful peer review program is reported in Chapter 14.

Self-evaluation according to stated goals and objectives or job description is a useful process strategy. Certainly, self-evaluation is an important component of any individual CNS performance appraisal. Depending upon the goals established, it may have more or less importance than other strategies. In practice, however, it is difficult for anyone immersed in a role to objectively evaluate her or his own activities. Because of this inherent subjectivity, self-evaluation should be coupled with another strategy.

There are numerous advantages to process evaluation. Although an indirect measure of the CNS's impact on quality of care, process evaluation directly examines the activities of the caregiver, which may be especially relevant to the question of whether proper practice has occurred (Donabedian, p. 169). For the individual CNS attempting to implement a broad, unstructured role, process evaluation can give needed validation of the scope, appropriateness, and effectiveness of her or his practice. For the researcher examining the overall role, process measures can directly evaluate CNS impact on staff behavior or on staff perception by yielding descriptive data that give concrete information. Process evaluation strategies that utilize other caregivers as data sources can contribute to the development of uniform expectations of the CNS. Presently, the process method is the most practical means of CNS evaluation. A number of tools are available to measure quality of nursing process (Barney, 1981; Hegyvary, Haussman, Kronman, et al., 1981; Wandelt & Ager, 1974). Use of written records, direct observation, or questionnaires are relatively straightforward data collection methods. In addition, most nurse administrators and CNSs are familiar with evaluation according to objectives and goals.

The major disadvantage of process evaluation is that it is not a direct measure of the quality of care rendered. For example, simply influencing a staff's perception of quality nursing care (a classic process measure) does not automatically raise the level of care that staff provides. There is insufficient research correlating patient care processes with outcomes to permit us to conclude that positive changes in nursing process result in positive patient outcomes (Hegyvary & Haussmann, 1976). Finally, one can question whether patients are able to accurately evaluate the activities of health care providers. Hardy raised this concern after finding that the patients she interviewed did not feel that such important nursing care functions as discharge planning were even necessary (1977, p. 331). (The issue of using patient opinions has been explored by French, 1981.) These drawbacks point to the fact that an accurate, comprehensive evaluation of the CNS role requires the use of all three of Donabedian's evaluation categories. In spite of these problems, however, process evaluation alone can yield relevant data concerning CNS effectiveness.

OUTCOME EVALUATION

Outcome evaluation examines the results of care in terms of changes in the recipient of the care; for the CNS, outcome evaluation measures CNS impact on patient care outcomes. (The reader should note that indirect CNS activities such as change agent can lead to positive changes in knowledge, attitudes, and behavior of staff nurses that could technically be considered "nursing outcomes." Because these changes are measured by process strategies, and because Donabedian's model deals only with *patient* outcomes, the author has chosen to consider the CNS effect on nursing staff as part of process evaluation, rather than outcome evaluation.) Outcome is the only direct measure of provider effectiveness and clinically is the most important measure of quality (Bailit et al., p. 154). The most obvious example of an outcome evaluation is one that measures changes in the patient's health status. In this type of evaluation, physical parameters such as presence or progression of disability or alleviation of symptoms are measured. Number of hospital days and number of hospital readmissions have been used as outcome measures, with a reduction in both indicating improvements of the patient's health status. As previously noted, Bloch (1975) identified additional categories of cognitive, psychosocial, and behavioral outcome. An example of evaluation according to cognitive objectives would be measuring the increase in patient knowledge after institution of a teaching program. Psychosocial variables such as improved social interaction or family understanding and participation in a patient's treatment may also be the focus of an outcome evaluation. In behavioral evaluation, items such as patient adherence to a therapeutic regimen are examined.

When an individual CNS works intensively with one client group, it should be possible to use outcome measures to document her or his impact. The nursing profession is developing outcome criteria for a variety of patient problems (Inzer & Aspinall, 1981; Mason, 1978; Zimmer, et al., 1974). Unfortunately, measurement of these criteria has proved to be a difficult problem. Development and testing of some outcome measurement tools have begun (Horn & Swain, 1977; Hover & Zimmer, 1978; Jette, 1980; Krueger, Nelson, & Wolanin, 1978), but further testing of instruments for reliability, validity, and feasibility remains a pressing need (Bloch, 1980).

Although it is clearly recognized that improved patient outcomes should be an important result of CNS practice, measuring this relationship has proven to be technically difficult. The necessity for careful selection of nurse-dependent variables within the control of the CNS, coupled with nursing's relative inexperience with developing such variables has undoubtedly limited efforts to research the role. The results of the few studies attempting to relate positive patient outcomes with direct CNS intervention have been disappointing. Little and Carnevali (1967) studied the effect of CNS care on tuberculosis patients, and Murphy (1971) studied the effect of CNS intervention in preoperative teaching on the level of postoperative patient complications. Both of these studies found no difference in the health status of patients cared for by CNSs compared with those cared for by other nurses. A major problem in both of these studies was that the patient responses observed (such as cardiac arrhythmias and X-ray findings) were highly doctor-dependent rather than nurse-dependent. Because the studies included variables beyond the control of the CNS, one should question the significance of their findings (Padilla, 1973). These findings indicate the need for improved measurement of outcomes as well as more thorough investigation of the relationship between CNS intervention and improvement in patient health.

There are other serious difficulties in implementing an outcome evaluation specifically for the CNS. In the tertiary health care setting where most CNSs practice, many variables influence the patient's health state besides the quality of nursing care. It is difficult to identify outcome criteria solely attributable to nursing care, much less to one CNS's intervention. Cognitive, behavioral, and psychosocial variables can be more difficult to measure than health state but may often be the realm in which nursing makes its unique contribution to patient welfare.

Patients with chronic disease present additional problems. One is the difficulty of knowing at what point in the course of the illness changes in outcome can be tested (Given, Given, & Simoni, 1979). It is also hard to know what outcomes are indicative of positive intervention for this population. Other impinging variables in patients who are managed on an outpatient basis over a long period of time complicate the process of identifying cause and effect relationships. Reliable outcome criteria in the complex patient with multisystem involvement are the most difficult to develop, yet this is the client population with which most CNSs deal.

A further disadvantage of patient outcome evaluation is that CNS performance in indirect functions such as consulting or teaching cannot be evaluated by examining changes in patient outcomes despite their importance to the CNS role. When the CNS is acting as a consultant or teacher, her or his effect on patients is mediated through other nurses or other health care professionals, and consequently is too far removed from the selected patient outcome to measure. In these situations, one would be more interested in examining changes in nursing behavior, knowledge, or attitude attributable to CNS intervention. This point strengthens the argument for combining structure, process, and outcome variables in researching the impact of the role. "Finally, although outcomes might indicate good or bad care in the aggregate, they do not give an insight into the nature and location of the deficiencies or strengths to which the outcome might be attributed" (Donabedian, p. 169). Given these difficulties, outcome evaluation should probably not be used as the sole means for evaluating the CNS. Combining process and limited outcome measures is certainly feasible, however, and may be preferable to evaluation by process measures alone.

USE OF THE MODEL IN INDIVIDUAL PERFORMANCE APPRAISAL

Clearly, any evaluation strategy should be based on the role components the CNS has emphasized in her or his practice. A newly hired CNS endeavoring to establish a strong consultant base in a hospital unfamiliar with CNSs will need quite a different evaluation plan from an established CNS working to strengthen discharge planning on her or his unit(s). Table 12-2 suggests a procedure for developing a method for evaluating individual CNSs. The first step is to identify the focus (or foci) of the CNS's practice. This focus can easily change over time, so that an evaluation procedure utilized in the first year of one's practice might not be appropriate by the third year. On the basis of these practice emphases, one can then define the desired goals or end products. These goals will determine whether structure, process, outcome, or a combination of these categories should be employed in making the evaluation and what measures or standards would be appropriate. Finally, one determines who should conduct the evaluations and at what intervals.

Use of such a procedure can enable one to consider the following points. First, what is the focus of the evaluation? It is as unrealistic to expect that any one evaluation measure can encompass all aspects of the CNS role as to expect that one CNS can simultaneously practice all aspects. In individual performance appraisal, it is more reasonable to select a few components that a given CNS has emphasized and evaluate those thoroughly. Different measures (structural, process, or outcome) and different evaluators (peers, patients, or nursing administrators) may be indicated depending on one's goals (see the examples in Table 12-2). If the institution has a strong quality assurance program that evaluates patient outcome criteria, outcome evaluation may be practical. Correlating such outcome evaluation with concurrent process evaluation would be ideal. If no such program exists, it may be unrealistic to attempt a large-scale outcome evaluation, regardless of its advantages. It may still be possible to obtain statistics from the business office, such as patient hospital days prior to the beginning of a CNS project or specific goal and after completion. Such information could be correlated with other data to yield information related to the CNS's effect on patient outcomes. If one is most interested in examining indirect functions, then structure and process components may yield the needed information (see the second example in Table 12-2).

Table 12-2
Guidelines for Developing an Evaluation Strategy for Individual CNSs

Steps in Process	Example #1 (One Major Focus)	Example #2 (One of a Number of Foci)
1. Select focus (or foci) of practice	1. CNS to develop teaching program for spinal cord-injured patients	1. CNS to identify educational needs of surgical nurses and provide appropriate in-service education for all shifts
2. Set goals, desired end results	2. CNS sets two goals: a. Nursing staff will accept and implement program (nursing staff outcome) b. Patients will have increased knowledge and increased ability to perform self-care (patient outcome)	2. 80% of all staff will participate in in-service programs at least once a month
3. Determine whether structure, process, or outcome evaluation is indicated	3. a. Structure b. Process c. Outcome—cognitive and behavioral objectives	3. a. Structure b. Process
4. Determine appropriate method and measure(s)	4. a. (1) Record of numbers of staff available for program (2) Administrative support—materials, time, etc.	4. a. (1) Time schedule—adequate staffing to allow attendance (2) Administrative support—materials, setting

(3) Audit reward system of unit—positive reinforcement for staff implementation

    b. (1) Questionnaire to staff—to determine attitude(s) about program

      (2) Evaluate nursing records (process audit)—to determine number of staff implementing and number of documented teaching sessions

    c. (1) Questionnaire to patients—test knowledge

      (2) Test self-care abilities and compare with patients before the program was implemented

    b. Audit nursing records—program topics, attendance; questionnaire to staff—to evaluate topics appropriate for their educational needs

5. Determine appropriate evaluator(s)

    5. CNS—to collect audit data, business office data survey nursing staff test patients

    5. CNS to collect audit data, survey nursing staff

6. Determine appropriate intervals for measurement

    6. One year after program implementation

    6. Six-month intervals

The second point to consider is the time required to implement an evaluation method. It is important to determine which data related to an individual's performance are easily accessible. Outcome evaluation is generally a slower method because of time elapsed before patient outcomes manifest themselves. If a program for CNS performance appraisal must be quickly implemented, process or structural evaluation may be most feasible in the short run. For example, if other CNSs in the institutions are willing to attempt peer review, then this may be the preferable method. Other practical constraints, such as expense or numbers of people involved in evaluation, may dictate the method chosen by the individual CNS. For example, a non–unit-based CNS interested in staff evaluation must elicit the cooperation of a group of staff nurses and spend adequate time with them for the method to yield reliable data (Hamric, Gresham, & Eccard, 1978, p. 23–25). It may be more realistic for this CNS to evaluate the effectiveness of her or his interventions according to outcome criteria for a select client group.

Visibility of the CNS's activities is an important factor in utilizing any evaluation method requiring direct observation of the CNS's practice. If a CNS is not observed enough for the evaluator to get some feeling for her or his skills and priorities, the observer cannot evaluate the CNS fairly. If one consistently gets feedback from an evaluator to the effect that "I never see you; I can't evaluate you," then the CNS must question what kind of impact she or he is having on the quality of care in that institution. In that instance, negative appraisal can be feedback leading to needed change in the CNS's activities.

The CNS should have significant input in determining both the method and the content of any performance appraisal. Constructing an evaluation tool is a valuable exercise in self-analyzing role performance. It also allows for modification as one matures and changes priorities within the position, thus preserving flexibility to meet the needs of one's client population.

Lastly, a thorough self-evaluation should accompany any evaluation by others. It is the author's personal belief that such evaluations should occur annually, both to document performance for the individual's record and the institution and to provide directions for professional growth.

ISSUES IN RESEARCHING THE IMPACT OF
THE CNS ROLE

As previously noted, some researchers have used process evaluation methods to examine the CNS's impact on nursing staff attitudes and behaviors. Others have utilized outcome criteria to examine CNS impact on patient care. The Girouard study (1978) identified cognitive and psychosocial outcome criteria in one hypothesis but reported only process data in discussing the study results. Only the Little and Carnevali study (1967) reported both process variables and outcome variables, but no relationship between the two was established.

Padilla (1973) did a thorough analysis of six experimental studies on CNS role effectiveness: Ayers (1971); Georgopoulos and Jackson (1970); Georgopoulos and Sana (1971); Little and Carnevali (1967); Melber (1967); and Murphy (1971). The reader is referred to Padilla's excellent in-depth discussion of the strengths and weaknesses of these research efforts. (The Melber study contains methodological weaknesses; its findings are open to question and consequently have not been included here.) Padilla concluded that, taken together, the studies she reviewed indicated that the CNS role was effective in improving certain *nursing* behaviors, such as recording clinical statements on the nursing Kardex. In contrast to these findings, Padilla stated that the effectiveness of the CNS in relation to *patient* responses seemed closely tied to the area of patient care to which she is directing her attention and is limited to nurse-dependent patient responses. . . . Thus far, clinical specialist research has not adequately shown that CNS nursing practice or leadership positively affect patient responses" (p. 330). Padilla also noted that the organizational context in which the CNS practiced influenced the findings of the studies she examined. She recommended that certain structural variables such as job description and organizational position be studied to determine the conditions within which the CNS role is most effective (Padilla, p. 329).

Research which examines selected direct and indirect aspects of the CNS role is valuable and needs to continue.

Thorough research of CNS role effectiveness, however, must go beyond process or outcome evaluation to examine and measure relationships between CNS practice, staff nurse practice and patient outcome, with structural components controlled or included. "Studies which attempt to document the linkages between process variables and patient outcomes represent a more comprehensive approach to health care evaluation than those which attend only to measures of process *or* measures of outcome" (Given, Given and Simoni, 1979, p. 87). In process-outcome evaluation, outcomes must be explicit, measurable, and based upon clearly desirable, predetermined goals. Structural and process data are collected to explain outcome attainment or its lack (Abramson, 1979, p. 212-3). Some process-outcome studies have been attempted. Two examples are Given, Given, and Simoni (1979), who studied hypertensive patients in an ambulatory care setting, and Hegyvary and Haussmann, who did a limited study of patients with congestive heart failure and patients undergoing abdominal hysterectomy (1976, pp. 18-21).

Studies that attempt to demonstrate a cause and effect relationship between process and outcome are extremely complex. Although numerous research methods are available (Waltz & Bausell, 1981; Isaac & Mitchell,

1981; Cook & Campbell, 1979; Campbell & Stanley, 1963), the lack of sophisticated tools to measure complex relationships, and the need to measure and correlate multiple variables pose serious challenges for the researcher. As Abramson notes, "In practice . . . difficulties usually abound, and such evaluations should not be undertaken lightly . . . Evaluation and service frequently make competing demands, and the requirements for a well-substantiated evaluation of effectiveness may be difficult to meet in 'the turbulent setting of the action program' " (p. 215). Regardless of these difficulties, collecting process data from CNSs and staff nurses and comparing these data with selected patient responses for a target population is within nursing's current research capability. An increase in beginning process-outcome evaluation studies using CNS practice will lead to greater sophistication in methodology and more reliable research. The reader contemplating such research would be well-advised to seek the counsel of someone with expertise in design, methodology, and statistical measurement—in short, an experienced nurse researcher.

Further discussion of the difficulties of process-outcome evaluation research is beyond the scope of this chapter. (The interested reader is referred to "Evaluation Research: Assessment of Nursing Care", *Nursing Research*, Vol. 29, March/April, 1980, for additional exploration of these issues. Until linkages between processes of care and outcomes can be demonstrated, it is premature to assert that process-outcome evaluation is the key to demonstrating the impact of the CNS role on nursing practice. It may represent, however, one possible avenue for future exploration.

CONCLUSION

If the CNS role is to survive, sound documentation of the effect of this practitioner on nursing practice and patient care must replace individual conviction that the role is viable. Cost-effectiveness of the CNS cannot be adequately addressed until such documentation occurs. Strategies for evaluation of aspects of CNS role performance are available, although development and measurement of process and outcome criteria must develop further before the impact of the CNS can be researched. Increased efforts at individual performance appraisal can generate data which can lead to more sophisticated research methodology. CNSs should welcome evaluation of their activities rather than viewing such examination as a restriction of their freedom. Creative experimentation with specialist input can only serve to clarify and strengthen the role.

REFERENCES

Abramson, J.H. The four basic types of evaluation: clinical reviews, clinical trials, program reviews, and program trials. *Public Health Rep*, 1979, *94*, 210–215.

Ayers, R. Effects and development of the role of the clinical nurse specialist. In R. Ayers, ed, The clinical nurse specialist an experiment in role effectiveness and role development. Duarte, CA: City of Hope National Medical Center, 1971.

Bailit, H., Lewis, J., & Hochheiser, L., et al.: "Assessing the quality of care. *Nurs Outlook*, 1975, *23*, 153–159.

Barney, M. Measuring quality of patient care: A computerized approach. *Superv Nurs*, 1981, *12*, 40–44.

Barrett, J. The nurse specialist practitioner: A study. *Nurs Outlook*, 1972, *20*, 524–527.

Bloch, D. Evaluation of nursing care in terms of process and outcome: Issues in research and quality assurance. *Nurs Res*, 1975, *24*, 256–263.

Bloch, D. Interrelated issues in evaluation and evaluation research: A researcher's perspective. *Nurs Res*, 1980, *29*, 69–73.

Campbell, D.T. & Stanley, J.C. *Experimental and quasi-experimental designs for research.* Chicago: Rand McNally, 1963.

Cook, T.D. & Campbell, D.T. *Quasi-experimentation: designs and analysis issues for field settings.* Boston: Houghton Mifflin, 1979.

Colerick, E.J., Mason, P.B., and Proulx, J.R. Evaluation of the clinical nurse specialist role: Development and implementation of a dual purpose framework. *Nurs Leadership*, 1980, *3*, 26–34.

Donabedian, A. Evaluating the quality of medical care. *Milbank Mem Fund Q,* 1966, *44*, 166–206.

French, K. Methodological considerations in hospital patient opinion surveys. *Int J Nurs Stud*, 1981, *18*, 7–22.

Georgopoulos, B.S., Jackson, M. Nursing kardex behavior in an experimental study of patient units with and without clinical nurse specialists. *Nurs Res*, 1970, *19*, 196–218.

Georgopoulos, B.S. & Sana, M. Clinical nursing specialization and intershift report behavior. *Am J Nurs*, 1971, *71*, 538–545.

Girouard, S. The role of the clinical specialist as change agent: An experiment in preoperative teaching. *Int J Nurs Stud*, 1978, *15*, 57–65.

Given, B., Given, C.W., & Simoni, L.E. Relationships of processes of care to patient outcomes. *Nurs Res*, 1979, *28*, 85–93.

Gold, H., Jackson, M., Sachs, B., Van Meter, M.J., et al.: "Peer review—A working experiment." *Nurs Outlook*, 1973, *21*, 634–636.

Hamric, A.B., Gresham, M.L., Eccard, M. Staff evaluation of clinical leaders. *J Nurs Adm*, 1978, *8*, 18–26.

Hardy, M.E. Implementation of unit management and clinical nurse specialists: Patient's perception of the quality of general hospital care and nursing care. *WICHE Commun Nurs Res*, 1977, *8*, 325–335.

Hegyvary, S., & Haussmann, R.K.D. Quality assurance. *J Nurs Adm*, 1976, *6*, 3–27.

Hegyvary, S.T., Haussman, R.K.D., Kronman, B., Burke, M. *User's manual for rush-medicus nursing process monitoring methodology.* Springfield, Va: National Technical Information Service, Stock #HRP0900638, 1981.

Horn, B.J. & Swain, M.A. *Development of criterion measures of nursing care.* Hyattsville,

Md.: U.S. National Center for Health Services Research (NTIS PB. #267004 & 267005), 1977.

Hover, J. & Zimmer, M.J. Nursing quality assurance: The Wisconsin system. *Nurs Outlook*, 1978, *26*, 242–248.

Inzer, F., & Aspinall, M.J. Evaluating patient outcomes. *Nurs Outlook*, 1981, *29*, 178–181.

Isaac, S. & Michael, W.B. *Handbook in research and evaluation*, 2nd Ed. San Diego, CA: EDITS Publishers, 1981.

Jette, A.M. Functional status index: Reliability of a chronic disease evaluation instrument. *Arch Phys Med Rehabil*, 1980, *61*, 395–401.

Krueger, J.C., Nelson, A.H., Wolanin, M.O. *Nursing research: Development, collaboration, and utilization.* Germantown, Md.: Aspen Systems Corporation, 1978.

Little, D.E., Carnevali, D. Nursing specialist effect on tuberculosis. *Nurs Res*, 1967, *16*, 321–326.

Luker, K.A. An overview of evaluation research in nursing. *J Adv Nurs*, 1981, *6*, 87–93.

Mason, E.J. *How to write meaningful nursing standards.* New York: Wiley, 1978.

Melber, R. The maternity nurse specialist in a hospital clinic setting. *Nurs Res*, 1967, *16*, 68–71.

Murphy, J.F. If P (additional nursing care): then Q (quality of patient welfare)? *WICHE Commun Nurs Res*, 1971, *4*, 1–12.

Padilla, G.V. Clinical specialist research: Evaluations and recommendations, conclusions and implications. In J.P. Riehl, & J.W. McVay (Eds.), *The clinical nurse specialist: Interpretations.* New York: Appleton-Century-Crofts, 1973.

Phaneuf, M.C. The nursing audit for evaluation of patient care. *Nurs Outlook*, 1966, *14*, 51–54.

Shaefer, J.A. The satisfied clinician: Administrative support makes the difference. *J Nurs Adm*, 1973, *3*, 17–20.

Simms, L. The clinical nursing specialist: An experiment. *Nurs Outlook*, 1965, *13*, 26–28.

Taylor, J.W. Measuring the outcomes of nursing care. *Nurs Clin North Am*, 1974, *9*, 337–348.

Wandelt, M.A. & Ager, J.W. *Quality patient care scale.* New York: Appleton-Century Crofts, 1974.

Waltz, C.F., & Bausell, R.B. *Nursing Research: Design Statistics and Computer Analysis.* Philadelphia: F.A. Davis, 1981.

Zimmer, M.J. principal investigator. Wisconsin Regional Medical Program. *Development of sets of patient health outcome criteria by panels of nurse experts*, Final Report, Project Number 17, Jan. 1-June 30, 1974. Milwaukee, Wis., The Program, 1974.

13. Evaluation of the CNS: Using an Evaluation Tool

Shirley Girouard
Judy Spross

The role of the clinical nurse specialist (CNS) has received much attention in the nursing literature. As defined by MacPhail, the CNS is "a graduate of a master's program in nursing, with a major in a clinical specialty, who is responsible for increasing her own clinical knowledge and competence and for enhancing the quality of nursing care and the quality of the organizational climate for learning and research." (1971, p. 5). Various components of the CNS role have also received much attention in the nursing literature. The five components most frequently identified are that of teacher, therapist/practitioner, consultant, researcher, and change agent.

Despite the attention given to the role of CNS, nursing literature provides little guidance as to how to evaluate the performance of the clinical specialist. Because the CNS role is often not well defined, performance evaluation is essential to provide direction to the individual specialist. Also, as stated by Colerick, Mason, and Proulx, "Evaluation is of paramount importance to nursing directors as it is at this top level of administration that the CNS needs to be evaluated if nursing directors are to be able to justify the hiring of such specialists" (1980, p. 29). Colerick et al. mention peer review, self-evaluation, administrative review, and nursing audits as methods that can be used to evaluate the performance of the CNS (p. 29).

The "dual purpose" framework proposed by Colerick et al. (a paradigm that is intended to serve as both a job description and an evaluation tool for the nurse administrator) has limitations. The framework is intended for use as an evaluation guide by the nurse administrator, but many of the behaviors identified in this model are ordinarily observed by the staff with whom the CNS is working rather than by the associate director or director of nursing doing the evaluation. The model's utility is further limited as an evaluation guide because, as the authors state, different hospitals employ CNSs in different ways, and thus expected behaviors can vary from institution to institution. Moreover, Colerick et al. do not discuss congruent goals between CNS and department and the role of these goals in administrative evaluation of the specialist. The interpersonal and collaborative skills of the CNS are also significant factors in success or failure of the CNS role and thus should be part of an evaluation guide for administrators, but in this model there is no expectation of collaborative interaction with other disciplines. Finally, the model includes no recognition of the fact that it is impossible to fulfill all the expectations described in service, education, consultation, and research at a given time. Some years the CNS may be primarily a reseacher, other years a teacher; the role components emphasized depend on the needs of the staff and the patients as well as the goals of the department.

Hamric, Gresham, and Eccard describe a type of evaluation in which the nursing staff in the specialty area(s) of the CNS evaluated clinical leaders' performance (1978). Such a tool enabled the CNS, along with other clinical leaders, to receive objective feedback about her or his performance and to specify behaviors that seemed to be important for effective implementation of the role. Since both the head nurse and the specialist were evaluated in this way, there was the added benefit of clarification of these leadership roles for the staff. The Hamric tool for CNS evaluation was constructed on the basis of the institution's job description, the literature on the CNS role, and the authors' experience in implementing the role.

As the time for the our own annual evaluations approached, in 1978 we began to investigate methods to meaningfully evaluate our performance. Weekly meetings with the associate director of the nursing department, our immediate supervisor, did not seem adequate to provide us with sufficient data about our performance. As Hamric et al. have stated, "Attempts by leadership personnel to evaluate one another are hindered by such factors as lack of direct observation of performance . . . and differences in role perception and emphasis" (p.18). With the encouragement of the associate director, we sought a method for obtaining input from those persons with whom we had the greatest contact—the staff and leadership people on our assigned units. It is important to point out that this is only one component of CNS evaluation. No attempt was made, for example, to evaluate the effects of the specialist on patient outcomes. (See also, Chapter 12.).

Del Bueno has asserted that judgments regarding performance should be based on a measurement of observed behavior compared to a performance standard (1977, p. 21). We felt that the unit leaders and staff, who saw the CNS on a day-to-day basis, were in a better position than the associate director to observe and evaluate certain aspects of our performance. With these thoughts in mind, we identified three objectives of the evaluation process to be done by the unit leaders.

First, we wished to determine the congruence between the unit leaders' perceptions of the CNS role and our own perception of it. Incongruence between perceptions would make it difficult to effect changes that would improve the quality of nursing care. We thought evaluation of the authors' performances by unit leaders would give us insight into misperceptions, unrealistic expectations, and any need to reexamine our own priorities in relation to those of the unit leaders. It would also facilitate self-evaluation of the change agent aspect of CNS performance. Secondly, we sought feedback about some of the clinical aspects of the role, including teaching and role modeling. Because the unit leaders are responsible for evaluating the performance of the nursing staff, we believed that the unit leaders could provide valuable information concerning our effectiveness as role models and teachers for staff nurses. The third objective of the unit leaders' evaluation of the CNS was to use their responses to set personal goals and unit goals. The latter would be done jointly with the unit leaders and staff.

Having established the objectives of the evaluation process, we needed a tool that the leaders could use in making their evaluation. This evaluation form was based upon our job description and was an adaptation of the tool for performance evaluation developed by Hamric et al. The tool was modified so that it was consistent with our institution's CNS job description and included a scale which the unit leaders could use to rate importance of CNS role components.

At Mary Hitchock Memorial Hospital, Hanover, New Hampshire, where the authors are employed, the CNS's job summary incorporates the components of the role addressed in the nursing literature. The job description includes 51 operational statements. These statements are grouped under the following broad categories:

1. Provide direct care to select patients;
2. Assist and guide staff in providing quality nursing care;
3. Participate in developing and effecting standards of nursing care practice;
4. Organize and participate in educational programs for staff;
5. Encourage the development of leadership skills in members of the nursing staff;
6. Work collaboratively with other members of the nursing department, other health care professionals, and other departments;

7. Investigate problems of nursing practice;
8. Maintain a high standard of professional responsibility and performance.

Thirty-five of the statements were reworded so that a scale similar to the Likert scale could be used by the leadership staff to rate both the importance of each item to the evaluator and the performance of the CNS on each item (Figure 13-1). The remaining statements, we felt, would be best evaluated by the associate director and were submitted separately to her (Table 13-1). In both questionnaires, scales for rating the importance of items ranged from "extremely important" (5) to "not a function of the clinical specialist" (1) (See Figure 13-2). The rating scale for performance evaluation was that described by Hamric et al. (Figure 13-3). Both rating scales included a "does not apply: do not know" category, which was assigned a "0" rating.

	Importance to You	CNS's Performance
Provides Direct Care to Select Patients:		
She regularly and systematically provides direct care to select patients.	5 4 3 2 1 0	5 4 3 2 1 0
When performing direct care, she is a role model for the staff.	5 4 3 2 1 0	5 4 3 2 1 0
She works effectively with other health professionals to assess, plan, implement, and evaluate patient care.	5 4 3 2 1 0	5 4 3 2 1 0
She enhances continuity of care when patients are transferred to other units.	5 4 3 2 1 0	5 4 3 2 1 0
She provides effective health teaching to select patients	5 4 3 2 1 0	5 4 3 2 1 0
She incorporates the role of patient advocate in clinical practice.	5 4 3 2 1 0	5 4 3 2 1 0
Assists and Guides the Staff in Providing Quality Nursing Care:		
She encourages and helps nurses to obtain and record a comprehensive and useful nursing data base.	5 4 3 2 1 0	5 4 3 2 1 0

Figure 13-1. Mary Hitchcock Memorial Hospital CNS evaluation tool.*

	Importance to You	CNS's Performance
She assists us to identify patient's problems and plan their care.	5 4 3 2 1 0	5 4 3 2 1 0
She stimulates us to try various approaches to the problems of patients.	5 4 3 2 1 0	5 4 3 2 1 0
She assists us to evaluate the quality of our care.	5 4 3 2 1 0	5 4 3 2 1 0
She is a good person to go to with patient care problems: if she doesn't have the answers she will try to find them.	5 4 3 2 1 0	5 4 3 2 1 0
She assists us in developing our patient care skills.	5 4 3 2 1 0	5 4 3 2 1 0
She encourages us to use the Problem Oriented Record effectively.	5 4 3 2 1 0	5 4 3 2 1 0
She participates actively in helping the staff to develop discharge plans for patients.	5 4 3 2 1 0	5 4 3 2 1 0

Participates in Developing and Effecting Standards of Nursing Care Practice:

She assists the head nurse to develop standards of care, communicate them, and holds staff accountable for meeting them.	5 4 3 2 1 0	5 4 3 2 1 0
She identifies needs for patient teaching outlines, procedures, protocols, and policies and works with the staff to develop them.	5 4 3 2 1 0	5 4 3 2 1 0
She supports and participates in the quality assurance program.	5 4 3 2 1 0	5 4 3 2 1 0

Organizes and Participates in Educational Programs:

She encourages continued learning and professional self-development.	5 4 3 2 1 0	5 4 3 2 1 0

(continued)

Figure 13.1 (continued)

	Importance to You	CNS's Performance
She guides the head nurse and assistant head nurses to develop and revise an orientation plan and follow-through of the plan.	5 4 3 2 1 0	5 4 3 2 1 0
She contributes to nursing student learning through informal and planned contacts.	5 4 3 2 1 0	5 4 3 2 1 0

Encourages the Development of Leadership Skills in Members of the Nursing Department:

She guides the head nurse and assistant head nurses in developing, presenting, and implementing changes in nursing practice.	5 4 3 2 1 0	5 4 3 2 1 0
She identifies staff nurses with leadership and/or teaching potential and helps to develop their skills.	5 4 3 2 1 0	5 4 3 2 1 0

Works Collaboratively with Other Members of the Nursing Department, as well as Other Disciplines:

She is effective in working with other services (physician, social workers, etc.) to enhance the quality of patient care.	5 4 3 2 1 0	5 4 3 2 1 0
She is an effective representative of nursing to other health care providers.	5 4 3 2 1 0	5 4 3 2 1 0
She interprets issues in health care and its delivery to staff, patients, and the community.	5 4 3 2 1 0	5 4 3 2 1 0
She works with the head nurse and supervisor in planning the budget.	5 4 3 2 1 0	5 4 3 2 1 0

Investigates Problems of Nursing Practice:

She investigates specific problems of nursing practice and uses the results to improve patient care.	5 4 3 2 1 0	5 4 3 2 1 0

(continued)

	Importance to You	CNS's Performance
She presents findings from research and ideas from the literature and suggests appropriate ways to implement these.	5 4 3 2 1 0	5 4 3 2 1 0
She collects descriptive or statistical data when needed to assess practice.	5 4 3 2 1 0	5 4 3 2 1 0
Maintains a High Standard of Professional Responsibility and Performance:		
She is able to perform patient care with a high degree of clinical competence.	5 4 3 2 1 0	5 4 3 2 1 0
She has the knowledge and clinical base which allows her to be a resource to the unit.	5 4 3 2 1 0	5 4 3 2 1 0
She is knowledgeable about nursing and health care issues.	5 4 3 2 1 0	5 4 3 2 1 0
She maintains flexible work patterns according to unit needs.	5 4 3 2 1 0	5 4 3 2 1 0
She respects the contributions of all health care workers while maintaining her commitment to the role of nursing in health care.	5 4 3 2 1 0	5 4 3 2 1 0
She is what a clinical specialist ought to be.	5 4 3 2 1 0	5 4 3 2 1 0

*Adapted from Job Description of CNS, Mary Hitchcock Memorial Hospital, Hanover, N.H. and from Hamric, A., Gresham, M., & Eccard, M. Staff evaluation of clinical leaders. *J Nurs Adm*, 1978, *8*, 18–26.

Figure 13.1 (continued)

Like Hamric et al., we also used open-ended questions to allow unit leaders to address issues of particular concern to them and to see if they had identified any improvements that had occurred on the units since the CNS had been employed. Evaluators were also asked to identify areas in which they felt the CNSs should be involved and were not.

Having developed the tool, we began to experience some anxiety about actually undertaking this—our first—evaluation as CNSs. We felt like Alice in Wonderland as she fell down the rabbit hole:

> Down, down, down. Would the fall never come to an end? "I wonder how many miles I've fallen by this time . . . I must be getting somewhere near the center of earth. Let me see: that would be four thousand miles down. I think—" (For, you see, Alice had learnt several things of this sort in her lessons in the schoolroom, and though this was not a very good opportunity for showing off her knowledge, as there was no one to listen to her, still it was good practice to say it over) (Carroll, 1976, p. 19).

After a year working in the clinical environment the authors were "down". It seemed too difficult to apply the knowledge we had learned in the ideal setting of graduate school to the real work setting in which we found ourselves. Though we had established good interpersonal relationships with our unit leaders, we believed the evaluation had the potential to provide us with more negative than positive feedback. We felt the need for feedback, however, to identify some possible etiologies for our feelings of frustration, to determine whether we were meeting our units' needs, and to explore some future directions. These rationales outweighed the anxiety we felt about soliciting our unit leaders' evaluations of us, so we forged ahead and requested their input. We hoped later to use staff as evaluators, but it seemed easier to use the unit leaders for our first evaluation attempt.

The evaluation forms were distributed to the head nurses and assistant head nurses on the three units for which we had direct responsibility. We distributed 3 forms to the oncology unit and 7 forms to the medical-surgical units. The leaders were told that signing the forms was optional. All of the leadership staff returned the forms and signed them. The three head nurses indicated that they had also received input from the staff on the units in completing the evaluation.

The responses rating the importance of various aspects of the CNS's role indicated that most items were considered to be very or extremely important to the respondents. Providing patient care on a regular basis, working with student nurses, interpreting issues in health care, and presenting research and ideas from nursing literature were rated as moderately or slightly important. Two or more respondents reported that they did not know what the CNS's role was in relation to quality assurance, involvement with student nurses, and budget planning. The results indicated that unit leaders agreed that most of the role components specified in the CNS job description were important. The unit leaders also felt that their respective CNS was performing above average in her role.

The responses to the open-ended questions were numerous. Both of the authors were mentioned by a majority of the respondents as having contributed by developing an orientation program for new staff. The CNS with two units received comments regarding the need to be more totally available to her units, two units being too much, and the need for the unit

Table 13-1
Items Evaluated by Associate Director

Provides Direct Care to Select Patients:

Identifies the learning needs of certain groups of patients and families and selectively assumes teaching responsibilities with them.

Participates in Developing and Effecting Standards of Nursing Care Practice:

Participates in nursing department efforts to develop and revise standards of nurse performance, nursing department philosophy and goals, and other forms of standards-setting.

Organizes and Participates in Educational Programs for Staff:

Fosters an environment in which inquiry and application of new knowledge are an integral part of nursing practice.

Participates in planning and offering educational programs sponsored by the nursing department.

Participates selectively in educational programs sponsored by the nursing department.

Encourages the Development of Leadership Skills in Members of the Nursing Staff:

Collaborates with the supervisor to evaluate the effectiveness of the head nurse's performance and to write her performance appraisal.

Identifies staff nurses with leadership or teaching potential and, with others in the nursing department, plans ways of helping them develop these skills.

Works Collaboratively with Other Members of the Nursing Department, Other Health Care Professionals, and Other Departments:

Plans change in a way that considers persons and departments who may be affected by it.

Collaborates with others who are planning change or new programs to determine an appropriate and dynamic nursing role.

Develops and maintains collegial relationships with physicians to enhance patient care decisions.

Supports and implements changes, programs, and goals of the nursing department and the hospital.

Understands the nursing and hospital structures and appropriately relates to others within them.

Participates in decision making, planning, and problem-solving operations of the nursing department through membership on committees, working groups, and ad hoc task forces.

Works collaboratively with the administrative supervisor to solve problems and plan new programs.

Discusses problems, job-related objectives, trends in care, and needed change with the director of nursing, the associate directors, and other CNSs.

Assists in the screening and selection of candidates for CNS, head nurse, and unit

(continued)

Table 13.1 (continued)

---

teacher positions.

Maintains a High Standard of Professional Responsibility and Performance:

Sets realistic short- and long-term goals for her own performance and appropriately evaluates her progress in attaining them.

---

staff to better understand the role of the CNS. No other trends were noted in the response to the open-ended questions.

The expectations and priorities of the unit leaders expressed by their responses to the questionnaires were congruent with those the CNSs had of themselves. The evaluation tool did, however, identify a few noncongruent expectations on the part of the unit leaders. For example, as already mentioned, they identified the CNS's function in providing direct patient care on a regular basis as a less important function. We explained the importance of this aspect of the role if we were to maintain our skills and have the opportunity to function as role models. Similar clarification was necessary regarding the CNS's role with students, in interpreting health care issues, and in presenting research and ideas from the literature. These misperceptions regarding the role of the CNS did not, however, significantly affect the appraisal. The first objective—establishing congruence between unit leaders' and clinical specialists' ideas about the role—was met.

Since we had received considerable positive feedback, we were encouraged regarding our ability to function as change agents. As measured by the evaluation tool, we were perceived to be effective as role models and teachers, thus meeting the second objective. The unit leaders identified this through their responses to the scaled items as well as in the comments they wrote to the open-ended questions.

The third and perhaps most important objective of the evaluation was that of data collection aimed at establishing personal and unit goals. The data collected from the evaluation tool enabled us to proceed to develop

---

5—Extremely important

4—Very important

3—Moderately important

2—Slightly important

1—Does not see this as part of clinical specialist's role

0—Does not apply; do not know

Figure 13-2. Importance scale.

5—Almost always does this, is consistently good at this, ranks high.
4—Usually does this, is usually good at this, ranks above average.
3—Sometimes does this, is occasionally good at this, ranks average.
2—Seldom does this, is not good at this, ranks fair.
1—Never does this, is not good at this, ranks poor.
0—Does not apply; do not know.

Figure 13-3. Performance scale.

goals for ourselves and the unit. The areas of CNS practice receiving average ratings were made the focus of the next year's goals. Since these were also aspects of the role that we felt to be important, the decision was compatible with our own job expectations. For example, quality assurance issues became a focus, and we worked with the unit staffs to develop criteria and methods for evaluating patient care. With input from the unit leadership group, it was possible for us to focus our time and energy meaningfully. The unit leaders also assigned priorities to the goals identified and methods for meeting the goals. The evaluation results were also used in addressing day-to-day matters. For example, the CNS with two units recognized the need for greater exposure to her units and accomplished this by structuring her time so that a regular time was scheduled for each unit and each shift.

The director and associate director were able to use these evaluations and the consequent goal setting to integrate specialty area goals into the broader goals of the department. This was an important outcome, since some unit goals may have implications for the budget. The associate director used the information to better advise and support the CNSs in pursuit of these goals and role implementation generally. Finally, the evaluations of the unit leadership group were used by the associate director in writing a formal performance appraisal of the CNSs. Use of this data probably enabled her to evaluate their performance more objectively than would have been possible otherwise.

For the neophyte CNS, the thought of being evaluated by staff may be threatening to self-esteem and self-confidence. The risk of employing this type of evaluation must be acknowledged, and a method of seeking support if such evaluation is undertaken should be planned. Going through the process with a colleague, we found, diminished the feelings of threat. The associate director was also available and supported this type of CNS evaluation. It is important to point out again that this evaluation method should be only a part of CNS evaluation. The authors also relied on self-evaluation and the associate director's evaluation for additional feedback.

Performance evaluation of the CNS should be multidimensional. The effect of the specialist on patient care outcomes, staff attitudes and performance, and interdisciplinary collaboration are other areas of evaluation that need exploration. The experience of evaluation by unit leaders, however, was a meaningful one for us and we have continued to use it as one component of our evaluation. The method was simple to implement and yielded valuable information. The thoughtful and honest evaluations of our performance solidified relationships, identified areas of mutual concern, and enabled the leaders to set mutually desired goals. Now that we have been provided with judgments based on observed behavior, we feel able to more effectively implement the CNS role.

REFERENCES

Carroll, L. *Alice's Adventures in Wonderland*. In *The Complete Works of Lewis Carroll*, 1st Vintage Books ed. New York: Random House, 1976, p. 19.

Colerick, E., Mason, P., & Proulx, J. Evaluation of the clinical nurse specialist role: Development and implementation of a dual purpose framework. *Nurs Leadership*, 1980, *3*, 26–33.

Del Bueno, D. Performance evaluation: When all is said and done, more is said than done. *J Nurs Adm.* 1977, *7*, 21–23.

Hamric, A., Gresham, M., & Eccard, M. Staff evaluation of clinical leaders. *J Nurs Adm*, 1978, *8*, 18–26.

MacPhail, J. Reasonable expectations for the nurse clinician. *J Nurs Adm*, 1971, *1*, 5–7.

14. Peer Review

Susan Leibold

EVOLUTION OF THE CONCEPT

Peer review—an exciting, relatively new, and evolving concept in performance appraisal—is currently defined as the critical review of one's clinical practice by colleagues who are equal in education, qualifications, and/or position and therefore are able to make qualitative judgments concerning clinical performance. The concept has undergone considerable evolution since it first appeared in medical literature in the 1960s. It originated, in part, from public demand for an organized form of medical review to ensure standards of medical care. Following the trend of medicine, the nursing profession realized that accountability for one's practice was an important step toward the development of professional status. In 1972, the American Nurses' Association (ANA) stated that one of its priorities was the promotion of peer review as a means of maintaining standards of care (Hauser, 1975, p. 2204). Unfortunately, peer review was not defined in this statement, and no actions were taken to develop a model.

Passos (1973) and Ramphal (1974) viewed peer review as a hallmark of professionalism. They saw it as a means of establishing collective strength in decision making among nurses that would help nursing to become less vulnerable to non-nurses' decisions about nursing practice yet also hold

Special thanks to the Medical College of Virginia Hospitals Clinical Nurse Specialist Group.

nurses accountable to society. Again, the authors were concerned with nursing practice in general, not on an individual level. The new idea that emerged from these two articles is that nursing must define its own practice and develop its own standards for care if it is to attain professional status.

Stronger support for peer review became evident in 1976 when the ANA published a discussion of quality assurance and the peer review process entitled *Issues in Evaluation Research*. Zimmer wrote that the standards for nursing practice should be set by a group of peers and that application of these standards through a nursing audit of discharge records would influence and develop social and professional values (1976, p. 64). In subsequent writings Zimmer has shown continued support for the development of nursing standards and the use of the peer review process, but her model provides only a global evaluation of the impact of nursing care, not the evaluation of individual practice that is reflected in the current concept of peer review.

The ANA further supported the peer review concept in the revised code for nurses published in 1976 (*Perspective on the Code for Nurses*). This was the first revision of the nursing code since 1968. The fourth point in the revised code is relevant to peer review. It states that "the nurse assumes responsibility and accountability for individual nursing judgments and actions" (p. 51). Further, evaluation of one's performance by peers is a hallmark of professionalism, and it is primarily through this mechanism that the profession is held accountable to society (pp. 51–52). This code defined the concept more clearly than before, indicating that peer review identifies specific behaviors of a particular nurse. These behaviors affect the nursing profession, instead of the profession's influencing the practice of the individual nurse. The code stresses that accountability for practice begins with the individual.

Furthering the idea of professionalism and accountability, between 1977 and 1979 numerous authors supported the development of a review system in which the individual nurse's actions are evaluated by peers (Lamberton, Keene, & Admoanis, 1977; Mullins, Colavecchio, & Tescher, 1979; Page & Loeper, 1978; Spicer & Lewis, 1977). Peer review, they asserted, not only holds the individual nurse accountable to her or his patients but also provides an educational process for nurses' self-actualization or professional growth. This is an important development within the peer review concept, reflecting a new awareness that change in nursing practice must be accomplished at the level of the individual nurse. Since peer pressure is a powerful motivator for change in a person's behavior, peer review, these authors felt, can help to promote the assimilation of professional standards. In this way peer review stimulates professional growth as well as promotes accountability.

Peer review is particularly appropriate for the CNS, since this specialist has special responsibility for improving the quality of nursing care and fostering the professionalization of nursing. CNSs who successfully learn to use peer review to improve their performance at the same time demonstrate the value of peer review to other nurses, who may in turn adopt the process to improve their own performance. Thus the groundwork is completed for improved nursing care.

Peer review can provide an important addition to the yearly evaluation process for the CNS. Because of the autonomous nature of the CNS role, the nursing administrator who evaluates the CNS does not observe the specialist's practice frequently. An ongoing peer review system supplements the yearly performance appraisal made by the administrator, as well as offers a growth experience for the CNS.

PEER REVIEW AND OTHER EVALUATION PROCESSES

Several types of evaluation for the CNS are described in nursing literature. Two of these—the nursing audit and the patient care audit—have sometimes been described as forms of peer review, but neither process fits the current definition.

The nursing audit was developed by Phaneuf (1972). It is a method of evaluating the quality of nursing care through "the appraisal of nursing process as it is reflected in the patient care record of the discharged patient." The audit evaluates quality of nursing care and reflects the standards of practice developed by the nurses within a given unit (p. 15). Because the standards used in the nursing audit are developed by nurses, this form of evaluation has been described as a form of peer review. It does not, however, provide for individual accountability for nursing practice and therefore does not fit with the current concept of peer review. Also, a closed chart audit does not reflect the totality of the role of the staff nurse and even less that of the CNS. The CNS role interfaces with those of many other nurses and auxilliary staff members, and the CNS's interventions and information sharing are not necessarily documented in any given patient's record. The nursing audit, therefore, while effective in evaluating quality of nursing care on a unit or within an institution, is not effective in evaluating an individual's performance.

The patient care audit is similar to the nursing audit in that it evaluates the quality of patient care in a nursing unit, department, or institution. It is different from the nursing audit because it is conducted while the patient is still in the hospital. The audit consists of direct observation, patient and nurse interviews, and chart review of a percentage of the patient population. The audit is conducted by nurses, using standards developed by nurses.

Since it is not a discharge chart audit, current quality of care on the unit reviewed is revealed. Like the nursing audit, however, it does not evaluate the quality of care given by the individual nurse. Because it focuses on the quality of care in an organizational whole, the patient care audit is inadequate as a mechanism for evaluating the quality of care provided by the individual specialist. Many CNSs are responsible for a patient population not confined to one unit. For such CNSs, the patient care audit will not cover the CNS's entire case load and so may not fully reflect the CNS's achievement in delivering patient care. The patient care audit is a useful tool, but it is not peer review.

While the nursing audit and patient care audit evaluate the quality of patient care, the administrative review or yearly performance appraisal is designed to evaluate the quality of job performance. Administrative review is the most common form of evaluation process utilized today for the CNS. This form of evaluation enables the CNS and the nursing administrator to establish goals and objectives for the upcoming year and review progress toward the goals and objectives established for the previous year. This is an important mode for meeting personal and departmental needs. The major flaw in administrative review, already mentioned, is that the patient care actions of the CNS are rarely witnessed by the person doing the evaluation. The nursing administrator gathers her or his information from other nursing employees and from the CNS's progress report. Accountability to the nursing department is maintained by this form of evaluation, but accountability to patients may be lost. Peer review is a natural complement to the administrative review process, since it provides the nursing administrator with documented behaviors recorded as the CNS's activity is evaluated by peers.

Finally, self-evaluation complements the administrative review and peer review processes. In making a self-evaluation, the CNS evaluates her or his progress toward established goals and objectives. If self-evaluation is used as the sole means of evaluation, however, it provides only a singular view of the situation and identifies no alternative courses of action. Self-evaluation is most useful when used in conjunction with administrative and peer review processes.

A MODEL FOR PEER REVIEW

Several tools for peer evaluation have been described, but these were designed to be utilized by staff nurses, nursing supervisors, and nursing faculty. There was no tool specific for the CNS. Models for peer review to date have been limited to a written self-evaluation and group interactional review (Gold, Jackson, Sachs, & VanMeter, 1973); a case presentation with a review committee gathering data for discussion and evaluation (Hauser, 1975, pp. 2206–7); and direct observation of a nursing faculty member with a pre- and post-conference (Page & Loeper, 1978, p. 22). These models appeared to be either too subjective or not congruent with the model of nursing practiced at the Medical College of Virginia Hospitals. Consequently, the CNS group undertook to develop a new, more specific tool.

The approach used to develop an objective peer review tool involved four steps. In the first step, we identified the essential aspects of CNS practice from the literature. Second, we developed a narrative tool based on the commonalities. Third, we analyzed the results from utilizing the narrative tool and identified specific behaviors defining the essential aspects of CNS practice in our hospital. Fourth, we developed an objective tool based on these results which the CNS group plans to use in future peer reviews. Each step will now be discussed in detail.

Development of the Narrative Tool

Before an objective tool could be developed, it was necessary to identify commonalities of CNS practice as described in CNS literature, and gather behaviors defining those commonalities. The common factor utilized as a starting point was the nursing process.

Components of the nursing process—assessment, planning, implementation, and evaluation—are part of every nurse–patient interaction, and the level on which these steps are performed can distinguish the CNS from the staff nurse. A subjective, narrative peer evaluation tool was developed (Table 14-1) as a form to be used by evaluators in assessing CNS practice in this first phase of our peer review process. With this subjective tool we hoped to be able to gather data to use in formulating an objective evaluation form appropriate to our setting. The term "narrative" was used because the evaluation was hand-written in an anecdotal or narrative description. It appeared that advanced use of the nursing process was one of the major commonalities of the CNS role. We were interested in determining whether this characteristic could be demonstrated in an observation experience. The narrative tool thus reviewed the use of the nursing process in two important components of the CNS role: clinical practice (either directly with patients, or indirectly in consultation with staff) and education (i.e., patient teaching or formal lectures given to staff).

In developing the narrative tool, we assumed that: (1) the percentage of time to be given to each aspect of the CNS role cannot be specified because each CNS has a different focus and therefore spends different amounts of time in the various components of the role. (2) The effectiveness of the CNS cannot be measured solely on the basis of patient outcomes because there are too many other variables that affect a patient's condition and

Table 14-1
Narrative Peer Review Tool

Situation	Strengths	Weaknesses or Suggested Approach
Clinical Situation		
What is purpose of activity?		
Assessment		
Planning		
Implementing		
Evaluating		
Teaching Situation		
Objectives		
Method		
Evaluation		
Ability to answer questions		

satisfaction. The Medical College of Virginia Hospital is a 1200-bed metropolitan teaching complex. Many students and professionals within the teaching hospital interact with patients. This fact increases the difficulty of evaluating the impact of the CNS solely on the basis of patient outcomes. Therefore the assumption was made that the basis for a CNS peer evaluation tool should be the essential aspects of role performance, a process method. (3)A nurse with a similar educational preparation is qualified to make subjective judgments about the practice of another nurse. This assumption was made after acknowledging the difficulty in measuring objectively the quality of the CNS's nursing actions. Many actions, including nursing process, reflect functions of the staff nurse. The CNS may practice these with a greater depth than the average staff nurse, however, making the CNS reluctant to have the staff nurse evaluate her or his performance. In addition, a staff nurse may only see a small portion of the CNS role. The subjective judgment of a peer, however, may add the depth to evaluation that is otherwise unattainable. Subjective data, it was felt, can be reliable and valid when the basis for the judgment is made by a peer and is made according to previously established criteria.

In preparation for the implementation of the narrative tool we undertook a two-part educational plan. First a large group discussion for all CNSs was arranged in which the concept, benefits, and pitfalls of peer review were reviewed. During a lively conversation concerning the definition of peer review several unsettling questions arose, such as "What makes a CNS different from other nurses?" and "Just what does a CNS do?" These questions led to small-group discussions. The small-group discussions produced concrete answers to the questions and helped to uncover commonalities, as opposed to differences, within CNS practice. A growth of group cohesiveness and a sense of trust were additional benefits from these group discussions. This was viewed as a solution to one of the major pitfalls of peer review, that of reluctance to give peer criticism. Difficulty in eliciting constructive suggestions for altering behavior is a problem cited in the literature; some reviewers lacked the personal security needed to give criticism (Gold et al., p. 635).

Gold notes that reviewees can feel threatened and defensive when faced with peer evaluation. Care was therefore taken in designing the peer evaluation process to make it less threatening. Even though the reviewee knew by whom and when she or he was being observed, the summary comments were anonymous and received in writing and privacy rather than before a committee or review board. Thus a personal encounter was avoided, and the reviewee had ample time to read, evaluate, and assimilate the comments of the observers.

Implementation of the Narrative Tool

Five clinical specialists volunteered to be evaluated. All had been practicing as CNSs for at least one year. It is not recommended that a newly employed CNS be evaluated until she or he has been practicing for at least six months. Waiting one year is preferable. It may take six months to one year for the CNS to establish the role and become oriented to the environment. The additional stress of a peer evaluation would be unfair to an already stressed new employee. Two other CNSs were randomly selected to observe each volunteer. In addition, faculty members from the university medical center school of nursing were asked to participate as evaluators. Each faculty member was chosen from an area of specialization similar to that of the volunteer, in keeping with Gold's suggestion that "peer review . . . be primarily specific to a clinical area or discipline, with the nurse specialists in that area having the option to involve nurses from other clinical areas as appropriate" (Gold et al., p. 636). The idea is both important and valid, but since it was not practical within our agency we decided that a faculty member with a master's degree in the reviewee's discipline could validate any clinically related questions that the two other reviewers might have. The evaluation team was thus composed of 2 CNSs and one faculty member.

Each of the 3 observers was asked to spend approximately 4 hours during a 3-month period observing the respective reviewee. The observation times were scheduled by the reviewers with the reviewee and were to include activities involving direct clinical practice or consultation, and education. A total of 12 hours of observation was accumulated by the evaluation team. During the observation periods, observers utilized the narrative tool by taking notes on the activities of the reviewee under the appropriate heading for each component of the nursing process. The observer also noted strengths or weaknesses of the CNS in the activity in the appropriate columns. At the completion of the observations, the three observers met, discussed their findings, and sent a written summary to the CNS reviewee. Anonymous copies were utilized for the development of the final tool.

Reactions to the Use of the Narrative Tool

The reviewers' comments about this reviewing procedure were very positive. It was thought that observing the specialists over a period of weeks gave a more accurate overall view of their practice than observing them within a one-week period. In all five review groups, consistency of observations was noted (i.e., one activity observed one week was consistently seen in the reviewee's practice by subsequent observers the following weeks). This held true for both strengths and weaknesses of activities observed.

Because the written summary was anonymous, the reviewers were free to give constructive suggestions for desirable changes in behavior. The constructive suggestions did not include references to purely personal differences in technique and style. This commitment by the reviewers to minimize personality differences added to the freedom to give constructive suggestions.

The reviewers made only one negative comment, concerning the written summary of the peer review experience. Writing the summary was found to be time-consuming and no clear recommendations had been given on how it should be structured. Consequently each summary was written differently.

This type of peer review process benefitted the CNS reviewers by allowing them to share their expertise with peers practicing in different specialities. This proved to be an unexpected bonus for the reviewers. Because CNS reviewers participated outside of their areas of expertise, they were exposed to an unfamiliar practice. All reviewers expressed pleasure in learning about another's practice.

The reviewees' comments about the experience were equally positive. Many had expressed apprehension prior to observation, and some feared that their performance would not meet colleagues' expectations. As the observations continued, however, apprehension subsided. Relief, associated with feeling good about one's performance, was expressed at the conclusion of each observation. Unexpectedly it was discovered that each reviewee had done an unwritten self-evaluation following each observation, consisting of reviewing the rationale for the nursing interventions made and exploring possible alternative actions. The self-evaluation was identified as an additional bonus of this experience. Reviewees found the written summary and comments valuable. A general feeling of satisfaction with this form of evaluation was expressed.

Analysis of the Narrative Tool

Content analysis was the next step. Analysis of the content was accomplished by the author and an independent coder separately and independently identifying all of the different behaviors presented in the written summaries. These different behaviors were then grouped on the basis of similarity and a definition was developed for each group of behaviors. A descriptive title was assigned to each group of behaviors which then became the categories. Each analyst read the summaries and used the category definitions to identify and classify all behaviors into one of the categories. In content analysis, categories are exhaustive (so that all data can be classified into a category) and mutually exclusive (no over-lapping among them). If the two coders reach an agreement rate greater than 65 percent, the reliability of the coders is satisfactory. An agreement rate of less than 65 percent indicates that the definition of the categories is unclear or that the coders do not understand and agree upon how the coding is to be done (Rubin and Erickson, 1977, p. 160).

The purposes of the coding are:

1) to develop categories that are representive of the behaviors of CNSs;
2) to determine if the categories were representative of the data (that is, the behaviors described in the summaries).

Eight categories of CNS practice were initially identified. They were assessment, problem solving, communicating, providing care, supporting, coordinating/collaborating, teaching, and evaluating. Each category was further defined in terms of specific actions performed by the CNS. The CNS's actions were assumed to be directed toward one of four groups: patients, patient's significant others, nurses, and other staff, and the membership of each group was carefully defined (Table 14-2).

The agreement rate between the author and the independent coder for coding actions into categories was 80 percent or above for all of the categories except coordinating/collaborating. We concluded that the

Table 14-2
Categories Derived from Content Analysis

Definitions of Categories of CNS Practice

Assessment: gathering of information and forming a judgment about the information.

Problem solving: an organized process that develops a potential solution to the problems identified.

Communicating: sharing of information, facts, or knowledge wittingly or unwittingly through spoken, written, or nonverbal language.

Providing care: performing some aspect of physical care.

Supporting: providing emotional care to identify feelings and to help work through those feelings.

Teaching: providing instruction either on an informal basis or in a formal group setting.

Evaluating: examining outcomes to see if desired results have been obtained.

Definitions of Groups Interacting with CNS

Patients: individuals, children or adults who are receiving an evaluation or treatment.

Significant others: support person(s) designated by the patient, including parents, spouses, other relatives, or close friends.

Nurses: the nursing assistant, licensed practical nurse, staff nurse, head nurse, nursing administrator, community health nurse, nursing student, nursing faculty, or other CNSs.

Other staff: the attending physician, resident, intern, occupational therapist, physical therapist, chaplin, social worker, school teacher, dietician, recreational therapist, volunteer, pharmacist, dentist, radiologist, respiratory therapist, speech therapist, or rehabilitation counselor.

coordinating/collaborating category was too broad and that the definition overlapped with several of the other categories—assessing, problem solving, supporting, and communicating. The actions previously coded into the coordinating/collaborating category were recoded into the seven remaining categories (Table 14-2).

Development of the Objective Tool

The seven remaining categories became the aspects of CNS practice to be specifically assessed in the second stage of our peer review process and formed the basis for the objective tool (Table 14-3). The term "objective" was chosen because the tool was based on content analysis, and could be quantified (see summary form rating scale, Table 14-4). The specific actions identified within each category represented parameters for qualitatively evaluating the CNS's clinical practice. For the convenience of the reviewer,

Table 14-3
Objective peer review tool.

	Patient	Significant Other
PATIENT CARE		
Assessing		
Areas assessed		
Psychosocial status		
Physical comfort needs		
Specific physical problems		
Method		
Direct observation		
Interview		
Chart review		
Comments:		
Problem solving		
Identifying problems		
Identifying alternatives		
Identifying consequences of alternatives		
Setting priorities		
Developing plans for care		
Comments:		
Communicating		
Rapport building		
Sharing information: Verbally		
Written		
Active listening		
Providing feedback		
Comments:		
Providing Care		
Establishing contract for care		
Physical comfort measures		
Specific treatments		
Comments:		
Supporting		
Measures offered to decrease:		
Anxiety		
Fears		
Fantasies		*(continued)*

Table 14.3 (continued)

	Patient	Significant other
Crisis intervention initiated		
Listening		
Empathetic understanding		
Referring to other support services (i.e., chaplain, social work, other CNS)		
Comments:		
Evaluating		
Uses return demonstration		
Questions to identify level of understanding		
Retrieves data from chart/lab		
Modifies/updates plan of care		
Modifies/updates teaching plan		
Comments:		
Teaching		
Process		
Assesses learner's needs		
States objectives		
Clinical application of theory/research		
Feedback to participants		
Method		
Variety of teaching methods employed		
Manages time		
Answers questions		
Visual aids		
Handouts		
Comments:		

COORDINATION OF CARE	Nurse	Other Staff
Problem solving		
Identifying problems		
Identifying alternatives		
Identifying consequences of alternatives		
Developing plans for care		
Discharge planning		
Comments:		
		(continued)

Table 14-3 (continued)

	Nurse	Other Staff
Communicating Rapport building Information sharing: Verbally Written Active listening Providing feedback Documentation Comments:		
Supporting Listening Reinforcement of decisions made Empathetic understanding Comments:		
Evaluating Uses return demonstration Questions to identify level of understanding Retrieves data Modifies/updates plan of care Modifies/updates teaching plan Provides formal evaluation form Comments:		

Teaching
 Process
    Assesses learner's needs
    States objectives
    Clinical application of theory/research
    Feedback to participants		

Methods
    Variety of teaching methods employed
    Manages time
    Answers questions
    Visual aids
    Handouts
 Comments:		

Table 14-4
Rating Scale used on summary form

5	4	3	2	1	0
Always	Almost Always	50/50	25/75 Seldom	Rare	N/A

the evaluation form was divided into two sections: patient care and coordination of care. The patient care section evaluates the actions directed to a patient or a patient's significant other. The coordination of care section evaluates actions directed toward nurses or other staff.

Plans for Implementing the Objective Tool

Our plans for implementing the objective tool in the future are based on the successful method used in implementing the narrative tool. Each CNS will be evaluated every 3 months by a different reviewer. After 9 months, the 3 reviewers will meet to prepare a joint summary, which will be sent to the CNS who was evaluated. To spread peer review activity over the year and because there are 12 CNSs in our group, each CNS will randomly select 2 other CNSs to observe and a month in which to conduct the review. It will be the responsibility of the reviewer to set observation times with each reviewee during the month. It will be the reviewee's responsibility to contact the faculty member, since she or he is not part of the random process, set up the observation time, and notify committee members when all observations have been completed so that the summary can be prepared. Activities observed will include both activities of the CNS in the clinical setting and those in an educational session (that is, patient/family teaching or formal group teaching).

During an observation session the observer will place a check mark on the observation form in the proper position to indicate the action observed and the type of person to whom it was directed. More than one check mark may be used beside an action. Reviewers are encouraged to use the "comments" area to identify specific behaviors and strengths or weaknesses observed. When all 3 reviewers have completed their observations of a CNS, a group meeting will be held to fill in a summary form for the reviewee. The summary form consists of the observation tool with the addition of a qualitative scale providing a rating for each action (Table 14-4). The completed summary form is sent to the CNS observed. The decision to communicate or not about the summary evaluation with an appropriate nursing administrator is up to the CNS.

Conclusion

The objective tool has not been tested for validity and effectiveness, and one can expect that adjustments will have to be made as more experience is gained with its use. The initial experience of peer review using a narrative tool demonstrates that peer review can be a positive experience, and similar results from the objective tool can be anticipated.

REFERENCES

American Nurses' Association, *Perspectives on the code for nurses.* Kansas City, Mo: ANA, 1978.

Gold, H., Jackson, M., Sachs, B., & VanMeter, M. J. Peer review—A working experiment. *Nurs Outlook*, 1973, *21*, 634-636.

Hauser, M. A. Initiation into peer review. *Am J Nurs*, 1975, *75*, 2204-2207.

Lamberton, M., Keene, M. & Admoanis, A. Peer review in a family nurse clinician program. *Nurs Outlook*, 1977, *25*, 47–53.

Mullins, A., Colavecchio, R., & Tescher, B. Peer review: A model for professional accountability. *J Nurs Adm*, 1979, *9*, 25-30, 25–26.

Page, S., & Loeper, J., Peer review of the nurse educator: The process and development of a format. *J Nurs Ed*, 1978, *17*, 21-29.

Passos, J. Y. Accountability: Myth or mandate? *J Nurs Adm*, 1973, *3*, 21–29.

Planeuf, M. *The nursing audit: Profile for excellence.* New York: Appleton-Century-Crofts, 1972.

Planeuf, M. A concluding paper. In ANA (Ed.), *Issues in evaluation research.* Kansas City, Mo: ANA, 1976.

Ramphal, M. Peer review. *Am J Nurs*, 1974, *74*, 63–67.

Rubin, R. & Erickson, F. Research in clinical nursing, *Maternal-Child Nurs J*, 1977, *6*, 151–164.

Spicer, J., Lewis, E. Intensive care staff nurses develop peer review criteria. *Nurs Adm Q*, 1977, *1*, 57–61.

Zimmer, M. Quality assurance for nursing care. In *Quality assurance for nursing care: Proceedings of an institute jointly sponsored by the American Nurses' Association and the American Hospital Association.* Kansas City, Mo.: ANA, 1974.

Zimmer, M. Evaluation using patient health/wellness outcome criterion variables and standards. In ANA (Ed.), *Issues in evaluation research.* Kansas City, Mo: ANA, 1976.

V. FUTURE DIRECTIONS

15. Current Trends in Education and Implications for the Future

Lucy Feild

History of CNS Education

The historical development of education for clinical specialization parallels that of nursing in general. "Postgraduate" courses offered by hospitals in the early part of the century comprised the first formal educational preparation for nurses who desired advanced knowledge in specific areas of practice. These courses, however, were known more for their recruitment value than for substantive content (Smoyak, 1976).

The Goldmark Report in 1923 proposed major reforms for nursing education in the United States (Goldmark, 1923). The majority of recommendations dealt with the need to end the apprenticeship approach to nursing education promulgated by service institutions to meet staffing needs. Goldmark further recognized the need for "postgraduate" programs within university settings in nursing administration and education, public health nursing, and private duty practice (Kalisch & Kalisch, 1978). Matejski's analysis of the gradual and modest effect of the Goldmark report on nursing education, in comparison to the swift and revolutionary impact of the Flexner report on medical education, provides important insight into the professional, political, social and economic differences between nursing and medicine. At the time of the Flexner report, medicine had been clearly established as an autonomous profession, and the widely publicized study findings helped to generate strong societal support for changes in medical education that had long been sought by physician leaders. The results of the Goldmark report, on the other hand, were not widely circulated in the

237

public sector. Nursing lacked both the functional autonomy and the distinct theoretical base to substantiate a professional image and to generate public support for educational improvements. Nursing practice and education occurred primarily in physician-controlled hospital settings where physician–nurse relationships were characterized by the inequalities in male–female relationships that were customary at that time. Furthermore, maintenance of hospital-based apprentice education for nursing was an effective cost containment measure that perpetuated the labor force. There was little resistance to the long hours and hard physical labor associated with nursing education when the Goldmark report was released. Students typically represented the lower socio-economic class, had been socialized into the prevailing work ethic, and viewed nursing as an opportunity for upward mobility. Such factors substantially impeded the implementation of changes in nursing education, no less needed than those in medicine (Matejski, 1981).

University-based programs in nursing administration and education eventually followed, but advanced preparation in clinical practice was not accorded the same priority by either service or education. This may be attributed to a variety of factors, including a poorly defined clinical nursing knowledge base, the lower level of status accorded to clinical practice, and the pressing need for adequately prepared nurses in administrative and teaching positions.

The nursing programs that developed in university settings in the forties at times had difficulty distinguishing between graduate and undergraduate curriculum content. Students enrolled at both levels found themselves in the same classes at some schools. There was early consensus on the need for specialist training at the master's level. First discussed in 1949, this recommendation won further support in 1952 at a work conference on graduate education in nursing sponsored by the National League for Nursing (NLN). There it was agreed that the purpose of baccalaureate education was to prepare nurse generalists, while master's education should be devoted to the preparation of nurse specialists (Smoyak, 1976, p.677). Six years later, the National Working Conference on Graduate Education in Psychiatric Nursing developed suggestions for educational preparation of psychiatric CNSs (National League for Nursing, 1958). Broad recommendations for future curriculum development included master's-level preparation designed to promote the development of expert skills, an in-depth knowledge base, and a commitment to lifelong learning and inquiry. More specific recommendations for educational preparation of CNSs were advanced in 1969 by the NLN's Council of Baccalaureate and Higher Degree programs (National League for Nursing, 1969). These included curriculum content that would enable students to acquire a broad foundation in psycho- or patho-physiology, specialized clinical practice, research and teaching skills, leadership and change-agent skills, and an understanding of the societal forces that influence health care delivery.

The first graduate program to prepare CNSs solely for advanced practice was begun in 1954 at Rutgers' University for psychiatric nurses (Smoyak, 1976, p. 678). Since then, numerous programs for the preparation of CNSs have appeared at universities throughout the country, the majority of these between 1972 and 1982. Of the 91 master's-level nursing programs accredited by the NLN in 1980– 1981, 81 stated that they offered clinical specialist preparation. The apparent lack of uniformity among curricula in these programs has been noted in the past (Schlotfeldt, 1974). Variations among program offerings may in part be explained by the lack of universal agreement regarding fundamental philosophical and theoretical issues central to the nursing profession itself and the continually evolving and varied nature of role implementation in clinical practice. The American Nurses' Association's (ANA's) *Nursing: A Social Policy Statement*, published in 1980, is an example of the work being done within the profession to lessen the ambiguity about the nature of nursing so characteristic of this stage in the profession's development. As the philosophical and theoretical bases of nursing become clearer, issues relative to role implementation of clinical specialists should also become easier to resolve.

ROLE-SPECIFIC COMPETENCIES

If the central objective of the CNS is to assure quality nursing care for clients, then nursing educators have the responsibility to prepare these expert practitioners to assess and respond to both current and future client needs. Curriculum content and learning strategies must be designed to ensure that graduates can develop and implement new roles as well as anticipate nursing care requirements for clients in a continuously changing and increasingly complex health care system.

Nursing does not clearly identify the role-specific competencies of CNSs who have completed programs; such education is designed to follow baccalaureate preparation with an upper-division major in nursing. Several works, however, address competencies of master's-prepared nurses in general. McLane (1978) developed a 68-item Process Competency Scale to determine a common core of nursing process competencies that all master's-prepared graduates should demonstrate regardless of functional role preparation. Of 286 questionnaires distributed to a sample of deans of schools of nursing, directors of nursing service, and directors of graduate programs in nursing, 118 were returned and usable. Twenty-five core competencies were identified, which fell into seven categories: inter-personal competence, researcher, accountability for nursing practice, change agent, educator, ability to articulate a philosophy of nursing, and humanizer. Of interest was the high rate of agreement among responders that educators should demonstrate high-level clinical skills and that clinicians should demonstrate teaching competence.

In 1978, the NLN Division of Baccalaureate and Higher Degree Programs published *Characteristics of Graduate Education in Nursing Leading to the Master's Degree*. Offered as a statement of accountability of educators to both students and clients, this document outlined nine central behaviors, consistent with McLane's process competencies, that students should expect to demonstrate as a result of graduate study in nursing. These are shown in Table 15–1.

The development of specific criteria to measure competency acquisition for CNS practice is clearly needed. Once completed, these should serve as a basis for evaluation of the adequacy of curricula by faculty, students, and clinical administrators. Awareness of existing deficits should help to guide decision making for curriculum revision. Nursing educators must anticipate, however, that as the needs of the health care delivery system and society's need for nursing care both change, so may the competencies required for CNS practice. For instance, the increasing average age of the U.S. population, coupled with increasing chronic illnesses and diminishing social resources, is likely to increase the need for gerontology nurse specialists whose health-maintenance and illness-prevention skills are complemented by well-developed counselling skills to assist the elderly to make individual decisions about issues such as desired quality of life. In addition, as nursing evolves as a profession, priorities among competencies may be reordered and expected levels of mastery may increase, signalling the need for further curriculum revision.

ISSUES RELATED TO COMPETENCY ACQUISITION

Delineation of expected competency attainment at the master's level should provide both a framework for curriculum planning and a basis for curriculum evaluation. While specific curriculum content may vary considerably among programs according to variables such as specialty choices and faculty expertise, student outcome attainment should nevertheless be fairly consistent among schools if standards are clearly defined and maintained. Interestingly, mechanisms to compare student outcome attainment across programs do not currently exist at the graduate level, although in the furture this could be partially rectified if certification of CNSs were to become a standard for practice at that level.

The future education of CNSs will be affected by a number of issues that have a direct relationship to competency acquisition.

Table 15-1
Characteristics of Graduate Education in Nursing*

Graduate Education in Nursing is Designed to Enable Students to

● Acquire advanced knowledge from the sciences and the humanities to support advanced nursing practice and role development.

● Expand their knowledge of nursing theory as a basis for advanced nursing practice.

● Develop expertise in a specialized area of clinical nursing practice.

● Acquire the knowledge and skills related to a specific functional role in nursing.

● Acquire initial competence in conducting research.

● Plan and inititate change in the health care system and in the practice and delivery of health care.

● Further develop and implement leadership strategies for the betterment of health care.

● Actively engage in collaborative relationships with others for the purpose of improving health care.

● Acquire a foundation for doctoral study.

*Reprinted with permission from National League for Nursing Division of Baccalaureate and Higher Degree Programs. *Characteristics of graduate education in nursing leading to the master's degree* (Publ. No. 15-1759). New York: NLN, 1978. Copyright 1978 by NLN.

Program Issues

Program issues include focus and length of programs, and socio-economic factors that affect both the university and the student.

Focus

Despite the fact that the vast majority of NLN-accredited master's level programs claim to provide CNS preparation, there seems to be a significant variation in the focus of curricula. Three options appear to predominate:

1. Clinical specialization (or advanced nursing practice) as a major curriculum focus, with both a clinical and a functional role practicum.

2. Clinical specialization as a major curriculum focus, with the opportunity to elect functional role preparation in another area such as teaching, management, or research.

3. Clinical specialization as a functional role minor in a specialty area such as medical-surgical nursing.

Such options may be confusing at best for potential applicants who take the time to compare and contrast program offerings at different schools. One could hypothesize that such confusion extends to both clinical nursing administration and graduate faculty whose definition of the role of the CNS is ambiguous. The relative dearth of master's-prepared nurses in clinical practice settings sometimes contributes to the CNS's being utilized in a variety of ways to meet important service needs related to quality-of-care issues. This is particularly likely to occur when job descriptions are vague, CNS predecessors and peers are few or nonexistent, and institutional needs for advanced nursing knowledge and skills are great. In response, educators may attempt to prepare the CNS to be "all things to all people."

If the CNS is to function as an expert in clinical practice, it is logical to expect that educational preparation for this role be based on a foundation designed to develop the knowledge and skills required to assure clinical competence in the "diagnosis and treatment of human responses to actual or potential health problems" (ANA, 1980, p. 9). Programs that fail to prepare CNSs to skillfully carry out the complex components of the clinical decision-making process do a disservice not only to their students but also to employing institutions and to clients who have a right to expect no less from those who present themselves as experts in nursing practice.

While some programs may purport to prepare CNSs who can also teach and/or manage, it is difficult to imagine how such differing objectives can all be adequately accomplished within the one to two years allocated to master's education in nursing. Each of these three areas, although not mutually exclusive, does in fact require specific knowledge and skills that take considerable time and effort to master. Nurses whose goals are exclusively nursing education or nursing administration would do well to consider programs designed to prepare them for these roles which are fundamentally different from that of the CNS. Nurses who intend to function in dual roles, such as that of practitioner-teacher, should plan to obtain sufficient preparation in both functional areas.

Length

There is considerable variation in the length of NLN-accredited master's programs that prepare CNSs. Comparison is complicated by inconsistent definitions of semesters. Some schools are on a quarter system, while others define program length in terms of semesters or months of full-time study. A more appropriate common denominator is the number of credits required for graduation, but this information is neither readily available nor necessarily equivalent. The shortest period alloted for CNS preparation is two semesters plus one summer session, reported by four schools, while the longest program extends for 24 months. Approximately one-third of the accredited programs are four semesters long, and an equal number vary according to specialty or role focus (NLN, 1980).

Socioeconomic Factors

A number of socioeconomic factors can be expected to have a measurable impact on the future education CNSs.

University related factors.   Many schools are faced with the possibility of declining enrollments coupled with continually escalating operating expenses. In the last 16 years (1965-1981), the financial pressure has been eased for schools of nursing by federal assistance given through the Nurse Training Acts and Research Funds that have provided a total of over $1.5 billion in institutional support, student traineeships, and research grants (Institute of Medicine, 1981). A dramatic shift in economic priorities in the United States seriously threatens the continuation of this aid. The temptation to reduce or eliminate expensive programs with low faculty-student ratios (typical in graduate nursing programs) may appear to be the most viable option to administrators at some financially troubled universities. Nursing faculty who will be directly affected by such proposed budget cuts have a responsibility to evaluate their programs as objectively as possible and to influence decision making about allocation of scarce financial resources in favor of those programs that meet high standards of excellence and are justified in view of present or projected societal need. Efforts to sustain programs of mediocre quality or those with limited potential value to society cannot be justified.

Student-related factors.   Potential applicants take a number of factors into account when choosing a graduate program, including course offerings, reputation of the school and faculty, tuition, geographic location, length of the program, and the option for part-time study. They also consider a host of personal factors, including personal and professional goals, availability of financial aid, family obligations, and the means to survive a loss of income if work must be curtailed while studying.

In 1980, there were 14,130 students enrolled in master's degree nursing programs in the United States. Fifty-one percent of these were engaged in part-time study, while 49 percent were enrolled full time. Fifty-five percent of the part-time students and 75 percent of the full-time students had a functional area of clinical specialization (NLN, 1981, p. 84). This preference for CNS preparation is an indication of the growing interest in clinical practice as a priority among those who are planning long-range careers in nursing. It should serve as a signal to both education planners and clinical administrators of a trend that bears watching.

Although enrollments in graduate nursing programs have been climbing steadily since 1961, there is good reason to be concerned that this trend could soon reverse itself. The precipitating factor is likely to be a federal cutback in nursing traineeships, loans, and scholarships, which have totalled $636.4 million since 1965 (Institute of Medicine, 1981, Appendix 1). In addition, the current well-publicized nursing shortage and attendant reports of widespread job dissatisfaction in clinical practice may discourage otherwise interested persons from entering nursing. This, in combination with the widening range of career options open to women and the prevailing assumption among many that nursing is a woman's profession, may discourage from entry those persons with the potential to be clinical nursing leaders of the future.

Nursing is learning the importance of influencing the legislative process on key issues that affect funding for educational programs needed to supply nursing resources for future leadership. Part-time programs and tuition reimbursement benefits will undoubtedly become more important in the future to nurses who wish to continue their education. Equally important are the changes that must occur in the practice setting to enable nurses to realize their full potential in health care delivery (National Commission on Nursing, 1981). As these changes begin to evolve, nursing should be in a better position to begin to attract men and women who choose clinical nursing practice as a lifelong professional career commitment.

Curriculum Issues

Organizing Framework

The majority of graduate programs in nursing offer clinical tracks in some or all of the following broad areas: medical–surgical, parent–child, psychiatric–mental health, and community health nursing. Some are divided into more specific subspecialties, such as cardiovascular or developmental disabilities nursing. Newer programs in areas of identified need, such as primary care and gerontology nusing are appearing with the assistance of special grant funding.

Current specialty-track divisions provide for the acquisition of critical content and skills unique to each area. Whether this particular delineation will prevail is the future in difficult to predict. As a theoretical framework for nursing evolves, it is possible that specialty areas will be derived instead from its components. If CNSs are to function collaboratively with other health care providers, however, areas of common knowledge must still be addressed. For example, the medical model, for many years the principal framework for most nursing curricula, has become less functional for nursing education as nursing theory development has progressed. The medical model is still useful and appropriate in organizing disease-related course content, however. It is also the prevailing categorization in clinical practice setting, especially in acute care.

Theoretically, graduate education should build on undergraduate preparation. As Stevens (1981) points out though, the concept of articulation among phases or aspects of nursing preparation is not clearly defined, and therefore the related issues are difficult to resolve. Articulation issues of particular interest to educators in CNS programs include the question of whether the graduate curriculum should articulate with a specific baccalaureate program, and the question of how courses within a specific program are integrated. Many programs require core courses that all graduate students must take, which may be pre-requisites to specialty-area theoretical and clinical courses. Stevens notes that while core courses are appealing from the standpoint of logic and savings in time and cost, their value has not been clearly substantiated; in fact, some faculty find that students have difficulty applying abstract concepts to which they were exposed in core courses and need review of these concepts in specialty courses before application and synthesis of their knowledge can occur (p. 701-702) The issue of articulation is not likely to be resolved in the near future, but educators need to address its advantages and disadvantages such as those outlined by Stevens (p. 703), as they work to strengthen graduate education for clinical specialization.

Theory Content

If CNSs are truly the experts in nursing practice, then the body of knowledge and the range of skills that they possess must be solidly based on nursing theory to provide a scientific basis for practice. This will become more feasible as theory development in nursing progresses. Content common to all clinical specialty groups should include analysis of theories and concepts relevant to nursing.

The hallmark of the CNS should be expertise in the clinical judgment process in nursing. This demands advanced skills in data collection, nursing diagnosis, projection of expected outcomes, planning, intervention, and evaluation. If the CNS is expected to demonstrate expertise in this process, then the curriculum must provide both theory and practice for skill development. Regardless of specialty, these clinical experts should be well grounded in the range of human responses to actual or potential health problems, such as those outlined in the ANA's Social Policy Statement (ANA, 1980, p. 10). These responses will be the principal focus of intervention in clinical practice and include areas of nursing concern such as self-care limitations, impaired functioning and self-image changes grievings and deficiencies in decision-making and the ability to make personal choices.

Of critical importance to nursing is the delineation of a universally accepted data base for nursing from which nursing diagnoses can be derived. This will not occur until there is general agreement on the philosophical foundation and theoretical components of nursing. It has become evident to many that as nursing develops its own identity the medical model is both insufficient and inappropriate for the practice of nursing, although its utility for defining collaborative aspects of nursing is acknowledged. A trend toward a distinct but complementary nursing focus on a functional patterns data base, as suggested by Gordon (1982) and reflected in the ANA's Social Policy Statement (1980), seems to be increasingly advocated. The data base issue is crucial because it not only reflects philosophical beliefs, values, and goals of nursing, but it also determines the diagnoses that nurses are expected to treat and for which they will be held accountable.

McLane's descriptive study of the integration of nursing diagnosis into baccalaureate and graduate education suggests that educators still have much to do to ensure acquisition of competency at both levels (1981, p. 105–113). Her idea for the future is that demonstrated ability to diagnose and effectively treat common nursing diagnoses could be a prerequisite to entry for graduate study; education preparation for clinical specialization would then focus on development of competency in making complex nursing diagnoses. As nursing's own body of knowledge expands, specialization in clinical practice may eventually be determined according to categories derived from functional patterns, such as mobility patterns or coping patterns, rather than by the present, more medically aligned categories, such as cardiovascular disease.

Additional theoretical content should be expected to include advanced-level science courses appropriate to the specialty area. Advocates of a stronger nursing focus in graduate curricula may tend to minimize the role of biophysical science, but a strengthened knowledge base in this area is vital to the specialist who in the future will be increasingly accountable for nursing decisions and who will practice in an increasingly collaborative role, particularly in acute care settings where a large number of clinical specialists are likely to continue to be employed.

Although there is a general trend in education away from the humanities in favor of science and technology, this redirection may not be in the best interest of nurses or the recipients of nursing care. Nursing is predicated on humanistic values and beliefs, and it should be possible to arrange the inclusion of humanities courses at the graduate level. Use of elective credits in these area should at least be an available option and encouraged by faculty.

Other theory courses, currently offered in many programs, will continue to be important in the future. These include content related to the CNS role, the change process, and concepts specific to the specialty area. Many schools are beginning to place a priority on content in ethical decision making and legislative issues; both trends are likely to continue as the need for such knowledge escalates.

Clinical Practice Content

Both the amount and focus of clinical practice courses in the CNS curriculum vary among programs at this time. It seems logical to expect that at least two separate and sequential courses will be required in the future, as is the current norm in many schools. The first course affords the opportunity to increase competence in practicing nursing at an advanced level by applying newly learned theory to practice; the enhancement of nursing diagnostic and therapeutic skills is likely to become a more clearly defined priority at this stage. The second course focuses on developing competence in the CNS role. Future trends are likely to include increased opprotunities in collaborative practice arrangements such as are described by Siegel and Elsberry for the primary care setting (1979). Emphasis on developing consultative, change-agent, and leadership skills will continue as students learn how to enhance quality nursing care delivery.

Research Content

In considering the future direction of educational preparation for CNSs one must first consider the future direction of nursing. Juanita Murphy recently articulated "the gnawing concern that we have not been recognized as colleagues in either the academic or practice arenas" (1981, p.649). She attributes this to the inadequate development of a unique, scientifically acquired nursing knowledge base that provides a sound rationale for clinical practice decisions. A major portion of the research required to provide a scientific basis for practice must be carried out in the clinical setting. This is particularly true in regard to high-priority studies recommended at an ANA conference on evaluation research for the assessment of nursing care (Lang & Werley, 1980). These recommended studies included the identification and validation of a taxonomy for nursing diagnoses and exploration of the impact of nursing interventions on patient outcomes. Those in the best position to participate in such studies are the practice experts—CNSs. In fact, one could argue that if CNSs expect to survive as viable entities in clinical practice in this era of cost containment and changing values that seem to deemphasize quality, they must be able to unequivocally demonstrate their effect on improving patient outcome attainment. Graduate education must provide them with the necessary research skills to accomplish this.

Research skills expected of the master's-prepared nurse, as noted by Hodgman in Chapter 5, can be acquired through several sequential courses. A course in the research process, with an undergraduate-level statistics prerequisite (currently not a standard admission requirement but increasingly expected) should provide a beginning theoretical basis for research. The ideal research experience at the master's level, and that expected in many other disciplines, is the thesis. It is essential that students who write theses have adequate guidance and supervision, preferably by a doctorally prepared faculty member with research experience beyond the dissertation. Unfortunately many nursing programs lack sufficient numbers of doctorally prepared faculty to meet this standard. As a result, students may be forced to choose between thesis work with less well-prepared faculty and alternatives to the thesis.

The lack of consensus on the thesis requirement, documented by Yeaworth in 1973, appears to continue to prevail. Information available from the NLN (1980) indicates that of the 91 NLN-accredited master's programs in nursing, 24 require a thesis; 4 of these also require comprehensive examinations. Fifty-seven programs provide the option of an alternative project, such as a clinical paper, clinical project, independent investigation, or comprehensive examination. Nine programs did not list a position on the thesis, and one school stated that neither a thesis nor an alternative project is expected.

Improvement in and standardization of the research component of graduate education is of critical importance, not only because of the need for research skills among CNSs but also because of the role of research in the future development of the nursing profession. The resolution of the issue of the level of research experience required in master's education depends to a large extent on the upgrading of educational and continuing research requirements for nursing faculty in university settings.

Faculty Preparation

Educational preparation and clinical expertise are the two most serious issues that must be addressed in regard to the faculty who will teach in CNS programs in the future. Perry (1982) argues convincingly that both a doctorate and continuing research productivity must be established as requirements for nursing faculty positions in the university setting if professional equality based on scholarship is to be achieved. Faculty who teach clinical courses, however, must be expert clinicians who can serve as effective role models for CNS students. Simultaneous excellence and productivity in teaching, research, and clinical practice may be almost impossible to maintain when one considers the typically heavy work loads that accompany positions in both academic and clinical settings.

Data profiling faculty who teach in CNS programs are not available, but preference for or expectation of doctoral preparation is now routinely addressed in faculty recruitment advertisements. While such a requirement can be readily justified from an academic viewpoint, schools that prepare CNSs must also have clinical preceptors who are actively involved in clinical practice to serve as expert role models.

The "unification model," proposed by Powers (1976), may be a feasible mechanism for distributing work loads realistically so that all three areas of professional nursing can be pursued. Nayer's (1980) and Gresham's (see Chapter 9) descriptions of the implementation of this model at Rush University suggest exciting possibilities for the utilization of CNSs in practitioner/teacher roles as preceptors for students enrolled in clinical courses. Helmuth and Guberski (1980) describe the role of the nurse practitioner with an academic appointment who serves as a clinical preceptor in the primary care setting. Such innovations are likely to be seen with increasing frequency in the future. Liaisons between practice settings and academic institutions will be mutually enhancing and probably essential in view of trends in nursing's growth toward professionalism; the CNS will probably be the key person to bridge the gap between theory and practice that presently exists in many settings.

Student Admission Requirements

Admission criteria for master's programs in nursing vary, but most schools take into account the applicant's baccalaureate preparation, grade point average, experience in nursing, standard test scores, letters of recommendation, and goal statements. Issues in regard to selected admission standards are discussed below; included are pertinent descriptive data about the present requirements of NLN-accredited master's programs.

Most programs require a baccalaureate in nursing, although a few will accept a degree in another area from the exceptional registered nurse applicant. Several generic master's programs have recently evolved; these graduate curricula provide college graduates who have earned degrees in fields outside of nursing with both basic and clinical specialist nursing education.

The weight that NLN-accreditation of baccalaureate programs carries is variable. Thirty-eight CNS programs require it, while 20 others are willing to make exceptions. The remaining schools do not specify NLN accreditation of the baccalaureate program as an admission requirement, although many indicate other type of accreditation, such as state or regional. The value of NLN accreditation rests in the fact that it sets standards against which baccalaureate programs can be judged. The fact that so many schools do not mandate such accreditation as a requirement raises concern about the adequacy of the applicant's preparation for graduate study. Moxley and White, however, urge that admission requirements be more flexible to meet individual student needs (1975), and Lenburg and Yeaworth (1975) argue that students with non-nursing baccalaureates can meet master's-level graduation criteria when appropriate learning experiences are required in the master's program. The National Commission on Nursing (1981) recently urged in its preliminary report that nursing explore alternate pathways for educational advancement in nursing. Nursing educators have a responsibility to ensure that standards are not sacrificed for the sake of flexibility along the way.

Requirements for clinical experience among the NLN-accredited master's programs are low. Approximately one-third specifically state that no experience is required, while the maximum amount currently expected prior to matriculation is two years, as cited by several programs. The argument against an experience requirement is that it may discourage scholarly pursuits among those with significant potential. One must also consider, however, the effect of limited experience on the development of clinical judgment skills. Gonnella and Veloski (1982) recently studied the impact of early specialization on the clinical competence of resident physicians and concluded that general knowledge and skill levels were weaker as a result. One could anticipate similar findings among nurses who become CNSs with minimal clinical experience. In addition, the value of the personal maturity usually gained as a result of life experience should not be underestimated, for it enables the clinical specialist to cope more effectively with the complex client situations encountered on a daily basis at this level of practice. Of equal importance is the fact that credibility as a CNS is predicated on demonstrated clinical competence, which is gained through both experience and education. Neophyte nurses who wish to advance rapidly to specialist positions would be wisely counselled by both clinical leaders and educators to gain several years of clinical experience prior to matriculation in a graduate program.

Admission standards will determine the caliber of students engaged in clinical specialist preparation, and the level of competency attained by graduates will have a significant impact on the future of nursing practice. Adjustment of admission requirements to maintain enrollments could be superficially appealing and easily rationalized in view of potential student interest in graduate study and the need for leaders in this role. The long-term consequences of such a move for the future of professional nursing, however, are largely negative in view of projected role responsibilities. Maintenance of high admissions standards would therefore seem to be both reasonable and justified.

FUTURE EDUCATIONAL NEEDS

Doctoral Education

Data available from the NLN indicate a growing interest in doctoral education in nursing (1981). Less than one percent of all nurses are now doctorally prepared, but enrollments are climbing steadily. Of the 1964 nurses with earned doctorates in the United States in 1979, the vast majority were employed in university settings. In 1979, 22 institutions offered doctoral preparation in nursing, and 12 others had programs for nurses in related fields such as education or public health. Mullane's survey done in 1978 found that 28 universities were planning new doctoral programs in nursing and predicted that approximately 50 programs would be functioning by the end of the century.

Downs (1978) discussed the issue of differences in the variety of degrees offered for nurses interested in doctoral education and urged that the distinctions among various degrees and what they prepare nurses to do be clarified as soon as possible to minimize confusion and mistaken decisions. The debate about the differences among degrees continues, but research preparation and theory development is generally agreed to be the primary orientation in the Ph.D. program whether the focus is in nursing or in a related field. The DNS is described as more practice-oriented in its reseach focus, while the Ed. D. provides preparation for teaching and educationally focused research.

Cleland (1975) has urged that new doctoral programs in nursing be developed carefully and cautiously to ensure that quality not be sacrificed in the haste to upgrade academic credentials. Nursing lacks sufficient numbers of seasoned, experienced faculty/researchers needed to respond to the current demand. Cleland sees this as a temporary situation that will resolve itself in due time if academic institutions do not overreact by proliferating doctoral programs prematurely.

Doctoral preparation for clinical specialization is currently unrealistic in view of the limited availability of doctoral educational opportunities, the even more limited demand by most clinical settings for nurses prepared at this level, and the economic constraints within the health care system that mitigate against the need for more expensive personnel. The most important consideration, however, is the inevitable tradeoff of clinical expertise for research competence that would occur in the transition process if doctoral preparation were to become the norm for CNS practice.

The need already exists, however, for clinically oriented nurse researchers who can design and lead investigations in the practice setting and are also qualified to hold senior faculty positions in the university. The percentage of time that such individuals could devote to direct clinical practice is likely to be considerably less than that of the CNS with a master's degree, but the latter's clinical background can provide an invaluable link between practice and scientific inquiry. As established CNSs consider long-range plans for personal and professional growth, clinically oriented doctoral education is an option that deserves careful consideration and is likely to assume increasing importance in the future.

Education for the Practicing CNS

One distinguishing characteristic of a professional person is a commitment to lifelong learning. The practicing CNS functions in a constantly changing and increasingly complex health care environment and holds membership in a discipline that is undergoing fundamental changes that will significantly shape its future as a profession. Consequently the knowledge base that the CNS requires is continually growing. Educational preparation at the graduate level provides a foundation for lifelong learning, but accountability for the acquisition of additional knowledge and skills rests with each individual and requires deliberate, goal-directed planning.

RECOMMENDATIONS FOR FUTURE CNS EDUCATION

The following recommendations are premised on the belief that excellence in the educational preparation of CNSs is not only achievable but required if individuals who graduate from these programs are to function competently and cost effectively in clinical practice.

First, specific criteria must be developed to measure competency acquisition for clinical nurse specialization, particularly in regard to the clinical judgment process, where levels of expertise can be distinguished. It is advisable that this process be undertaken at the national level to ensure wide-ranging input, consensus, and applicability.

Second, standards within graduate CNS programs should be more consistently operationalized across programs to enhance both the student selection process and program comparison for evaluation purposes. Clearer definition of the CNS role and development of criteria of competency should be helpful in developing standards for both student selection and program evaluation.

Third, the length of educational preparation for clinical specialization must be determined by the amount of time required for acquisition of competency. Numerous variables influence competency acquisition, including student abilities and experience, faculty preparation, curriculum content, and teaching strategies. It is hard to believe that all students are comparably prepared when so much variability among programs exists. Given the content that should be covered and the desire that at least a beginning level of synthesis occur prior to graduation, it seems reasonable to hypothesize that programs two years in length are required. Before such a recommendation can be entertained, however, two relevant research questions must first be answered:

1. What is the relationship between length of the curriculum and competency achievement among program graduates?
2. What other variables affect competency achievement; what is their effect?

The economic and professional implications of program length are critically important and therefore deserve serious attention by future planners.

Fourth, nursing faculty have a responsibility to participate at appropriate levels in financial decision making regarding resource allocation. They must: (1) be knowledgeable about financial matters affecting both the school of nursing and the university; (2) ensure that the school of nursing is fairly represented on university committees that have input into administrative financial decisions; (3) justify faculty resource allocation for the preparation of CNSs to both administrators and the legislature, and (4) demonstrate cost-effective resource utilization.

Fifth, both educators and clinical administrators must continue to explore innovative and flexible options to assist students who wish to pursue graduate education for clinical specialist preparation. Educators, however, have an important responsibility to maintain high academic standards in the process.

Sixth, efforts must be directed to resolve the multidimensional issue of program articulation in order to establish and maintain more consistent educational standards.

Seventh, CNS programs must focus on the development of expertise in the clinical judgment process in nursing. Graduates must clearly understand the unique philosophical basis of nursing practice, be well grounded in the evolving theoretical components of nursing, and demonstrate competence in identifying and treating complex nursing diagnoses regardless of specialty area. Such a focus could facilitate specialization in unique areas of nursing concern, and thus enhance the development of nursing as a profession.

Eighth, the issue of role development for clinical specialization requires careful deliberation. Clinical role models are essential, but equally critical are learning experiences designed to allow students to acquire skills in role implementation. If curricula remain short and experience requirements are not increased, it is reasonable to expect that graduates' abilities to function adequately in CNS positions will be considerably hampered. Possible alternatives to insufficient role preparation in the academic setting include the development of clinical fellowships for neophyte CNSs for defined periods, to assist with role transition and role development; however, the cost of such a proposal may render it unfeasible in the short run.

Ninth, CNSs must be able to participate actively in the research process, particularly in regard to quality assurance activities that measure and attempt to improve patient outcomes. An adequate research background is a prerequisite. It is therefore recommended that the thesis become a requirement as faculty resources increase. An undergraduate elementary statistics course would then become an admission requirement.

Tenth, it is strongly advised that admission requirements, particularly those that reflect the adequacy of undergraduate education and the amount of clinical experience, be reconsidered to ensure that students entering CNS programs have the necessary foundation for advanced knowledge and skill development.

Finally, it seems clear that doctoral preparation for full-time faculty positions will evolve and that this trend is essential from a professional perspective. Options for utilizing expert CNSs to assist with role development and the applications of theory to practice will then be even more important.

Nursing is undergoing constant and rapid changes as it evolves in its professional development. Nurse educators in CNS programs must keep in mind that their mission is to prepare nurses to competently assume leadership in the clinical arena to improve, maintain, and account for the quality of nursing care. This responsibility mandates the need for CNS educational preparation of the highest quality.

REFERENCES

American Nurses' Association. *Nursing: A social policy statement* (Publ. No. NP-63). Kansas City: ANA, 1980.

Cleland, V. Nursing research and graduate education. *Nurs Outlook*, 1975, *23*, 642–645.

Downs, F.S. Doctoral education in nursing: Future directions. *Nurs Outlook, 26*, 56–61.

Flexner, A. *Medical education in the United States and Canada.* New York: Carnegie Foundation, 1910.

Goldmark, J. C. Nursing and nursing education in the United States: Report of the Committee for the Study of Nursing Education and report of a survey by Josephine Goldmark. New York: MacMillan, 1923.

Gonnella, J.S., & Verloski, J.J. The impact of early specialization on clinical competence of residents. *N Engl J Med*, 1982, *306*, 275–277.

Gordon, M. *Nursing diagnosis: Process and application.* New York: McGraw-Hill, 1982.

Helmuth, M.R. & Guberski, T.D. Preparation for preceptor role. *Nurs Outlook, 28*, 36–39.

Institute of Medicine. *Six month interim report by the Committee of the Institute of Medicine for a Study of Nursing and Nursing Education.* Washington, D.C.: National Academy Press, 1981.

Kalisch, P.A., & Kalisch B.J. *The advance of American nursing.* Boston: Little Brown, 1978.

Lang, N.M., & Werley, H.H. Evaluation research: Assessment of nursing care. *Nurs Res, 29*, 68.

Lenburg C.B., & Yeaworth, R.C. Who shall be admitted to graduate study? *Nurs Outlook*, 1975, *23*, 633–637.

McLane, A. Core competencies of masters-prepared nurses. *Nurs Res*, 1978, *27*, 48–53.

McLane, A.M. Nursing diagnosis in baccalaureate and graduate education. In M.J. Kim & D.M. Moritz (Eds.), *Classification of nursing diagnosis: Proceedings of the third and fourth national conferences.* New York: McGraw-Hill, 1981.

Matejski, M.P. Nursing education, professionalism, and autonomy: Social constraints and the Goldmark Report. *Adv Nurs Sci*, 1981, *3*, 17–30.

Moxley, P.A., & White, D.T. Fitting the graduate program to the student. *Nurs Outlook, 23*, 625–629.

Mullane, M.K. (Research reporter) survey of doctoral programs in the USA conducted by AACN. *Nurs Res*, 1978, *27*, 315.

Murphy, J.F. Doctoral education in, of, and for nursing: An historical analysis. *Nurs Outlook*, 1981, *29*, 645–649.

National Commission on Nursing. *Preliminary report.* Chicago: The Hospital Research and Educational Trust, 1981.

National League for Nursing. *The educational preparation of the clinical nurse specialist in psychiatric nursing.* New York: NLN, 1958.

National League for Nursing. *A review of the preparation and roles of the clinical nurse specialist: Extending the boundaries of nursing education.* New York: NLN, 1969.

National League for Nursing. *Master's education in nursing: Route to opportunities in contemporary nursing, 1980-81* (Publ. No. 15-1312). New York: NLN, 1980.

National League for Nursing. *Nursing data book: 1980* (Publ. No. 19-1852). New York: NLN, 1981.

National League for Nursing Division of Baccalaureate and Higher Degree Programs. *Characteristics of graduate education in nursing leading to the master's degree.* New York: NLN, 1978.

Nayer, D.D. Unification: Bringing nursing service and nursing education together. *Am J Nurs*, 1980, *80*, 1112–1113.

Perry, S.E. A doctorate—Necessary but not sufficient. *Nurs Outlook*, 1982, *30*, 95–98.

Powers, M.J. The unification model in nursing. *Nurs Outlook*, 1976, *26*, 482–487.

Schlotfeldt, R.M. On the professional status of nursing. *Nurs Forum*, 1974, *13*, 16–31.

Siegel, H.J., & Elsberry, N. Master's preparation for joint practice. *Nurs Outlook*, 1979, *27*, 57–60.

Smoyak, S. Specialization in nursing: From then to now. *Nurs Outlook*, 1976, *24*, 676–681.

Stevens, B.J. Program articulation: What it is not. *Nurs Outlook*, 1981, *29*, 700–706.

Yeaworth, R.C. Alternatives to the thesis. *Nurs Outlook*, 1973, *21*, 335–338.

16. Future Directions in Administrative Utilization of the CNS

Duane D. Walker

The nurse administrator has the ultimate responsibility for utilization of the clinical nurse specialist (CNS) in the acute care setting. Because of the many rapidly moving social forces affecting the role that the CNS will play in the future, planning for utilization of the CNSs must be an ongoing process engaged in jointly by nurse administrators, nurse educators, and, of course, CNSs. Conscious decisions based on analysis of changing forces must be made, with subsequent development and implementation of strategies for utilization of the CNS. Because the nurse administrator has the key role in establishing positions in the acute care setting, CNSs must communicate their potential contributions to these administrators.

A MODEL FOR PLANNING FUTURE UTILIZATION

The model suggested here for planning future utilization of the CNS integrates two frameworks for sorting out elements of this complex question. The first consideration is how to plan for future changes. For this aspect, the model is developed on the basis of Lewin's change theory (Lewin, 1951). For the second consideration, administrative utilization, Fayol's classical Functions of a Manager framework are added (Fayol, 1949). This part of the model is essential because it explains the nurse administrator's responsibility for utilization of the CNS in terms of the administrator's management functions. Integration of change theory with the nurse administrator's functions provides a model through which to explore how the nurse administrator may facilitate changing what is now (current forces) to what is desired (goals).

Change Theory

Any consideration of the future is a consideration of change. Change is the difference between what is now and what will be at some future point in time. Change can be expressed as shown in Figure 16-1. The change process does, therefore, provide a useful framework with which to consider the future—with the obvious need to also consider the "now" or "what is."

Lewin's theory of change looked at the tendency of systems to maintain a status quo. "Forces" are factors affecting the system. The forces may be either driving (tending to move) or restraining (tending to remain immobile). When balanced, the forces are "in equilibrium"—the field is "frozen," and there is no change. An alteration of the relative strength of certain forces causes disequilibrium ("unfreezing") and movement. During the "moving" phase, change takes place. When forces come to a new balance, equilibrium is reestablished, and the field is again said to be "frozen." Any further shift of the forces will again cause disequilibrium and result in change. The phases of change may be thus expressed as shown in Figure 16-2. Lewin's theory is useful as a tool for managing change because on can manipulate individual forces in such a way as to "move" a social process in a desired direction and "refreeze" when a desirable field is achieved. If Lewin's phases of change are utilized as a tools for strategizing change for the future, Figures 16-1 and 16-2 are integrated as shown in Figure 16-3. This model can be used to plan future directions for the CNS by further defining the "now" and the "future" aspects of the model. "Now" is simply the state of the art—what currently exists, or the state of the forces that affect the CNS. The "future" element of the model is simply a goal for CNS utilization (the word *goal* replaces *future* in the model). Without this goal, the other aspects of the model will be undirected.

Obviously not all the forces that will affect the future can be determined, and an in-depth exploration of those that might be determined is beyond the scope of this chapter. Five major forces within society, health care institutions, and the nursing profession will be identified , however, and strategies for goal-directed use of the CNS in the future will be considered in light of these forces.

Fayol's Function of Manager Theory

The second half of the model is based on Fayol's classic, *Functions of a Manager (1949)*, diagrammed in Figure 16-4.

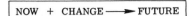

NOW + CHANGE ⟶ FUTURE

Figure 16-1. Change.

CHANGE

Unfreezing ⟶ Moving ⟶ Refreezing

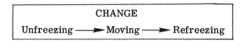

Figure 16-2. Phases of change.

NOW + CHANGE (Unfreeze | Move | Refreeze) ⟶ FUTURE

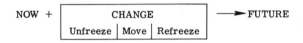

Figure 16-3. Planning change.

PLAN	ORGANIZE	DIRECT	CONTROL

Figure 16-4. Fayol's managerial functions.

Fayol identifies four stages of management by the individual manager. *Planning* involves considering problems or unmet needs and figuring out solutions or ways to meet those needs. *Organizing* involves defining the tasks and time frames necessary to achieve the solution. *Directing* people to do the task includes making assignments and structuring their responsibilities. The fourth function, *controlling*, implies providing necessary motivation throughout the process and evaluating results.

The nurse administrator, the CNS, and the nurse educator all have a role to play in implementing this management model. The nurse administrator has the responsibility for setting goals for utilization of the CNS within the acute care setting. It is therefore the nurse administrator who will plan, implement, and evaluate planned change within the overall institution. CNSs and nurse educators should, however, aid nurse administrators to identify forces that affect nursing practice to set goals, and to plan and effect change. A model that considers administrative responsibilities should utilize the power and expertise of the nurse administrator to facilitate integration of the CNS into the complex organization in an efficient and effective manner.

The ultimate responsibility for the success of the CNS role lies, of course, with the CNS. The CNS must make the nurse administrator aware of her or his potential functions and demonstrate her or his skills and knowledge of practice to patients, administrators, and colleagues to increase awareness of the worth of this relatively new role. Further, the nurse educator must know what education is needed to prepare the CNS to meet patient and staff needs not already met by staff nurses. Creativity and integration of ideas and goals are required of all three.

Integrating the Model

Integration of the change and management theories provides the needed framework for planning future utilization of the CNS. The integrated model is shown in Figure 16–5.

USING THE MODEL

"Forces" may be considered at any given point in time while the system is in equilibrium. A measurable goal is defined. Strategies are developed to unfreeze specific forces—the planning function. Strategies explain how these forces can be increased (made driving) or decreased (made restraining) to enhance the probability of reaching the goals. Such planning by managers often is done through committees or organizational processes. Plans are implemented—the organizing function. Functions and respons-

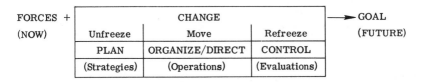

Figure 16-5. Integrated model for future CNS utilization.

ibilities are delegated under the direction of the nurse administrator—the directing function. Implemented plans (policies/procedures) are then evaluated in terms of preset goals—the controlling function. Often quality control groups are active in this latter function.

The results of the evaluation are fed back into the model which functions as a cybernetic (self-correcting) system. If outcomes are successful when measured against the goal, the strategies remain in the operational part of the system—the organize/direct stage. If outcomes fall short of goals, they are fed back as forces, to be replanned if possible. The model now looks as shown in Figure 16–6.

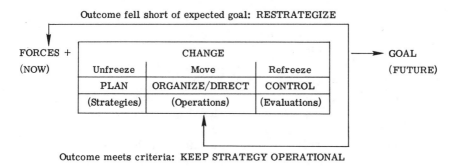

Figure 16-6. The model as a self-correcting system.

APPLICATION OF THE MODEL TO FUTURE UTILIZATION OF THE CNS

Identification of the forces

The forces that affect the CNS role today must be considered first as input into the model. The five forces to be considered here are:

1.   Economic growth
2.   Consumerism
3.   Scientific/technological advances

4.   Evolution of management
5.   Changes in education

Each of these forces will be considered as they affect society as a whole, health care organizations, and nursing. Before putting these forces into the model, however, one must state what one would like to come out of the model—in other words, what is the desired goal? What is a desirable utilization of the CNS in the future?

IDENTIFICATION OF THE GOAL

The process used by the nurse administrator in utilizing the CNS is to plan, implement, coordinate, evaluate, and adjust responsibilities and functions of the CNS within the organization. Although this is not a new idea, increased creativity in goal identification would expand current roles and identify new roles as forces shift and new needs arise. Clarifying or changing CNS roles and defining new goals should be carried out in cooperation with the CNS, including writing of the position description or contracting for services. The nurse administrator may first determine needs, or the CNS may determine needs and bring them to the attention of the nurse administrator.

A major goal of the nurse administrator is to provide for cost-effective, quality health care. This complex goal is made measurable in a specific organization by a variety of mechanisms, including quality assurance programs, staff–patient ratios, feedback from patients, and balanced budgets. The CNS may offer improved quality, but at what cost? The nurse administrator must recognize these costs and be able to defend them in terms of quality or must find a less costly way to meet the need without sacrificing quality. The goal of the nurse administrator in utilizing the CNS is to understand her or his abilities, match them with identified unmet staff and patient needs within the organization, and facilitate integration of the resulting newly created roles into the organization in a cost-effective manner.

Formulating Specific Objectives

Specific objectives of the above goals are developed and implemented by the nurse administrator through Fayol's "four functions" of management framework. These objectives form the strategy for utilizing the CNS in the acute care setting in ways that will enhance quality care within the cost-containment constraint. An example of an objective for each function, under the cost-containment/quality goal, is listed below:

1.   *Plan:* A need is recognized, and a possible approach for meeting that need is selected: for example, parents of children having open heart surgery are seen to need specialized education, and the administrator speculates that a nurse could teach and support the family.
2.   *Organize:* Through a committee or individual decision, possible ways of meeting this need are explored, with attention given to the cost and expected quality of possible alternatives. Each alternative is considered in terms of established cost and quality criteria.
3.   *Direct:* The person(s) to whom this responsibility will be delegated is selected. A job description or contract with this nurse is formulated, using a participatory style of management. In the above example, perhaps a CNS is hired to set up a plan within cost and quality constraints to meet the needs described.
4.   *Control:* Evaluation of how well the implemented plan met the established criteria is made. Resultant feedback is a new force—new information about the effects of the change.

Successful elements can be fed back to the "organize" and "direct" functions of the nurse administrator. These two functions are operational, and the nurse administrator will oversee, but the CNS will be accountable. Unsuccessful elements should not be allowed to remain in the field as negative forces but should be fed back and used in replanning the strategy for change.

Four Limitations of the Model

The first limitation of our model is that today's assumptions about the forces in the field may not be valid in the future. Should these assumptions change, the strategy should be readjusted.

Second, the specific forces considered in this chapter are derived from current CNS literature. Of course, any list of forces, unless exhaustive, would reflect some type of bias. The length of this chapter prohibits exhaustive listing, but the author considers the selected forces to adequately represent significant factors affecting the current CNS role.

Third, in deciding whether a force is a driving or restraining force, one sometimes has to make a subjective judgment. A disagreement with this judgment would necessitate replanning accordingly.

Fourth, this model produces new, untested strategies obviously not yet evaluated. In using a theoretical approach such as this, the proof is in the grounding or trial of the strategies. The model thus represents creative ideas, not established procedures.

MAJOR FORCES AFFECTING THE CNS

Economic Growth

The main impelling force behind our economic history has been expansion—the thrust of rapid growth has brought giant enterprise, big labor, and big government. Growth is now dangerously straining limited resources. Heilbroner, an American economist, predicts that growth of energy supplies and ecological safety margins will be near zero or even negative a century from now (1977).

With more imminent consequences on a national front, conservation is "in," government spending is decreasing, and budgets are being cut. Many economists believe that the days of "America can afford anything" are over. The American public is engaging in value spending. People want value for their money; the emotional spending is through. Historically, America has promised each generation a higher quality of life than that of their parents—this too is predicted to be at an end.

This economic development pattern has been reflected in hospitals. Rapid growth, fostered by the Hill/Burton Act, has dwindled to closing of hospitals, competition to fill beds, and imposed cost containment. The rudimentary or nonexistent budgets of one decade ago are becoming very sophisticated. Since 1971, with wage and price controls followed by state rate commissions and the cost containment push, hospitals have been under continual pressure to control rapidly escalating costs (Walker, 1982).

Nursing has been moving forward economically through various types of collective action, but the profession faces many of the money and image problems encountered in the twenties. There is money in health care, but the division of the health care dollar is inequitable, and nurses have not received a fair share. Since the economic pie is not likely to increase, nursing's best chance for economic advance is to go for a larger slice of the pie. Currently nursing is doing just that under the name of "comparable worth" (Sheridan, 1982).

The economic forces affecting CNS utilization, clearly are restraining forces. Limitations in economic growth, tight budgets, lack of substantial economic success for nurses during a more prosperous economic period— these factors paint a somewhat grim picture for nursing. The cost of the

CNS adds to this economic burden. Is the patient willing to pay more for specialized services? Can the nurse administrator justify the cost of the CNS within her or his organization? Will the 1977 American Nurses' Association's resolution (ANA, 1977) recommending that patient bills clearly identify nursing services rendered promote free market approaches, letting patinets directly choose whether or not to direct payment for CNS services?

Strategy

Currently, many CNSs practice in acute care settings as in-house consultants. This free-floating consultation service to nurses and patients, offering a variety of specialties, may be considered in light of the economic forces to be a luxury. Reinhardt believes in containing the costs of health care services through greater efficiency in production (Reinhardt, 1979). Free-floating consultation may not be efficient unless the CNS has a relatively steady flow of clients needing services that cannot be provided by a less well-educated—and presumably less costly—nurse.

The nurse administrator, for reasons of quality care, may want to utilize the CNS for direct patient care in high acuity areas or for other specific skills. This action may be justified for cost containment by considering which functions provided uniquely by the CNS are needed by the organization. Then the functions can be incorporated into a patient classification system with a special code indicating need for a CNS's skills. The patient classification system can thus be used as an indication of specific patient needs that require a CNS's knowledge and skills. This ability of the nurse administrator to quantitatively and qualitatively define unique staffing needs is a valuable tool for efficient "production" without sacrificing—in fact promoting—quality.

This strategy may be carried one step further. If the specific service provided to the patient is documented as needed and provided, the charge can be made directly to the patient. Does the patient want to pay for this sophisticated care? Doctors, laboratories, and many other health care professionals have successfully offered more sophisticated care to patients with correspondingly higher price tags attached. Nurses, if they can define and justify their service, should expect a similar response. Direct pay may thus make consultation a more viable option for the future.

Another approach to efficient use of the CNS in providing direct care is to add CNS functions and responsibilities to the top of the clinical nursing career ladder as a unique level. Such a position may contain other responsibilities besides direct patient care, such as consulting to patients or staff, teaching, or research, but essentially this would be a staff position of clinical expertise. This position is more easily justified for cost containment as a new part of an existing clinical ladder system than if a new role is introduced in a time of position cutbacks.

Consumerism

There was a time when consumers were quiet, they got what they bought, and they had little recourse if the service or item was less than expected. The choice lay in whether or not to purchase the good or service.

The 1960s ended the consumer's intimidation. Consumerism was called "the hot topic" of the seventies by Bloom and Geyser in *Harvard Business Review* (1981). Consumer protection legislation and regulations were pursued. Proconsumer positions received strong public support. Consumerism, although not as trendy and extreme, will probably be with us for some time to come. The government's involvement in consumerism may lessen, however, if the Reaganomics trend of the early eighties based on Friedman's "decrease government" continues (Friedman & Friedman, 1979).

Hospitals once were places to go to die. With the advent of insurance plans and antibiotics, hospitals also became places to be born and have surgery. Few non–health care workers other than patients entered the doors. With the advent of consumerism, however, Mr. Nader did. He attacked the system and the caretakers, with subsequent lawsuits filed and articles in local papers that could destroy a hospital's reputation and empty it beds—a costly effect. Consumers began to question the "sanctity" of hospitals and the "gods" of medicine—a movement still popular.

As government was questioned about federal spending by consumers— first in the late sixties—the government turned to hospitals, which were and continue to be big spenders of federal tax monies and demanded more fiscal accountability. Budgets became mandatory in order to receive government medicare funds. The *Joint Commission of Accreditation of Hospitals* gained momentum as a certifying body. Health care journals and articles on the cost of health care flooded the lay readers' market.

Consumer interest in health care is alive and well. It will probably outlive many movements because it involves not just consumer products but the consumer's own health and well-being.

Consumers want to know about their health care.

The patient education aspect of nursing is not new, many rural, non-hospital-based nurses have never stopped practicing it. In acute care settings it is alive and well again. This important function of nursing is now supported by formal courses in nursing education.

These consumer forces are driving forces favoring the growth of the CNS role. More sophisticated consumers will need more skilled nurses, and

CNSs can meet those needs. Cost again, is probably the greatest deterrent. If options for payment can be carefully pursued, the need for CNS expertise by consumers may be better met.

Strategy

The role of the CNS in relation to patient teaching is performed either directly to the patient or family or indirectly by teaching other nurses how to do patient education. One common theme in the literature is that the CNS teaches or consults with other nurse employees to improve quality care and so assists in staff development and has an effect on a large number of consumers. In the future the CNS may provide patient education from a more traditional, more easily justified position—in-service education. It is suggested, however, that she or he not assume this position without education in curriculum and teaching if the position demands use of this additional knowledge and skill.

One other role the CNS can play in relation to consumers is that of patient advocate. Although every nurse is considered a patient advocate, the CNS may provide this service in a unique way. Since many CNSs are specialized in one area, a patient with complex problems may need an advocate who understands in depth her or his unique situation, someone who can pull together the fragments of health care on behalf of the patient into a total care mode. Although this level of patient advocacy is a current CNS practice expectation, most CNSs function exclusively in the tertiary setting. A future strategy would be to extend their activities beyond this setting. An example might be to make a CNS responsible for her or his patients in the clinic as well as on the units. This would enhance patient advocacy, if CNSs followed patients after they left the hospital.

Scientific/Technological Changes

Much has been written about the fast-paced advances of the scientific community and technological advances affecting all phases of society. The effect of the changes is evident in health care, more specifically in hospitals as evidenced in monitors, scanners, chemotherapeutic agents, and many other innovations.

The rate of change is not slowing, although cost containment has dampened the onetime intensity of pursuit of technological gimmicks. In the early seventies large numbers of hospitals and doctors' offices purchased—rather than shared—exorbitantly expensive, quickly outmoded equipment. Extremely expensive technological purchases made health costs skyrocket, and no consideration was given to the effect on cost to the consumer. The institution of Health Service Agencies (HSAs) was an attempt to monitor the outrageous spending in health care. This system, however, was severly limited because it put consumers on the same boards with medical personnel. Because the consumer could not understand the technical language, representation was hardly equal. Also, health care institutions, mostly hospitals, spent much time and money preparing cases to get the equipment they wanted before presenting their case to HSA boards, thereby defeating the very purpose of the boards.

The extreme of the scientific/technological explosion, monitoring patients' every body function with the latest equipment, has been opposed by some. Holistic health movements, hospice movements, vitamin fads, health food, massages, and acupuncture alternatives followed the technological boom. The consumer was thereby offered more choices of health care, including some new nonmedical options.

The technological/scientific movement increased fragmentation of patient care by decreasing the number of generalists, for each part of an ailing body a specialist could be seen. Less common was care for the whole person. The tremendous expenses in a time of economic slump (the mid seventies), forced hospitals to prepare budgets to justify the use of sophisticated equipment and escalating health care bills to patients. For the first time hospital growth ceased, and some hospitals, deeply in debt, were forced to close.

In spite of many of the negative economic problems involving technological advances and related costs, the increased scientific/technological care offered and continues to offer many positive mechanisms for increasing lifespan and sometimes quality of life. The overall effect was, in fact, to provide more specialization than already existed in health care. This, of course, meant there needed to be more health care specialists.

The idea that "a nurse is a nurse"—that all nurses performed the same functions—was generally accepted until the 1970s. Keeping up with the technological advances, nurses also became more sophisticated in their specialist skills. As nurses continued developing throughout their careers, more and more unique opportunities to specialize became apparent.

Nursing itself was also reaching for professional status. Included in this was the development of increased autonomy in practice. CNSs and nurse practitioners were a predictable outgrowth of these forces—in fact, they have enhanced the driving forces toward position changes.

It is evident at this point that the scientific technological advances were positive forces in the development of the CNS role. Because of economic restraints, however, the justification of these positions in terms of cost containment has now become essential.

Strategy

Because of increased fragmentation of care, the role of the nurse was reinforced as the vital link between technological advances and a more desired, currently popular Gestalt-type care. It is the nurse who is in the position to meet many of the human needs of the patient—the patient who is an emotional, psychosocial being, who needs knowledge and skill to attain her or his highest level of functioning. These are the responsibilities of any nurse. With sophisticated medical treatment, however, it may be a CNS who needs to coordinate or teach a staff nurse to coordinate a complex plan of care.

To save costs to the consumer, the CNS should also be considered for some of the functions currently being performed by physicians, such as physical examinations. Many of these functions are already being performed by the nurse specialist, who is near the patient 24 hours a day, whereas the physician usually is not. Unfortunately, the Nurse Practice Act is usually not up to date in terms of describing what the nurse specialist is capable of and often actually doing. Instead the nurse performs the needed function for the patient, and a physician comes in afterward and "writes the order," Updating the Nurse Practice Acts might point out other needed CNS functions. These functions might be incorporated into the top level of the clinical ladder, as mentioned earlier.

Evolution of Management

Management has been evolving from a Theory X position, where a manager assumed people were lazy and used negative motivators, to a more currently accepted Theory Y assumption, a humanistic approach to management (McGregor, 1960). This is an international movement in management. It is evidenced in the United States through participatory management and in the growing economy of Japan through what is known as "bottom-up" management—or the Americanized "quality circles." Management can no longer give one-way directions: unions, the educated middle class, economic improvements, and higher standards have ended that era. Input is accepted, in fact sought and needed, from all levels of the organization—from the "bottom, up" (Ouchi, 1981).

The simple, classical pyramidal organizational structure (Fayol, 1949) has been adjusted by many organizations to match today's more complex society. This traditional organizational structure does not meet the need for input from specialists when complex problem solving and decision making must be done. Technological advances and specialization have increased the complexity of problem solving within organizations. Expert input from various sources is essential in complex decision making. Participatory management, a system for shared decision making, and other non-traditional organizational structures often promote necessary group inter-actions. This phenomenon is also evidenced by increased numbers of task forces and committees integrating specialties, through which work is accomplished in organizations.

Nurses, historically, drawn primarily from minorities, were suppressed in bureaucratic/authoritarian system. Although management has generally moved to a more participatory approach in most organizations, health care systems seem to be the last to implement management innovations. The changes toward the humanistic movement and collective action in nursing are two important factors that, when coupled with striving for professional status, are helping to move nursing from traditional authoritarian subordination in hospitals to a more asserted professional practice.

These new developments in management theory can be considered a driving force toward utilization of the CNS in the acute care setting. The CNS's role is often considered more autonomous than the usual nursing staff role. This autonomy is in congruence with participatory management. In other words, input from this speciality practitioner is more likely to be accepted by the organization.

Strategy

As participatory management becomes better accepted in the health care field, the nurse administrator can utilize this new environment to promote CNS positions. This management environment offers a forum for input from the CNS as an expert in a specific nursing area. During a nursing conference on a particular type of patient, for example, the CNS may offer input from her or his more in-depth knowledge and experience in that area. The patient is helped indirectly and the staff is helped developmentally by that sharing of expertise. The nurse administrator should also utilize complex organizational charts in a creative way to try out new staff or line positions that might increase overall quality care utilizing a nontraditional nursing role. An example is a CNS functioning in a staff position as a consultant to other nurses, a stress consultant, such as exists at Stanford University Hospital in California.

An important factor in today's high level of turnover in nursing and high number of nurses who leave the profession is job dissatisfaction. Through creative role development and responsibilities appropriately designated to CNSs job satisfaction can be increased and turnover of CNS positions decreased. Contributions made to staff by CNSs can also increase the job satisfaction of the staff nurse. CNSs can be used as experts to head committees and task forces involving their specific expertise. The results of a job satisfaction survey that would identify staff needs might help justify a position for a CNS who would help meet those needs.

Changes in Education

Not long ago most traditional three-year diploma nursing schools were indirectly dependent upon Blue Cross and other third-party payers for financial support. Now most three-year schools have closed and have been replaced by two-year asociate degree programs and four-year baccalaureate degree programs. The current debate involves the question of whether four-year programs should be the entry level into practice for registered nurses. Nursing education has increased in quantity and quality; theoretical frameworks are explored in school, and technical and practical experience follow. The move into academic centers and the increasing number of nurses with degrees, along with the movement toward professional status in nursing, prepared the way for increased numbers of master's-prepared nurses, some of whom pioneered CNS roles. Many other forces in the field were favorable during the early 1970s—increased technology, increased specialization, and other factors discussed earlier.

Health care organizations, during the time three-year diploma schools flourished, obtained free (or essentially free) labor through use of student nurses in a staff capacity. The advancement of the profession and the move into academic, nonhospital settings for preparation of nurses often had the side effect of decreasing the amount of clinical or hands-on education that the new nurse had experienced. This phenomenon led to the establishment of many preceptor programs, programs that provided additional technical practice "on the job."

The move of nursing education from three-year schools into academia was more than just a pragmatic move. it marked a major change from technologically based education to theory-based education, currently still emphasized in nursing education. This move was concurrent with nurses striving for attainment of professional status. Movement into the academic setting has not only increased the basic level of education of registered nurses but has also encouraged and increased the number of advanced degrees in nursing. Other advanced educational fields such as education and administration are also offered to nurses.

Certainly the move of nurses from technological training to professional, theory-based education is a driving force that has helped to develop the CNS role; in fact, the CNS role may be a direct result of this move. All CNSs are prepared at the master's and sometimes even doctoral level.

Strategy

The nurse administrator should provide input into the educational system for CNSs regarding specific learning needs. This would facilitate efficient utilization of these specialists upon graduation. Besides specific CNS roles, many CNSs will assume some type of dual responsibility in a hospital setting. If the CNS does want to assume this type of role, she or he must be prepared for both aspects of the position; hence CNS education must go beyond clinical skills.

Unique positions for the CNS can be created by the nurse administrator. Some examples include (1) CNS/nurse researcher: this person obviously would have to have additional education in the area of nursing research. A doctorate would be desirable. (2) CNS/stress manager: this professional (mentioned earlier) might deal with stress and reality shock found in the clinical setting—not patients' but nurses'. The justification for this person is in turnover and burnout statistics. The rationale is to provide care for the caretaker.

An obvious use of the CNS, appropriate to some hospital organizational structures, is the head nurse role. If the head nurse assumes management functions (hiring, firing, staffing, counseling, or budgeting), the role is CNS/manager. Management theory and skills are essential in this position to complement the clinical skills needed for the job. Some believe both management and clinical skills in the head nurse are important in such functions as directing staff nurses. A strong opposing view that the CNS should free the head nurse to be a manager seems equally represented. Barbara Stevens considers it an unrealistic expectation for a CNS in a line position to be held accountable for both management tasks and clinical outcomes (Stevens, 1976).

In addition, of course, the CNS may be well utilized as a clinical expert in her or his specific area of clinical expertise. The problem of justifying cost for what some consider a luxury position may possibly be solved through billing patients directly for services. Some hospitals are already billing for actual nursing care (Wood & Goldman, 1979, and St. Luke's Hospital). First, however, nursing care costs must be clearly differentiated from non-nursing costs. With clear billing for nursing care, perhaps some day patients will have more choices regarding the type of care they receive.

CONCLUSIONS

This chapter has explored the role of the CNS in light of the following points:

• *Current forces* of decreased economic growth, increased consumerism, scientific/technological management, and educational advances. (It is noteworthy that four of five forces are favorable to CNS development.)

• *The goals* for future utilization of the CNS in the acute care setting within the constraints of cost and quality.

• *Goal attainment strategies* that may be developed to fully utilize CNSs in acute care settings in the future.

The nurse administrator must consider the strategies suggested here in relation to the health care goals of her or his organization and plan now for the future utilization of the CNS. Such plans for potential utilization of the CNS must be shared with nursing educators so that the new CNS will possess marketable functions in this cost-conscious era.

Most important, it is the responsibility of CNSs as clinical nurse leaders, to raise awareness of their functions and contributions to health care. CNSs must prepare for roles useful in the total health care picture, base their practice and rationale for their functions on research, and be able to market themselves (with awareness of the current and future health care markets) into key roles. In this way the CNS can not only affect the health care of society in the future but can also be assured a place in the tight health care market on the horizon.

In the early seventies, master's-prepared nurses were often called "change agents." Many of these "change agents" were the first CNSs pioneering a new wave of professionalism. The CNS movement has helped nursing make great strides forward as a profession. CNSs continue to open new doors, advance clinical practice, and assume new and creative roles in health care. For continued growth as a profession, nurse administrators need to facilitate and encourage the CNSs—our entrepreneurs in clinical nursing.

REFERENCES

Bloom, P. N., & Geyser, S. A. The maturing of consumerism. *Harvard Business Review* 1981, *59*, 130–139.

Commission on Economic and General Welfare: Reimbursement for Nursing Services (Position Statement). Kansas City: American Nurses Association, 1977, p. 12.

Fayol, H. General and Industrial Management. New York: Pitman Publishing Corp., 1949.

Friedman, M. & Friedman, R. Free to choose. New York: Avon, 1979.

Heilbroner, R. L. The Economic Transformation of America. New York: Harcourt Brace Jovanovich, 1977.

Lewin, K. Field Theory in Social Change. New York: Harper and Row, 1951.

McGregor, D. The Human Side of Enterprise. New York: McGraw-Hill, 1960.

Ouchi, W. Theory Z: How American Business Can Meet the Japanese Challenge. Reading, Mass.: Addison-Wesley, 1981.

A Patient Classification System for Staffing and Charging for Nursing Services. Phoenix, Ariz.: St. Lukes Hospital Medical Center, p. 12.

Reinhardt, U. E. Health manpower policy and the cost of health care. *Nursing Dimensions*, *7*, 60–68, 1979.

Sheridan, D. R. The season for collective bargaining. *Nurs Admin Q,* *6*, 1–8.

Stevens, B. Accountability of the clinical specialist: the administrator's viewpoint. *J Nurs Admin, 1976*, *6*, 30–32.

Walker, D. D. The cost of nursing care in hospitals, in L. H. Allen (Ed.): Nursing in the 1980's: Crises, Opportunities, Challenges. Philadelphia: Lippincott, 1982, p. 131–142.

Wood, C. & Goldman, M. Interrelated programs in split-cost accounting prescheduling and peer review, in E. Schmied (Ed.): Maintaining Cost Effectiveness. San Francisco: Nursing Resources, 1979, p. 32–33.

17. The CNS and the Nurse Practitioner

Harriet J. Kitzman

Nursing is undergoing extensive change, and nowhere is that more in evidence than in the practice of the clinical nurse specialist (CNS) and the nurse practitioner (NP). NPs and CNSs are continuously changing their scope of practice in order to keep pace with the profession's expanding knowledge base and the ever changing health care needs of present and future consumers. As the scope of practice of these two groups of clinicians change, it is apparent that their relationships will change as well. While a chapter such as this, aimed at understanding the interrelationship between CNSs and NPs, risks being outdated before it is off the press, it is important to identify today's perspectives in order to make projections for the future.

During the 1960s and 1970s, advanced educational programs have been developed for these two types of specialists, and positions for the utilization of these newly founded nursing competencies have been developed within the health care system. During this period nurses have had to come to grips with the issues of leadership, accountability, and responsibility that accompany advanced professional preparation; physicians and other health team members have had to develop a basic understanding of what could be expected of nurses with advanced preparation and accept them as collaborators in the direct care of clients; and the public has had to grasp the notion that the same competencies and professional behaviors cannot be expected from all nurses because of differing levels of education and the ever-increasing body of knowledge with its concomitant specialization.

NPs and CNSs have contributed significantly to the evolution of one another's roles during this time, and because of the intertwining nature of their relationship it is difficult to identify which group has been responsible for any specific advance in the practice of nursing. While not the intent of this chapter, it can be argued that CNSs paved the way for the full recognition of the existence of an advanced body of clinical nursing knowledge and skills and the need to keep clinical practice central in the advanced study of the discipline. In similar fashion, NPs can be credited with paving the way for a new practice role for nursing that required new skills, new understanding, and, particularly, new behaviors, a role that acknowledged and demonstrated a more complete contribution of nursing to health care (Mauksch, 1968). While strides had been made by CNSs in the direction of new attitudes and behaviors long before NPs appeared (Fagin, 1981), the NP movement hastened the development.

It can also be argued that CNSs demonstrated the need for advanced academic and clinical preparation; NPs in turn, paved the way for the utilization of advanced preparation in providing care to a population (general ambulatory clients) that historically had had only limited access to nursing services because of the organization of health care delivery. In short, the evolution of the NP and CNS roles have been parallel and intertwined; each has had an impact on the other.

What is the nature of the practice of the NP and that of the CNS? Are there differences? NPs and CNSs both receive the same initial socialization into the profession of nursing. Both make use of advanced knowledge and skills in the clinical practice of nursing. They operate from a common understanding of the nature of nursing, a common value of humanitarian service, and a common goal of providing health services to people. They foster human behaviors in their clients or patients that lead to well being and optimal functioning (Donaldson & Crowley, 1978).

Both roles thus have made important contributions to the development of nursing. There is a need today, however, to create a common view for the public regarding the level of professional responsibility and accountability that can be expected of nurses with advanced preparation. With this in mind, let us examine the similarities and differences between the CNS and NP roles. In general this chapter will advance the central belief that the contributions of the CNS and NP must be combined if the profession of nursing is to grasp the current opportunity to fully utilize professional nursing services.

HISTORICAL PERSPECTIVE ON THE NP ROLE

Since the history of the development of the CNS role is given earlier in this book (Chapter 3), only the history of the NP role will be given here.

Overview

The first NP demonstration project was developed in 1965 at the University of Colorado under the codirectorship of Loretta Ford, R.N., Ed.D., and Henry Silver M.D. The goal of the project was to determine the safety, efficacy, and quality of a new mode of nursing practice—practice designed to improve health care to children and families—and to develop a new nursing role (Ford & Silver, 1967). In a paper presented in 1981, Ford described the framework for that project and the social circumstances that made it possible. Ford describes the first NP program as one based on a

> nursing model for the delivery of *health* care to essentially well populations of children and their families. The shortage of physicians at the time *provided the opportunity* to try new approaches for expanding the nurse's scope of practice, not changing the nature of nursing or extending medical services per se (Ford, 1981, p. 4).

As a nurse educator, Ford was interested in testing a new role for nurses that would, in turn, influence collegiate nursing curricula. The guidelines she used were based on basic values and commitments of the nursing profession. They included a commitment

> to care for and be accountable to people . . . ; to clinical nursing practice in managing *health* care problems; to colleague relationships . . . ; to inquiry into ways to improve nursing practice and health care delivery; and to the continuing development of nursing as a profession through increased scientific and humanistic education (1981, p. 4–5).

The guidelines for the new image of nurses used by Ford in the development of the first NP program served as a reference for the NP programs that were to follow. From time to time these guidelines were blurred by those involved because of their desire to find speedy solutions to the problems of matching nursing potential with health care needs—solutions that often required extensive compromise. Few would deny, however, that the well-qualified NP of today fulfills the image presented by Ford. From this origin, it seems appropriate for purposes of this chapter to define the well-qualified NP as that nurse who has met Ford's original conception of appropriate preparation—master's-level preparation in nursing.

Definitions of the NP Role

During the late sixties and early seventies, there was extensive experimentation in expanding the scope of nursing practice through the development and practice of the NP. The NP was considered a potential health care resource for people of all ages (Public Health Service, 1971). By the mid-seventies, conceptual and functional descriptions of the NP had been put forth that proved to be of tremendous consequence.

In 1976, guidelines for NP training programs were published in the *Federal Register*. These guidelines defined the NP as possessing the ability to

1. Assess the health status of individuals and families through health and medical history taking, physical examination, and defining of health and developmental problems;
2. Institute and provide continutiy of health care to clients (patients), work with the client to insure understanding of and compliance with the therapeutic regimen within established protocols, and recognize when to refer the client to a physician or other health care provider;
3. Provide instruction and counseling to individuals, families, and groups in the areas of health promotion and maintenance, including involving such persons in planning for their health care; and
4. Work in collaboration with other health care providers and agencies to provide and where appropriate, coordinate services to individuals and families (Guidelines, 1977, p. 3).

A statement on the scope of practice of the NP was also issued by the American Nurses' Association (ANA) in 1976. This states that the NP/clinician

> as a *primary care provider* [emphasis added] ... assesses the physical and psychosocial status of clients by means of interview, health history, physical examination and diagnostic tests ... ; interprets the data, develops and implements therapeutic plans, and follows through on a continuum of care of the client ... ; implements these plans through independent action, appropriate referrals, health counseling, and collaboration with other health care providers (ANA, 1976b, p. 3).

Ford, pioneer of the NP movement, summarized the characteristics of the NP when she wrote:

> The ideal nurse practitioner is conceptualized as one who is able to use sophisticated clinical knowledge, to demonstrate a high level of accountability to persons served and to teammates, and to assume roles commensurate with professional nursing preparation (Ford, 1979, p. 113).

While these definitions have much in common, they do differ. The differences reflect the history of the NP movement and the different concepts that are used when defining the term.

NP Education

While education in nursing at the master's level was originally envisioned as the appropriate approach in the preparation of NPs, alternate methods were found (Ford, 1979a, p. 113). Societal demands to rapidly meet primary health care needs and nursing's lack of momentum in establishing appropriate educational offerings in graduate programs within university schools of nursing created a milieu that encouraged the preparation of NPs through short-term continuing education programs. These short-term programs were rapidly conceived and generated, often with only limited reference to standards (Ford, 1981). Institutions providing health services (e.g., doctors' offices, health departments, and outpatient departments) as well as a variety of university professional schools (e.g., schools of medicine, public health, and nursing) joined the movement to prepare NPs to meet health care demands.

Exploration of and experimentation with different educational approaches were encouraged through grants from the federal government, foundations, and local agencies. Experimentation with different practice roles was also encouraged, and educational programs often were tailored to prepare NPs for unique roles. Commonality of prerequisites, goals, objectives, and content among the early NP programs was limited. Educational prerequisites ranged from a diploma or associate degree to a master's degree in nursing; length of program ranged from a few weeks to two years (Sultz, Henry & Carroll, 1977).

A call for standards soon came. In 1972 a joint statement of the ANA's Division on Maternal and Child Health Nursing Practice and the American Academy of Pediatrics was issued that identified guidelines for short-term continuing education programs to prepare pediatric nurse associates. These guidelines recommended that programs run for a minimum of four months and that they include classroom work and clinical practice. They also identified standard content to be included.

Questions continued to be raised regarding the appropriate organization to set standards for NP programs. The ANA Council on Continuing Education took the lead, and by 1974 a National Accreditation Board for Continuing Education was established. By 1975 the mechanism was in operation to accredit short-term continuing education programs (Allen, 1977; ANA, 1975).

Standardization of programs was also encouraged by the development of guidelines for NP programs issued by the Department of Health, Education, and Welfare under the Nurse Training Act of 1975. To receive funding as an NP program, a program had to meet guidelines in regards to length, objectives, and content. Since NP programs were costly to operate, modification of programs to meet these newly developed guidelines and thus make them eligible for funding soon occurred. NP programs then had to be a minimum of one academic year in length in order to receive funds, with at least four months of this academic year given to classroom instruction (Guidelines, 1976, p. 3).

NP preparation has increasingly become a part of the mainstream of nursing education. Systematic assessment skills have been incorporated into baccalaureate programs. Master's programs that prepare NPs have increased in numbers. Short-term continuing education programs for NPs that do not meet standards have all but disappeared because of both lack of funding and the risk of graduates being unrecognized by the professional credentialing system. Administrators and faculty of many short-term continuing education programs are exploring the potential of incorporating their offerings into graduate programs. NP preparation now requires one year, and, increasingly, potential students are considering investing the added time required to complete a master's program that also offers them the academic credential. If other certification programs follow that of the school nurse practitioner certification program and require completion of a baccalaureate in nursing after 1985, graduates from other than baccalaureate nursing programs will necessarily be eliminated from short-term NP programs because they will not be recognized through the certification mechanism. In short, NP preparation is increasingly within the mainstream of formal nursing education and is subject to the standards set by the profession's organizations.

NP Certification

Just as there was a call for standardization of NP programs, so too there was a call for a credentialing system that would recognize the professional competence of the individual practitioner. If the NP was prepared to provide services that could not be expected of every registered nurse, how was the public to identify the qualifications of that NP?

Different ANA Divisions on Practice had long been struggling with the issue of certification for excellence in practice versus certification for competence in practice. By 1976 an Interdivisional Council on Certification was formed by the ANA Divisions on Practice to "coordinate certification activities and to establish guidelines for recognition of specialties and relations with other organizations in regard to certification" (ANA, 1976a, p.1). Through the efforts of this Interdivisional Council, two types of professional recognition became available: certification for competence, and membership in the American College of Nursing Practice for Excellence (Allen, 1977, p.83–84). Certification as an adult, family, school, gerontologic, or pediatric NP has become available. It is important to note here that certification as NP is now separate from certification as CNS, a point that may have significant implications for the future.

During the early to mid-seventies, some NPs were encouraged by health care administrators to take the national certifying examination for the position of assistant to the primary care physician offered through the National Board of Medical Examiners. In some instances, reimbursement for services was made easier for the care provider recognized as a physician's assistant, and some NPs were pressured to become physician's assistants in order to retain their positions. Most NPs, however, recognized the loss of professional autonomy as nurses that they would suffer if they were to become physician's assistants and chose to remain in nursing and seek certification through the certification programs that the ANA was developing.

Since the certification program has been in effect, graduates of NP programs have increasingly sought certification as a method of demonstrating their competence. Given the potential importance of certification, this trend can be expected to continue.

Practice of the NP

The NP movement began in community-based ambulatory care. The codirectors of the first NP demonstration project were well aware of the unmet health needs of individuals in the community and saw a role for the nurse in meeting those needs. At the time, primary care was gaining a new level of recognition, and unmet needs in primary care were receiving extensive publicity.

Positions created for the early NPs were supported by demonstration programs in primary care within large organizations and by practice expansion in private practice. These newly founded positions allowed the NP to concentrate on direct care, relatively unemcumbered by the demands for nonpatient care activities and the policy restrictions on practice found at that time in many traditional staff nurse positions. Access and accountability to the patient and health team colleagues were increasingly possible within these new positions. Both of these factors reinforced the new behaviors inherent in the NP role. NPs who were unable to shape their positions to allow access and accountability to patients soon became dissatisfied about being "unable to practice as NPs" and sought other positions. This has resulted in high employment rates and high levels of job satisfaction among NPs. For example, the employment rate for NPs in 1977 was found to be 90 percent (Sultz, Zielezny, Gentry, & Kinyon, 1980, p. 85).

The NP role in traditional primary care settings has long since been institutionalized, however tenuously. In private practice, outpatient clinics, health maintenance organizations, and community health centers there are fairly common expectations of who the NP is and what services she or he can be expected to provide. Studies have documented the kinds of health and illness problems the NP can manage competently (Diers & Molde, 1979; Prescott & Driscoll, 1979; Sox, 1979). The range of problems managed has been found to be broad and the approaches to clients many and varied. Problems of health and illness that are associated with entrance into the health care system; primary prevention; the monitoring of chronic conditions; and alleviation of stress associated with growth and development from conception through death have all been demonstrated to be effectively managed by the NP in primary care.

The NP's practice in primary care is characterized as one where other health care providers are considered full professional colleagues. Whether involved in team practice or consultation and referral practice, the expertise of the different professionals is recognized and utilized in the planning and provision of services. Complex self-care problems are referred to the NP, and complex disease diagnosis problems are referred to the physician, with the recognition that many health and illness problems encountered in primary care can be successfully managed by either. In short, the NP's practice in primary care is both independent and interdependent.

Nurses prepared as NPs have gradually developed roles in acute and chronic care institutions, homes, schools, industry, and other settings within the community. Some of these new roles have been more successful than others, and the factors determining such success have been varied and complex (Goodwin, 1981). Demonstration projects have generally been successful from the point of effectiveness of services; however, long-term funding of essentially new positions has not always been forthcoming. Nevertheless, NPs can be found in a variety of settings providing care to patients at all points on the health and illness continuum.

As NPs begin to work with selective populations (e.g., the developmentally disabled), should they be prepared as and be referred to as CNSs? What implications does this have for their preparation and credentialing? Many nurses today are prepared to practice both as NPs and as CNSs. Some nurses have obtained preparation as CNSs and as NPs by completing two separate programs. Some nurses previously prepared as CNSs have entered NP programs, while others prepared as NPs have chosen to enter CNS programs. Still others have entered more recent programs that offer preparation as both NP and CNS. How does one then decide whether she or he is practicing as an NP or as a CNS? Does it make a difference? Because communications about NPs and CNSs may utilize different conceptualizations, confusion often ensues. In one instance, every advanced practitioner of nursing believes she or he should be referred to as an NP. In another, these same nurses find the title inappropriate. The same is true with the CNS.

CONCEPTUALIZATIONS OF THE NP AND CNS ROLES

Overview

The similarities and differences between the NP and CNS roles can be more completely understood if one examines them in terms of concepts common to both roles. Different conceptualizations of the roles have contributed to difficulty in clarifying these interrelationships. For example, Ford describes the NP as a nurse for all settings: "The nurse practitioner is fast becoming the norm for qualified professional nurses regardless of setting in which they find themselves" (Ford, 1979b, p.16). The ANA's *Scope of Practice* statement, however, describes the NP as a provider of primary care (1976b, p.3). If these two statements are considered simultaneously, the suggestion seems to be that all care by well-qualified nurses is primary care, regardless of the services provided, a statement few would accept. Such statements appear to represent differing fundamental conceptualizations of the two roles. Let us see what common definitions of the roles can be found in each of the areas normally referred to in definitions of advanced nursing practice: professional attributes, range of knowledge and skill, domain of services, interprofessional juxtaposition, and directness of services rendered.

Professional Attributes

Professional attributes include the knowledge, skills, attitudes, and behaviors of the nurse as a professional. The NP is often seen as one who is able to create a new image for the nurse, demonstrating the health services that can be offered by a nurse prepared with increased professional knowledge and skills as well as with new attitudes about role, responsibilities, and accountability within the organization of health services.

In terms of professional attributes, CNSs are not distinguishable from NPs. In order to be effective in professional practice and in interdisciplinary health care planning, implementation, and evaluation, both NPs and CNSs "use sophisticated clinical knowledge, . . . demonstrate a high level of accountability to persons served and to teammates, and . . . assume roles commensurate with professional nursing preparation" (Ford, 1979a, p.113).

The length and level of professional education for NPs and CNSs is becoming comparable. Since educational programs with the accompanying professional socialization are becoming comparable, professional recognition and accountability should also. Recognition for advanced practice competence is already established for both NPs and CNSs through the profession's certification programs. Such recognition is taking on increased importance as issues of reimbursement are discussed, since recognition of professional competence and accountability will be required in order to obtain direct reimbursement for professional services.

Range of Knowledge and Skills

Range of knowledge and skills can be considered in terms of two dimensions: (1) "breadth versus depth" and (2) assessment versus intervention—or the nursing process dimension. While both the NP and the CNS have a full range of knowledge and skills that enable them to retain a holistic approach to patient care, differences do exist with regard to the depth and application of knowledge and skills. The NP is expected to possess and utilize a broad range of physical, psychosocial, and environmental assessment skills; she or he is expected to respond to the full range of common health and illness problems of the population for which she or he provides care. The NP's assessment and intervention skills must be broad; they must be as complete in mental health as in physical health assessment and include interventions aimed at both socioemotional and physical well-being.

The CNS, while retaining a holistic approach to the patient, has more selective competencies because she or he focuses on specific populations that generally are characterized by both age and health care problems. As a result, the CNS has a narrower range of advanced assessment skills and intervenes in more depth with more complex problems within the defined population served.

Systematic assessment skills and high-level clinical judgment and intervention skills are required of both the CNS and the NP. The differences come in the range and depth in both of these activities.

Domain of Services

The concept of domain of services is frequently used in defining the NP role, since this specialist is frequently seen as fulfilling health care needs in the area of primary care. The CNS role, in contrast, developed originally in tertiary care settings (Schultz, 1979), and much of the literature on the role still emphasizes secondary and tertiary care.

There may be some historical and current practice relevance to the distinction of NPs and CNSs in terms of domain of services. For example, as stated earlier, the ANA's *Scope of Practice* statement identifies the NP as a primary care provider. Inconsistencies do exist, however. Nurses prepared in NP programs have chosen to provide specialty, non–primary care services, and CNSs have practiced and are still practicing in primary care settings.

Will domains of practice be used in the divisions of nursing specialties in the future? Is primary care a specialty in its own right or the core of all nursing specialties? Primary care is multifaceted and for some is basic to all specialties. For example, Fagin identifies primary care as the generic discipline, the academic discipline of nursing, and nursing's major focus (1978). For others, however, primary care is a specialty within nursing (Zagornik, 1979).

Curriculum experts have grappled with the issue, but no consensus has evolved. Some graduate programs have incorporated primary care preparation into existing CNS programs, while others have developed a separate primary care specialty program. Expansion of knowledge and clinical skills through research in all levels of care is increasing. NPs may have expanded that knowledge and clinical practice skill first in primary care, while CNSs expanded primarily in secondary and tertiary care; however, that distinction cannot readily be assumed for the future. The curricula of graduate programs, along with the research that is done and the practice that evolves, will shape or obliterate the distinction between levels of care. That exploration, however, goes beyond the confines of this chapter.

Interprofessional Juxtaposition

Because NPs carry out some medicotechnical functions traditionally found in medical practice, they often have been thought to require more physician dependence and interdependence in both education and practice. CNSs, in contrast, have been thought to be prepared and to practice exclusively in the tradition of nursing. Of all of the areas of role definition probably this one produces the most conflict, because from it challenges arise concerning professional role identity, value systems, and allegiance.

For example, the issue frequently arises when the legal aspects of NP practice are discussed. Most states now have provisions permitting nurses to practice in the expanded NP role (Leitsch & Mitchell, 1977). The portion of the practice that involves disease diagnosis and prescription functions require collaboration with a physician in many states. Early regulations developed to govern NP practice have fallen behind actual practice in regards to NP–physician relationships; nevertheless these laws still exist and support the idea of physician–nurse collaboration. In contrast, CNS practice has generally not required the utilization of such regulations.

Additionally, many NPs currently work in private practices of physicians. While some in these situations have full economic and legal partnership arrangements, most are still employees of the physician's practice. In contrast, CNSs have generally been assumed under the nursing practice budget of institutions and have not received direct reimbursement from the physician.

The literature abounds, however, with descriptions of well-qualified NPs practicing at a high professional level as independent practitioners or as copractitioners functioning as members of interdisciplinary teams. CNSs, in turn, have been described as practicing in a fashion requiring exceptional physician–nurse interdependence and collaboration, though employed by institutions. As one examines the complex nature of health care, it becomes clear that the NP and the CNS both must have effective colleagueship with physicians if the communication required to plan, implement, and evaluate clinical services is to exist effectively.

Directness of Service

NPs have generally defined their goal as "to provide patient care" (Ford & Silver, 1967, p.43), while CNSs have defined their goal as "to improve patient care" (Crabtree, 1979, p. 1). For example in discussing the role of the CNS in hospital nursing services, Crabtree suggests that "the majority of the clinical specialist's time should be devoted to evaluating implementation of the nursing process in the assigned area and taking corrective action as indicated" (1979, p.8). While these statements are oversimplifications, they do reveal the unidimensional focus of the role of the NP—to provide direct services—and the multidimensional role of the CNS—to provide both direct and indirect service—and the greater amount of time spent by the CNS in consultation, education, and general counseling of others who are providing direct care.

In reality, NPs find themselves responsible for many indirect services, and many CNS hold positions that allow them to spend the majority of their time providing direct services. Directness of services will be increasingly important as direct reimbursement for nursing services comes to the forefront. For example, which services will be directly reimburseable and which are expected to be the responsibility of the employing agency? Some scheme for making the distinction will be required.

The conceptualizations of these advanced nursing roles are not independent of one another. It takes a professional nurse with professional attributes and a broad range of knowledge and skill to provide primary care, while providing care to clients with complex restorative problems requires professional attributes and depth of knowledge and skills.

THE EVOLVING NURSING SPECIALTIES

Where does all of this lead? How is the NP to be distinguished from the CNS? Perhaps the question should be rephrased. What seems to be the major question today is how the responsibility of nursing is to be divided and how the procedures for articulation of these divisions of responsibility are to be developed.

The NP movement has ushered in new opportunities to make nursing services available to the population, across the health and illness continuum, regardless of setting. CNSs have contributed by expanding specialty services, thus improving preventive and restorative care. An advanced body of knowledge and skills supporting the full range of nursing services in primary, secondary, and tertiary care is now in evidence and ready to be incorporated into educational programs and expanded through clinical research.

In nursing as in other professional disciplines, specialization has become a necessity that has increased with new practice opportunities and increased knowledge and skills. The ever changing needs of the population to be served, the organization of health services, and the available body of knowledge and skills will continue to shape these specialties. The specialties, in turn, will have overlapping intradisciplinary and interdisciplinary boundaries. Whether primary care, with the practice opportunities, opened by NPs, will be a specialty in nursing or the core of other traditional nursing specialties is not yet clear. The potential for clinical research, pioneered by CNSs, to expand knowledge in primary health care is as great as that for secondary and tertiary care. Whether or not that potential is actualized will depend upon multiple factors, including the interests of individual nurse scholars, the potential for developing research methods appropriate for the primary care arena, and the political climate within the professional and the health care systems.

The divisions of specialty practice that evolve naturally from this advanced knowledge may be the same as they are currently. One cannot be certain, however. Time are changing, and so are the health care needs of the population nursing serves. Adhering to models developed in another era will stifle growth of more natural specializations.

Regardless of how the specialties are divided, advanced nursing practice cannot be setting-bound, because nursing needs are not exclusively setting-restricted. For example, high-level medicotechnical care, commonly perfected in the hospital setting, is now essential to meet the needs of some patients receiving complex treatments in the home. The institutionalized elderly and chronically ill are in need of superb primary care. Patients in intensive care units need care plans that reflect information available from the primary care nurse specialist/practitioner who may have provided years of care to the patient.

Nurses with specialty preparation must be free to move from setting to setting when the needs of the patient can be most efficiently and effectively met by doing so. For this to become a reality, however, a mechanism by which the individual nurse gains access and demonstrates accountability to the different health care settings will be required. Professional nursing practice privileges are being developed, and this system will need to be expanded. Any institution must be assured of the appropriateness of the qualification of those providing services. Granting practice privileges is one such mechanism; it not only ensures that providers are qualified but also provides a means by which their services can be orchestrated.

In addition, in order to move from setting to setting, new mechanisms for direct reimbursement for nursing services are essential. During this period of cost containment, expansion of services is unlikely unless such expansion can be demonstrated to reduce costs in other areas. With increased activities leading to improved client well-being and function, CNSs and NPs are demonstrating that their services are cost effective. Continued efforts in this area will be required, however, if mechanisms for reimbursement that facilitate flexible role development are to emerge.

As patients needs change, different specialists are required. The mechanisms for consultation and referral must be more fully developed. While some mechanisms, such as public health nurse referrals, have been in existence for many years, more intraprofessional mechanisms need to be developed for use both among specialists within the same health care setting and those in different settings. It is now not unusual for a patient to receive direct or indirect services from several CNSs. For example, a toddler hospitalized with burns may receive services from a CNS specializing in burn care, a pediatric CNS specializing in the care of the hospitalized toddler, a pediatric CNS specializing in pain management in children, and a medical–surgical CNS specializing in nutritional support. Each presumably has something unique to offer because of her or his advanced knowledge and skills. It is also not unusual for a patient at home to be receiving services from several CNSs and NPs. To ensure both efficient and effective communication between these specialists, processes of consultation, referral, and teamwork will need to be examined so that professional accountability is clear and services documented for professional practice and reimbursement purposes.

The current interrelationships between CNSs and NPs have been shaped by the social times and the stage of development of the nursing profession. It is now time to make the contributions of each come together and to use these contributions in the preparation of the next generation of nurses. Specialization in nursing should not be based on titles such as *practitioner* and *specialist*; it must be based on the natural specializations that emerge out of practice—specializations that are based on the unique knowledge and skills required to meet nursing needs that are naturally found together and are inherent in the nature of nursing.

This chapter sets the stage for the development of a model that would take advantage of the advances made by both CNSs and NPs. Chapter 18 will explore the implications of this analysis of the NP and CNS roles and the need to examine specialization for the future.

REFERENCES

Allen, E. Credentialing of continuing education nurse practitioner programs, In A. Bliss & E. Cohen (Eds.), *The new health professionals*. Germantown, Md.: Aspen, 1977.

American Nurses' Association. *Guidelines for short-term continuing education programs preparing adult and family nurse practitioners*. Kansas City, Mo., ANA, 1975.

American Nurses' Association. ANA divisions on practice: Recognition of professional achievement and excellence in practice. *Am Nurs*, 1976, *8*, 1. (a)

American Nurses' Association. *The scope of nursing practice*. Kansas City, Mo., American Nurses' Association, 1976. (b)

Crabtree, M. Effective utilization of clinical specialists within the organizational structure of hospital nursing services. *Nurs Adm Q*, 1979, *4*, 1–10.

Diers, D., & Molde, S. Some conceptual and methodological issues in nurse practitioner research. *Research in Nursing and Health* (No. 2). 1979, *2* 73–82.

Donaldson, S., & Crowley, D. The discipline of nursing. *Nurs Outlook*, 1978, *26*, 113–120.

Fagin, C. Psychiatric nursing at the crossroads: Quo vadis. *Perspect Psychiatr Care*, 1981, *19*, 99–106.

Fagin, C.M. *Primary care as an academic discipline*. Paper presented at the Robert Wood Johnson Foundation national program, nurse-faculty fellowship in primary care. First annual symposium, Nashville, Tenn., Apr. 21, 1978.

Ford, L., & Silver, H. Expanded role of the nurse in child care. *Nurs Outlook*, 1967, *15*, 43–45.

Ford, L. The future of pediatric nurse practitioners. *Pediatrics*, 1979, *64*, 113–114. (a)

Ford, L. A nurse for all settings: The nurse practitioner. *Nurs Outlook*, 1979, *27*, 516–521. (b)

Ford, L. *Practice perspective in primary care: Nursing.* Paper presented at the National Interdisciplinary Conference on Primary Care under the sponsorship of the Columbia University School of Social Work, Arden House, Harriman, N.Y., May 29–31, 1981.

Goodwin, L.D. The effectiveness of school nurse practitioners: A review of the literature. *J Sch Health,* 1981, *51,* 623–624.

Guidelines for nurse practitioner training programs. *Federal Register,* 1976, *41,* (16), 3.

Institute of Medicine. Primary care in medicine: A definition. Washington, D.C., National Academy of Science, 1977.

Leitch, C.J., & Mitchell, E.S. A state by state report: The legal accomodation of nurses practicing expanded roles. *Nurs Pract,* 1977, *3,* 19–22.

Mauksch, I. The nurse practitioner movement—Where does it go from here? *Am J Public Health,* 1978, *68,* 1074–1075.

Prescott, P., & Driscoll, L. A. Nurse practitioner effectiveness: A review of physician–nurse practitioner comparison studies. *Evaluation and the Health Professions,* 1979, *2,* 387–418.

Public Health Service. *Expanding the scope of nursing practice: A report of the secretary's Committee to Study Extended Roles for Nurses* (DHEW Pub No. [HSM] 73-2037). Rockville, Md., Department of Health Education and Welfare, 1971.

Reiter, F. The nurse clinician. Am J Nurs, 1966, *66,* 274–280.

Schultz, M. Primary nursing: How and why it works. In M. Kennedy & G. Pfeifer (Eds.), *Current practice in nursing care of the adult.* St. Louis, Mo.: C. V. Mosby, 1979.

Sox, H. Quality of patient care by nurse practitioners and physician's assistants: A ten year perspective. *Ann Intern Med,* 1979, *91,* 459–468.

Sultz, H., Henry, O. H., & Carroll, H. Nurse practitioners: An overview of nurses in expanded role. In A. Bliss & E. Cohen (Eds.), *The new health professionals.* Germantown, Md.: Aspen, 1977.

Sultz, H., Zielezny, M., Gentry, J., & Kinyon, L. *Longitudinal study of nurse practitioners, phase III* (DPH Pub. No. [HRA] 80-2). Hyattsville, Md., Department of Health Education and Welfare, 1980.

Zagornik, D. *The nurse as a primary care provider: Scope of responsibility.* Presented at the Fourth National Conference on Graduate Education in Psychiatric and Mental Health Nursing, American Nurses' Association Division on Psychiatric and Mental Health Nursing Practice. Pittsburgh, Pa., Apr. 2–4, 1979.

18. A Model for Future Clinical Specialist Practice

Judy Spross
Ann B. Hamric

The development of the clinical nurse specialist (CNS) role was nursing's response to numerous changes in health care delivery, among them the increased knowledge and skills required to deliver nursing care. There is every reason to expect that the position of the CNS will continue to evolve in response to changes in nursing and in health care. Indeed, the flexibility of the CNS role places this practitioner in an ideal position to adapt her or his practice to meet society's changing needs. Walker (Chapter 16) has described a model for examining the forces causing such change and for devising future strategies that CNSs and nurse administrators based in a tertiary setting might employ to respond creatively to these forces. Kitzman (Chapter 17) has examined the relationship between two types of advanced practitioners in nursing—CNSs and nurse practitioners (NPs)—and concluded that their contributions to health care must be combined if nursing is to effectively address the changing needs of society. This chapter proposes to build upon and elaborate the ideas advanced in the preceding chapters of Part V and, on the basis of the trends discussed, to propose one possible model for future CNS practice. The authors realize that such a proposition is hypothetical at best. No attempt is being made to assert that this is the ideal or only possible form for future practice. Indeed, the model is not entirely futuristic; most CNS readers will recognize aspects of their current practice in this description. It is the authors' belief, however, that developing a specific description of practice that arises from and extends the ideas advanced in this book (and elsewhere) will help focus and stimulate thought and encourage discussion regarding possible avenues for future growth of the CNS role.

BRIEF DESCRIPTION OF THE MODEL

Walker (Chapter 16) has described future strategies for the CNS role within the tertiary setting. In this setting the role is and will continue to be viable. Indeed, one can argue that the most central need for the CNS is in the acute, tertiary care setting. Another strategy for future practice is also feasible, however.

The CNS practice described here will be client-based rather than setting-based; that is, the CNS will interact with clients in primary and secondary as well as tertiary settings. She or he will combine the assessment skills of the NP with the complex clinical decision-making skills of the CNS for a specific client population—for example, elderly clients, individuals with long-term chronic illness, disability, or complex health maintenance regimens. The CNS will provide direct and indirect care to clients in hospitals, clinics, homes, and specialized community settings such as hospices or dialysis clinics. Depending upon the specialty, the CNS's practice base may be a tertiary facility such as a medical center, a primary care facility such as a public health department, or an independent practice.

Consistent with the authors' belief that in the future, the skills and strengths of NP and CNS roles need to be combined in one role for the clinically focused master's prepared nurse, the term advanced registered nurse practitioner (ARNP) will be used to describe this future role. This change in terminology seems a natural outcome of the evolution of nursing practice and efforts to minimize proliferation of role titles.

Before examining the role of this future practitioner in greater detail, it seems prudent to examine current trends that support this direction for the CNS.

TRENDS INFLUENCING THE FUTURE OF CLINICAL SPECIALIZATION

Previous authors have cited a number of societal, legislative, and professional trends that are potent forces shaping the direction of nursing practice. Among the driving forces supporting further development and refinement of the CNS role are increasing consumer involvement and sophistication in health care, scientific advances and increasing educational preparation of nurses, and evolution of resource management to reflect a less rigididly hierarchical, more participatory style (Walker, Chapter 16). The growing body of nursing knowledge and skills in all areas of patient care, from primary to tertiary settings (Kitzman, Chapter 17), and development of nursing frameworks that are distinct from but complement the medical model (Feild, Chapter 15) also support increased CNS autonomy and responsibility outside traditional hospital settings. It is clear that continued definition of nursing practice both within the profession and with other health care colleagues and consumers is a major priority of nursing (Sovie, 1978). It is somewhat disturbing to note that in two recent texts advocating holistic and interdisciplinary approaches to health care (Pelletier, 1979; Tubesing, 1979) the role of the nurse, when mentioned at all, is vague. These authors do not suggest that the nurse be eliminated. Some mention is made of the nurse's role in patient education and counseling, but there is no mention of the restorative and rehabilitative skills of the nurse, nor is the nurse portrayed as a full-fledged colleague on the health care team. Defining practice and giving an accurate portrayal of nursing services continue to be vital to the profession's growth.

Some other driving forces with particular relevance for the model being proposed deserve mention. These include the increasing proportion of the population over age 65, the increasing demand for home health services, and the increasing demand for hospice services. It is estimated that by the year 2000 the aged will account for 25 percent of the total population in this country. At the present time, the elderly constitute 10 percent of the population and account for 29 percent of health care expenditures. They also have the highest rates of hospitalization (Kotthoff, 1981, p. 24). Care of the elderly is one potential area for expansion of the CNS role and ties in closely with the increasing demand for home health services and hospice care. The current trend of early discharge means more clients and families are at home trying to cope with chronic illness and concomitant knowledge deficits, health risks, and comfort problems. At the same time that acute care is increasing in complexity because of technology, chronic illness requires complex adaptations to be made in the home. Thus the CNS role should become increasingly important in community health settings. Deinstitutionalization of mental health services is another factor encouraging the CNS to provide therapy to clients who find themselves in the community. It seems likely that in future health care systems nurses will be the primary health professionals managing chronic and terminal illness in homes, clinics, and institutions with physicians primarily treating patients in acute care settings (Christman, 1978).

The nursing profession foresees a strong role for the CNS in all settings. Supported by the Bureau of Health Professions, a (WICHEN) Western Interstate Commission of Higher Education in Nursing panel of nurse consultants developed projections for the number of CNSs and NPs needed by 1990 (U.S. Dept. of Health and Human Services, 1981). Among their estimates for CNS utilization are

1. 3–5 CNSs for each 100 patients in large teaching hospitals
2. 2–4 CNSs for each 100 patients in small long-and short-term hospitals
3. of all registered nurses (RNs) in ambulatory care and community health settings CNS to constitute 5–10 percent

This same report cites the need for master's-prepared NPs in

1. Hospital ambulatory care (10–13 percent of all RNs)
2. Physician's offices (15–25 percent of all RNs)
3. Community health (10 percent of all RNs)

While these figures seem overly optimistic, given the current economic climate, they support the fact that the need for nurses with advanced clinical knowledge and skills will continue to exist. By advocating placement of CNSs at all levels of care, the findings also suggest that there may be value in combining CNS and NP roles.

Economic constraints resulting in cost containment pressures and increased competition between hospitals for patients (Walker, Chapter 16; Sample, Chapter 8) are clearly major restraining forces on expansion of the CNS role. Other forces, such as the projected oversupply of physicians by 1990 (Ginzberg, 1979; Nichols, 1980) could either enhance or impede nursing's development. An enlarging population of physicians will certainly increase competition for fewer health care dollars. As Nichols noted, to the extent that "physician extenders" (he included NPs and physicians assistants (PAs) in this category) seek to diagnose and treat disease, "It would appear they are on a collision course with the medical profession" (p. 107). If nursing succeeds in defining its services to the public, however, and if mechanisms for direct reimbursement for nursing services are developed, the alternative of independent CNS practice that provides services sufficiently distinct from medical care could be viable. In either event, the projected oversupply of physicians will certainly affect health policy decisions as well as options available for CNSs and their professional colleagues.

One additional restraining force, the lack of direct reimbursement for nursing services, is a significant barrier to employment of NPs (Sullivan, 1978; Weston, 1980) and CNSs in independent practice (Felder, Chapter 4). The outcome of this issue will affect the development of the CNS role in its flexibility, its autonomy, and the nature of its interprofessional relationships. For these reasons, the issue deserves considerable scrutiny. Several arguments have been advanced regarding the need for third-party reimbursement. In institutions, separate identification and billing for nursing services would increase accountability of nurses for services provided and increase recognition of nursing as a distinct service. Fees for service paid directly to the nurse provider would increase access to nursing services for consumers and would increase nurse autonomy. There is some debate as to whether reimbursement would reduce costs. Some nurses advocate less costly charges for services, while others contend that similar services should be reimbursed equally regardless of provider (Archbold & Heiffer, 1981). The state of Maryland scored a victory in 1978 and 1979 when legislation was passed that paved the way for third-party reimbursement for nurse midwives and NPs (Goldwater, 1982). In a discussion of reimbursement of nurse midwives, Hackley points out that current policies requiring supervision by physicians increase the productivity and earnings of the physician (1981, p. 16). Her points regarding lack of direct reimbursement are as relevant for the nursing profession generally as for nurse midwives in particular. Lack of direct reimbursement is detrimental to the nursing profession she asserts, because

1. It implicitly denies the existence of the profession and the value of its services.
2. It fosters the collection of inaccurate data on types and cost effectiveness of providers.
3. By falsely claiming that doctors supervise NPs and midwives, it perpetuates fraud and promotes the belief that nurses serve merely in ancillary roles.
4. It limits the freedom of nurses with advanced education to set up practice (p. 16).

Direct reimbursement for nursing services is a stated goal of the profession (American Nurses' Association, 1977), and some strategies for achieving it are being developed (Griffith, 1982). The goal is a long way from being realized, however, and ranks as one of the most critical issues facing the nursing profession in the next decade.

BASIC ASSUMPTIONS

The model proposed by the authors is based on several assumptions concerning goals for nursing, most of which have already been articulated by the profession.

First, the model requires direct reimbursement for nursing services. Consequently it assumes that efforts to obtain third-party payment for nursing services will be successful and that CNSs will be able to contract with institutions to be directly reimbursed for their services.

Second, the model assumes that mechanisms for granting nurses practice privileges in various settings will exist.

Third, the model assumes that consumers clearly understand the services nurses provide and can contract directly with nurses.

Fourth, the model assumes that a mechanism for certification of advanced practitioners exists and is a standard for practice at this level.

Last, well-developed mechanisms for consultation, referral, and teamwork among professional groups and within nursing will need to exist if this model is to be fully realized. A climate of mutual respect and openness to inquiry and change among nursing groups is necessary to implement the independent and interdependent activities envisioned for the future CNS.

DESCRIPTION OF THE MODEL

Both the foregoing discussion and Kitzman's Chapter 17 support the convergence of the advanced clinical skills traditionally associated with the CNS and NP, into a new role, both to serve clients more efficiently and to clarify nursing roles. As baccalaureate programs incorporate health history taking and physical examination skills into their programs, the need for separate NP certificate programs will diminish. Moreover, the settings in which NPs practice today are also settings that require skills in effecting change; consultation; and the use or conduct of research. If Christman is correct in his belief that nurses will gravitate to primary care as an area in which they can function with autonomy (1978, p. 364), the combination of NP and CNS skills will be essential. The terms *clinical nurse specialist* and *nurse practitioner* will probably have to be exchanged for a title that more accurately describes the advanced clinician of the future, since there will probably be fewer CNSs aligned according to a body system or particular malady and more whose skills encompass a wide range of treatment and health maintenance behaviors for a select client population.

As Kitzman points out (Chapter 17), confusion concerning existing titles results from differing, often conflicting conceptualizations used to describe the CNS and NP roles. The ARNP title is currently in use in New Hampshire and other states for nurses with advanced clinical skills (New Hampshire Law RSA 326B, p. 2). Such a redefinition would prevent the perpetuation of conflicting conceptualizations and stereotypes associated with the CNS and NP roles. The ARNP title seems to be a more accurate description of the future clinician described in this model, who would possess skills currently within the domains of both the CNS and NP. In this model of future practice the ARNP title would replace the titles of CNS and NP; the roles and functions of these two current practitioners would be assumed by the future ARNP.

In describing the entry points in the health care system where the ARNP gains access to clients, we will use Aydellotte's descriptions of future primary, intermediate (or secondary), and tertiary care centers (1978). She predicts a three-tiered health care system, not unlike the one that exists today but whose services and functions are more clearly defined. Primary care centers will provide entry into the system, emergency care, health maintenance, long-term and chronic care, and treatment of temporary malfunctioning not requiring hospitalization. The intermediate center will provide treatment of temporary malfunctioning requiring hospitalization, evaluation of chronically ill patients to see whether a change in treatment is needed when such evaluation requires hospitalization; and provision of counseling and treatment not available in primary care centers. Tertiary care centers will treat patients with esoteric illnesses and provide health manpower, new knowledge, new programs, and demonstrations for the total health delivery system. All three centers will need master's-prepared nurses, with primary care centers providing clinical and administrative leadership in midwifery, long-term illness, chronic illness, and infant and child care.

In order for the reader to identify the distinctions between the proposed model for ARNP practice and current CNS practice, Kitzman's (Chapter 17) categories for conceptualizing the NP and CNS roles are used as a framework for a more detailed discussion of ARNP practice. The ARNP will therefore be described in terms of professional attributes, range of knowledge and skills, domain of services, directness of service, and interprofessional juxtaposition.

Throughout this discussion of possible conceptualizations of the ARNP role, some common themes can be identified:

1. The ARNP is both an independent and interdependent agent, rendering direct and indirect care to clients.
2. The ARNP is a clinical leader for staff nurses and students.
3. The ARNP is a clinical role that has the client as its focus.
4. The ARNP has ultimate authority over and autonomy for her or his practice of advanced professional nursing.
5. The ARNP has full professional parity with other caregivers.

PROFESSIONAL ATTRIBUTES

The ARNP will demonstrate an ability to use advanced clinical knowledge, will exhibit a high level of accountability, and will function both independently and interdependently with other providers. In a discussion of specialization in nursing practice, the American Nurses' Association (ANA) asserts that specialists must meet two primary criteria: (1) possession of an earned master's degree and (2) ability to meet eligibility requirements for certification (ANA, 1980, p. 23). ARNPs, as the specialists of the future, will need to meet these criteria. In addition, the ANA expects such specialists to participate in selected educational programs and research activities and to publish on topics related to their practice.

As Kitzman notes, the CNS and NP roles are presently comparable in these terms, since a high level of professionalism and accountability is required for all advanced practitioners of nursing. As nursing's knowledge base continues to expand and collegial and interdependent relationships among all health care providers are fostered, it is even possible that the clinical doctorate will become the educational standard for achieving this level of practice (Mundinger, 1980, p. 63).

RANGE OF KNOWLEDGE AND SKILLS

In *Nursing: A Social Policy Statement* (ANA, 1980), characteristic functions of specialists in nursing practice were identified. They include

1. Identification of populations at risk
2. Providing direct care to selected patients
3. Intraprofessional consultation
4. Interprofessional consultation and collaboration in planning total care for individuals and groups (ANA, 1980, p. 26).

The ARNP will build on basic history taking and health assessment skills learned in undergraduate school. This future practitioner will possess advanced skills in assessment, clinical judgment, and intervention for clients with biological and/or psychosocial dysfunction. Specialty divisions may occur along developmental lines (such as care of neonates, adolescents, or the elderly); in terms of categories of chronic disabling conditions (care of the spinal-cord–injured or of patients with chronic respiratory or renal diseases); according to health maintenance regimens (care of diabetics, patients with stomas, patients needing stress management); or in terms of some new specialization that represents "reasonable expansion of nursing's scope of practice" (ANA, 1980, p. 27). Type and range of knowledge, experience, and skills will vary greatly depending upon specialty area. Regardless of specialty, the ARNP will possess advanced knowledge of human response phenomena. In addition, advanced concepts in nursing theory, theories related to nursing practice such as role and change, skills in adult education, and research skills will also be required.

The research skills of the ARNP will be highly developed. Ideas for research that spring from the ARNP's practice will be similar to those in present CNS or NP practice, but the ARNP alone or in collaboration with nurse researchers will have increased ability to plan and implement studies based on those ideas.

DOMAIN OF SERVICE

Primary nursing has been advanced as an ideal model for professional nursing practice as well as for interdependent practice with physicians (Mundinger, 1980; National Joint Practice Commission, 1977). We believe this method of nursing care delivery is essential to the effectiveness of ARNP practice.

Because of the range of functions of the ARNP, this specialist cannot be confined to one setting. With the client as her or his central focus, the ARNP will move freely into various settings to consult, coordinate, facilitate, or deliver direct care. The ARNP may be based primarily in one major setting (primary, secondary, or tertiary) and gain access to clients through this setting but will be free to deliver care to the client as needed, regardless of setting.

In the primary care setting defined by Aydellotte (1978), an ARNP might engage in an independent practice devoted to health maintenance. Such a model has been described by Kinlein (1977) and others (Alford, 1976; VanScoy-Mosher, 1978). Such practices may become more common if it is demonstrated that planned health maintenance improves health and reduces health care costs.

One can envision group nursing practices caring for chronically ill patients. Such a model could develop in association with visiting nurse agencies or tertiary health care settings. An illustration would be the ANRP whose specialty is care of patients with sensory, motor, and perceptual deficits. This ARNP, through direct care of patients and clinical supervision (preceptorship) of baccalaureate-prepared nurses, could direct the primary care of patients who have suffered strokes or spinal cord injuries. Should such a patient develop a complication such as pneumonia, the patient would be referred to a physician and probably hospitalized in a secondary or intermediate health center. Here the ARNP or the patient's primary nurse would become a consultant to the nurses in the intermediate center.

Another role for the ARNP in primary care might be joint practice with physicians. This model exists today and is likely to continue, particularly in certain client populations. Oncology is an example where joint practice may be particularly effective. Clients on maintenance chemotherapy may require adjustments in doses or drugs for medical reasons. Concomitant alterations in comfort and nutrition, as well as ineffective coping, are areas amenable to nursing care. Effective nursing care as well as medical care can influence the patient's response to medical treatment.

The ARNP in an intermediate center would serve as primary nurse for a group of patients as well as preceptor for staff nurses. ARNPs in intermediate centers would tend to have a broader range of knowledge than in a tertiary setting. Depending on the population served and epidemiologic factors, some ARNPs might have expertise in areas that would meet special needs of the population served. Examples of patients that might be admitted to an intermediate health center include noncompliant diabetics or diabetics with acute problems requiring temporary changes in treatment.

In tertiary care settings where clients present with very complex physiologic and/or psychosocial problems, ARNP roles and implementation of the model will evolve somewhat differently than in primary and secondary settings. Aydelotte's (1978) predictions about future tertiary care settings as treatment centers for esoteric illnesses and as centers for health education and research demand a variety of organizational placements for ARNPs. In this setting the indirect functions of the ARNP will assume more importance than in other settings, although direct care will continue to be an important part of the role. Because of the teaching and research functions of tertiary care centers and the increased complexity of patient care needs, the ARNP will be expected to influence the care of a larger group of clients than she or he could possibly care for directly. The ARNP in this setting is thus likely to be more specialized and to have a smaller caseload than her or his counterpart in primary and secondary settings. Some of the indirect functions of the ARNP which will be important in tertiary health centers include those of consultant, coordinator, educator, and researcher. Several configurations for ARNP practice in tertiary settings are possible and in fact more than one may coexist in the same setting. Regardless of organizational placement, the ARNP would continue to follow clients after they leave the tertiary center.

One author predicts that the practitioner we identify as ARNP will be the clinical leader ("patient care specialist") of a unit, providing direct care to clients and indirect care through clinical supervision of staff (Farkas, 1982). As the clinical leader of a unit, role modeling by providing direct care to selected clients and clinical supervision of staff will be essential to the delivery of care to clients with complex biopsychosocial dysfunction. The ARNP in tertiary care may need to make a larger time commitment to evaluation of care and clinical nursing research than would be true in other settings, since she or he might be the only nurse with the expertise to adapt evaluation and research methods to the particular specialty.

The practitioner-teacher model has been described elsewhere in this book (Gresham, Chapter 9). This model is a component of the "unification model" which has also been advanced as a way of making expert care more available to clients (Christman, 1982). A service budget alone might allow only one ARNP to be hired. Unifying the budgets of service and education might enable four to be hired, each with commitments of 25 percent academic time and 75 percent service time. Christman uses oncology as an example. In the unification model, ARNPs in medical, surgical, pediatric, and geriatric oncology could be employed.

The authors believe that Farkas's model and the unification model are not mutually exclusive and are consistent with the WICHEN projections for 1990 and with the ANA's *Social Policy Statement*. We believe these models will become more common and that CNSs currently in staff development positions will diminish.

An ARNP whose specialty is medical oncology can serve as an example of ARNP practice in tertiary care. This ARNP would be unit based but would continue to monitor client progress through clinic and home visits. She or he would provide direct care to some clients and supervise or evaluate the care given to all clients. As consultant, the ARNP might be asked to see a surgical patient due to receive adjuvant anticancer chemotherapy. As teacher, she or he might have responsibility for graduate or undergraduate students during their clinical experiences. As a co-ordinator of client care, she or he might collaborate with a physician to introduce a technological advance in the clinical setting (e.g., continuous morphine infusion via an implantable infusion device). Such planning would include developing standards of care for these clients, education of staff nurses and communication with visiting nurses who would care for clients at home. As a researcher, the ARNP might develop and implement a study on psychoprophylaxis prior to emetic chemotherapy.

The flexibility of the current CNS role in responding to the needs of clients will be equally important to the future ARNP role.

A number of other organizational arrangements are possible for the ARNP. Decisions regarding type and location of organizational placement will be made on the basis of the setting, client needs, and the ARNP's knowledge and skills.

DIRECTNESS OF SERVICE

The balance of direct and indirect care activities of the ARNP will depend on the setting and the needs of the client population. As a direct care–giver, the ARNP will have responsibility for a group of patients (a case load) that is a subset of the larger group of patients whose care she or he must influence. For this larger patient group the functions associated with the CNS role that affect care indirectly (change agent, consultant, clinical teacher, supervisor, and researcher) will continue to be important. The ARNP may shift emphasis from direct care to indirect modes as the patient moves to a different point along the health–illness continuum. For example, an ARNP specializing in care of patients with chronic renal disease might have a renal unit in a tertiary care center as her or his primary base but would continue to work with clients at home, in community dialysis centers, or in ambulatory clinics as indicated. An ARNP specializing in care of the elderly might provide direct care to a client in her or his home, a nursing home, or an extended care facility. If this client became acutely ill and entered a tertiary care facility, the ARNP would provide consultant and liaison services to the nursing staff giving direct care. The complexities of the health care system dictate the increased need for a central practitioner who maintains contact with clients regardless of their health status. At the same time, the realities of specialization make it impossible for that practitioner to master the knowledge and varied skills required to give direct care in all circumstances. As a consequence, the consultative and collaborative skills of the ARNP (and other care providers as well) are vital to maintain continuity of care for clients as they need the services of various components of the health care system.

INTERPROFESSIONAL JUXTAPOSITION

Kitzman writes that practice complexities require that all advanced practitioners of nursing be both independent of and interdependent with other care givers. This independence/interdependence does not relate solely to the physician but also to other health care professionals such as social workers and physical and occupational therapists.

Christman envisions a health care system where shared power and responsibility are a major ingredient (1978). Interprofessional collaboration between nurses and physicians has been the focus of the National Joint Practice Commission (NJPC) (NJPC, 1977). This commission disbanded in 1981, but not before it had carried out demonstration projects in joint practice. Factors that appear to facilitate joint practice in hospitals are primary nursing, use of integrated patient records, and joint practice committees (NJPC, 1977, 2–3). The work of the NJPC can be used by ARNPs to more clearly define and develop interprofessional relationships.

The availability of direct reimbursement for nursing services, maturation of nursing theory development, and clear articulation of nursing practice to the public will promote interdependent relationships between nurses and other providers.

VALUE OF THE MODEL IN IMPROVING CARE

If this model is to be considered a feasible mode of future ARNP practice, it is important to speculate on the advantages such a model would have for clients. A risk for clients of professional specialization is fragmentation of care. The ARNP model, however, acknowledges specialization while specifying a client-centered focus. The unification of advanced professional nursing practice, blending CNS and NP roles, would also foster coordinated care, lessening the risk of fragmentation.

As ARNPs establish independent and collaborative practices in institutions and communities, expert nursing care will be more accessible to clients. As two NPs noted, their clients wanted someone who would treat them as individuals. Clients perceived them as taking more time with them and being more thorough, two factors which clients valued (Alford & Jensen, 1976, p. 1968).

One of the authors' clients identified her primary nurse (a staff nurse) as an "anchor" in the tertiary setting to which she came for chemotherapy. This client valued the consistency of care and coordination available to her through the primary nurse and stated that she felt she had *a* nurse just as she has *a* physician. As health care systems become more complex, having such an "anchor" may promote a wiser use of health resources than our current fragmented system allows. In addition, it is conceivable that expert care may prevent or limit hospitalizations by helping clients maintain and restore health and adapt to illness.

DIFFICULTIES AND CHALLENGES

The proposed model faces several challenges. Within nursing there is a degree of threat in the suggestion that two types of advanced practice roles combine their skills and emerge as one. Nurses in both the CNS and NP roles have explored and defined new areas of practice. In the new role, practice differences will be maintained depending on specialty, setting, client population, and other factors. Convergence of the CNS and NP roles will help unify advanced professional practice and extend nursing's power and influence.

Providing continuity of care may pose problems. Is it realistic to expect that an ARNP can follow a clilent who needs services in another setting? An ARNP might have a case load of 20–30 patients (an inflated figure, if one considers that the WICHEN projections do not allow for the convergence of NP and CNS roles or for clinical practice by faculty members). With such a case load ARNPs should, through direct and indirect methods, be able to facilitate continuity of care. In a rural setting, a home visit may mean the ARNP must travel quite a distance. If the catchment area of a setting is quite large, an ARNP might accomplish more for a client's continued care by providing continuing education for local nurses and maintaining phone contact. Regardless of the situation, the ARNP should have the freedom and authority to see how the needs of clients can best be managed.

Another difficulty presented by the model is the question of salary.

Should ARNPs rely on income from services provided, or should they be salaried? This issue is closely tied to methods of reimbursement for nursing services in general. It seems that for the time being most ARNPs will be employees. As direct reimbursement becomes available, however, ARNPs and nurse administrators should consider combining salaries with fees for services as compensation for ARNPS (e.g., a renal ARNP may receive a salary for being unit clinical leader and additional reimbursement from a client or third party payer for home visits.

Of 58 articles on the NP reviewed by Monteiro, 45 percent cited interdisciplinary conflicts or tensions as stressors in the NP role (1978, p. 336). The proposed model will not lessen the threat physicians may perceive. If attempts at independent or interdependent practice are perceived by physicians as "losing" clients or giving up "ownership" of clients, the ARNP may encounter as much (if not more) resistance to changing roles as NPs did when that role was introduced. Economic constraints and the probability of a physician glut in 1990 will not make it easier to reduce physicians' perceived threat and make them amenable to change.

Another challenge to the profession will be to provide the numbers of ARNPs that are suggested by the WICHEN figures and necessary for implementation of the model. The prospect of a physician glut and ARNP deficit in 1990 is an unfavorable omen for the profession, particularly if nursing roles continue to be vaguely identified by consumers and health professionals.

A final challenge presented by the model relates to accessibility of care. The current health care system is not designed to afford easy or equitable access to nursing care. The model requires that nursing care be more available to clients than it is today. If it is to be more accessible, changes in professional and consumer attitudes and in the reimbursement system would most definitely have to occur. Strategies for meeting these challenges might include, but are not limited to, (1) setting up projects to demonstrate that ARNP management of particular client populations (e.g., diabetics, hospice patients) improve health outcomes; (2) through accrediting agencies, setting standards of care for certain populations whose needs ARNPs are prepared to manage; and (3) establishing joint practices and joint practice committees both within and outside institutions.

CONCLUSION

An important responsibility of those currently in CNS positions is to formulate explicit descriptions of the scope and limits of their responsibility and authority. The CNS cannot be all things to all people. The role was developed primarily with a clinical focus, but this focus has shifted as institutions have used CNSs in other than clinical roles. The original mandate for the CNS to be an expert care-giver and improve nursing practice must remain central to the continuing development of the CNS role and its evolution to the role of ARNP. The ARNP should continue the successful work of CNSs and NPs in demonstrating both independent and interdependent clinical practice and in fostering clinical acumen in other nurses—both hallmarks of professional practice.

The ARNP can be a pivotal resource for her or his client population. Both as a direct caregiver and as a coordinator of the client's health care resources, the ARNP has tremendous potential to actualize nursing theory in a strong practice position.

The model presented here is one possible response to the forces shaping health care. The effectiveness of such a model is dependent upon the presence of such conditions as third-party payment and a clear definition of nursing practice. Other practice models are certainly possible and in fact need to be conceptualized if nursing is to remain a vital force in health care. The authors recognize that it is much easier to conceptualize future advanced practice than to do the difficult work necessary to establish such a practice. Individual CNSs and NPs who practice nursing today with interdependence, responsibility, and skill are laying the foundations for practice models of the future.

REFERENCES

Alford, D.M., & Jensen, J.M. Reflections on private practice. *Am J Nurs*, 1976, *76*, 1966–1968.

Archbold, P., & Hieffer, B. Reframing the issue: A debate on third party reimbursement. *Nurs Outlook*, 1981, *29*, 423–427.

American Nurses' Association. *Reimbursement for nursing services: A position statement of the Commission on Economic and General Welfare* (Publ. No. EC-139). Kansas City, Mo.: ANA, 1977.

American Nurses' Association. *Nursing: A social policy statement* (Publ. No. NP 63 35M). Kansas City, Mo.: ANA, 1980.

Aydellotte, M. 'The future health delivery system and the utilization of nurses prepared in formal educational programs. In N. Chaska (Ed.), *The Nursing Profession*. New York: McGraw-Hill, 1978.

Christman, L. Alternatives in the role expression of nurses that may affect the future of the nursing profession. In N. Chaska (Ed.), *The nursing profession*. New York: McGraw-Hill, 1978.

Christman, L. The unification model. In A. Marriner (Ed.), *Contemporary nursing management*. St. Louis: C.V. Mosby, 1982.

Farkas, N. The clinical specialist in hospital organizations. In A. Marriner (Ed.), *Contemporary nursing management*. St. Louis: C.V. Mosby, 1982.

Ginzberg, E. *Predictions and options for nursing and health care. Future Encounters in Health Care.* (NLN Publication 52-1815). New York: National League for Nursing, 1979.

Goldwater, M. From a legislator: Views on third party reimbursement for nurses. *Am J Nurs*, 1982, *82*, 413–414.

Griffith, H.M. Strategies for direct third party reimbursement for nurses. *Am J Nurs*, 1982, *82*, 400–411.

Hackley, B.K. Independent reimbursement from third party payers to nurse-midwives. *J Nurs Midwif*, 1981, *26*, 15–22.

Kinlein, M.L. *Independent nursing practice with clients.* Philadelphia: J.B. Lippincott, 1977.

Kotthoff, M.E. Current trends and issues in nursing in the U.S.: The primary health care nurse practitioner. *Int Nurs Rev*, 1981, *28*, 24–28.

Monteiro, L. Interdisciplinary stresses of extended nursing roles. In N. Chaska (Ed.), *The Nursing Profession.* New York: McGraw-Hill, 1978.

Mundinger, M.O. *Autonomy in nursing.* Germantown, Md.: Aspen Systems Corp., 1980.

National Joint Practice Commission. Brief description of a demonstration project to establish joint practice in hospitals. Chicago: NJPC, 1977.

New Hampshire Law RSA 326B.

Nichols, A. Physician extenders, the law, and the future. *J Fam Pract*, 1980, *11*, 101–108.

Pelletier, K. *Holistic medicine.* New York: Delacorte Press, 1979.

Sovie, M. Nursing: A future to shpae. In N. Chaska (Ed.), *The nursing profession.* New York: McGraw-Hill, 1978.

Sullivan, J.A. Overcoming barriers to the employment and utilization of nurse practitioners. *Am J Public Health*, 1978, *68*, 1097–2011.

Tubesing, D.A. *Wholistic health.* New York: Human Sciences Press, 1979.

U.S. Department of Health and Human Services. *Evaluation and updating of the criteria established by the WICHE panel of expert consultants* (DHPA Report No. 81–19). Annandale, Va.: JWK International Corp., 1981.

VanScoy-Mosher, C. The oncology nurse in independent practice. *Cancer Nurs*, 1978, *1*, 21–30.

Weston, J. Distribution of nurse practitioners and physician's assistants: Implications of legal constraints and reimbursement. *Public Health Rep*, (May-June, 1980) 95: 255–258.

Index

Index